CORNEA
Atlas

Commissioning Editor: Paul Fam
Development Editor: Tim Kimber
Project Manager: Kathryn Mason
Designer: Andy Chapman
Marketing Managers: Lisa Damico (US), Gaynor Jones (UK)

CORNEA
Atlas

SECOND EDITION

Jay H Krachmer MD

Professor and Chairman
Department of Ophthalmology
University of Minnesota Medical School
Minneapolis, MN
USA

David A Palay MD

Associate Clinical Professor
Department of Ophthalmology
Emory University
Atlanta, GA
USA

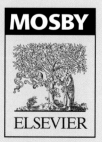

MOSBY

ELSEVIER

MOSBY
ELSEVIER

An affiliate of Elsevier Inc.

First edition 1995
Second edition 2006

ISBN 0323039626
EAN 9780323039628

British Library Cataloguing in Publication Data
A catalogue record for this book is available from the British Library

Library of Congress Cataloging in Publication Data
A catalog record for this book is available from the Library of Congress

---

Notice

Medical knowledge is constantly changing. Standard safety precautions must be followed, but as new research and clinical experience broaden our knowledge, changes in treatment and drug therapy may become necessary or appropriate. Readers are advised to check the most current product information provided by the manufacturer of each drug to be administered to verify the recommended dose, the method and duration of administration, and contraindications. It is the responsibility of the practitioner, relying on experience and knowledge of the patient, to determine dosages and the best treatment for each individual patient. Neither the Publisher nor the author assumes any liability for any injury and/or damage to persons or property arising from this publication.

The Publisher

Printed in China
Last digit is the print number: 9   8   7   6   5   4   3   2   1

Contents

Preface

It was a pleasure for us to have the opportunity to write a second edition of our *Cornea Atlas*. We feel that this edition is a significant improvement over the previous book. Again, finding the time to write this book was easy, we just slept less!

How does this edition differ from the first edition?

- Nearly all the figures from the first edition have been edited with improvements.
- Many figures have been eliminated or replaced.
- There are 215 new figures.
- In the first edition, 25% of the figures came from contributors. In this edition, 36% came from outside of our collections. Using the Internet, we were able to obtain contributions from Africa, Asia, Europe, and South America.
- There are a total of 93 contributors.
- We expanded examples of international anterior segment disease.
- There is a new chapter entitled "External Eye Manifestations of Chemical and Biological Warfare." Unfortunately, ophthalmologists need to be educated on this topic.

- New deep lamellar optical keratoplasty procedures are addressed.
- There is greatly expanded coverage of refractive surgery.
- There is a new chapter entitled "Iris Tumors."
- With the previous edition, there was a slide collection which quickly sold out. This edition comes with a DVD that contains all of the images. It is easy to bring them into a digital presentation. We personally created the search words for the DVD and feel that the user will enjoy its power and simplicity.

We hope that this edition is greatly improved but realize that we can still do better. As with the first edition, we ask that readers let us know how we can make a future edition an even greater contribution.

Jay H Krachmer, MD
David A Palay, MD

Acknowledgements

We are extremely grateful to our many colleagues, associates, and friends who helped with the preparation of this book. We would like to credit and thank the following contributors for sending us materials:

Wallace L M Alward, Iowa City, Iowa (7.38, 10.130)
William Basuk, Poway, California (1.7)
Allen D Beck, Atlanta, Georgia (15.5)
Mario Brunzini, Buenos Aires, Argentina (86.6)
J Douglas Cameron, Rochester, Minnesota (5.16, 10.111, 10.162)
Emmett Carpel, Minneapolis, Minnesota (10.125)
H Dwight Cavanagh, Dallas, Texas (7.6)
Naveen S Chandra, Walnut Creek, California (22.30)
Steven Ching, Rochester, New York (6.62, 6.63, 6.64, 6.65, 8.93, 8.94, 8.95, 10.165, 11.54, 20.71, 20.72)
Gary Chung, Seattle, Washington (5.13, 5.14, 5.15, 16.9)
David Cogan, Deceased (12.11)
Elisabeth Cohen, Philadelphia, Pennsylvania (8.24, 8.25)
Michael Conners, St. Louis, Missouri (4.7, 22.32, 22.33)
Elizabeth Davis, Minneapolis, Minnesota (22.37)
Michael Diesenhouse, Sun City, Arizona (8.110, 17.11, 17.12)
Claes Dohlman, Boston, Massachusetts (21.35, 21.36)
Donald Doughman, Minneapolis, Minnesota (8.101)
Richard Eiferman, Louisville, Kentucky (3.31, 8.79, 16.2, 17.1, 17.7, 20.51)
Robert S Feder, Chicago, Illinois (10.17, 10.18, 10.19, 10.34, 10.35, 10.53 (Lattice IIIA)
Sandy Feldman, San Diego, California (8.50, 8.51)
Richard K Forster, Miami, Florida (6.30, 6.31, 9.5, 9.6)
Herb Friesen, Deceased (3.24, 3.25, 6.35, 6.48, 9.1, 9.2, 9.3, 9.4)
Denise de Freitas, São Paulo, Brazil (11.75, 22.31, 22.34)
Lawrence Gans, St. Louis, Missouri (18.5)
W Richard Green, Baltimore, Maryland (3.23)
Michael R Grimmett, Palm Beach Gardens, Florida (5.43)
Hans Grossniklaus, Atlanta, Georgia (2.5, 2.10, 2.14, 2.18, 2.26, 2.29, 2.32, 2.34, 2.36, 5.28, 6.61, 7.15, 7.18, 7.28, 7.31, 7.41, 8.26, 10.3, 10.29, 10.30, 10.31, 10.47, 10.57, 10.88, 10.91, 10.113, 10.153, 10.166, 11.84)
M Bowes Hamill, Houston, Texas (15.38)
Stephen Hamilton, Atlanta, Georgia (8.38, 18.6, 21.37)
Kristen Hammersmith, Philadelphia, Pennsylvania (20.36)
David Hardten, Minneapolis, Minnesota (22.35)
Andrew Harrison, Minneapolis, Minnesota (1.6, 2.4, 8.78)
Koji Hirano, Nagoya, Japan (10.36, 10.37, 10.38, 10.53 (Lattice IV), 20.64, 20.65, 20.66, 20.67, 20.68)
Edward J Holland, Cincinnati, Ohio (2.35, 2.37, 4.23, 5.24, 5.44, 5.52, 6.36, 6.49, 6.77, 6.85, 6.86, 6.87, 8.10, 8.11, 8.15, 8.29, 8.87, 8.88, 8.89, 8.90, 8.115, 10.48, 10.49, 10.50, 10.53 (Granular II), 10.60, 10.61, 10.175, 11.11, 11.24, 11.34, 11.82, 14.20, 14.21, 14.26, 15.78, 15.79, 17.5, 19.3, 19.7, 19.13, 19.14, 19.17, 19.18, 20.18, 20.31, 21.14, 21.15, 21.16, 21.17, 21.18, 22.3)
Andrew Huang, Minneapolis, Minnesota (6.50, 6.53, 8.31, 10.51, 10.52, 10.176)
Infect Dis Clin North Am, 1992 (8.107)
Int Ophthalmol Clin 29:98–104, 1989 (8.114)
Joe Iuorno, Richmond, Virginia (5.3, 5.4, 5.32, 6.81, 8.124)
Tim Johnson, Iowa City, Iowa (19.12)
David Jordan, Ottawa, Canada (4.26)
Muriel I Kaiser-Kupfer, Bethesda, Maryland (12.12)
Jack Kanski, London, England (7.12, 7.35)
Kenneth Kenyon, Boston, Massachusetts (8.18, 8.30, 10.54)
William H Knobloch, Deceased (8.8)
David Knox, Baltimore, Maryland (8.47, 8.49)
Steven Koenig, Milwaukee, Wisconsin (15.7)
Regis Kowalski, Pittsburgh, Pennsylvania (11.1, 11.2, 11.3 (A,C,D,E,F), 11.4)
Burton J Kushner, Madison, Wisconsin (2.8, 2.9)
Ethan Kutzscher, Daly City, California (11.85, 11.86, 22.21, 22.27)
Peter R Laibson, Philadelphia, Pennsylvania (6.12, 6.58, 6.73, 6.74, 6.79, 7.8, 10.2, 10.4, 10.16, 10.46, 10.53 (Thiel-Behnke) 10.143, 11.21, 11.25, 11.28, 11.35, 11.49, 11.58, 11.59, 12.6, 12.7, 13.3, 13.4, 13.7, 15.32, 15.76, 21.9)
Ronald Laing, Boston, Massachusetts (7.4)

Scott Lambert, Atlanta, Georgia (19.16)
Michael Lemp, Washington, DC (4.1, 4.2, 4.3)
Mary Lynch, Atlanta, Georgia (7.32, 7.36, 7.37)
Marian Macsai, Chicago, Illinois (21.26, 21.27, 21.28, 21.34)
Mark Mandel, Hayward, California (15.82)
Mark J Mannis, Sacramento, California (3.3, 4.18, 4.20, 6.60, 10.64, 10.65, 20.15)
Daniel F Martin, Atlanta, Georgia (5.5, 18.17)
Darlene Miller, Miami, Florida (17.3B)
Andrew Moyes, Kansas City, Missouri (4.27)
Jeffrey Nerad, Iowa City, Iowa (2.17)
David Park, Stillwater, Minnesota (22.36)
Charles Pavlin, Toronto, Canada (5.26, 5.27)
Louis Probst, Ann Arbor, Michigan (22.9, 22.10, 22.13, 22.18, 22.19)
John J Purcell, Jr, St. Louis, Missouri (10.32, 10.33)
Christopher Rapuano, Philadelphia, Pennsylvania (10.20, 18.13, 21.7, 21.8, 21.12, 21.13, 21.23, 21.24, 22.14, 22.22, 22.24)
Merlyn Rodrigues, Potomic, Maryland (10.80, 10.112, 10.157)
Roy Rubinfeld, Chevy Chase, Maryland (10.5, 20.74, 22.11, 22.12, 22.15, 22.16, 22.17, 22.20, 22.26, 22.28, 22.29)
Alan Sadowsky, Fridley, Minnesota (8.86, 8.91, 8.92)
Steven Schallhorn, San Diego, California (22.7, 22.8, 22.25)
Ivan Schwab, Sacramento, California (8.123)
Wendell J Scott, Springfield, Missouri (8.14)
Gilbert Smolin, San Francisco, California (8.9, 8.12, 8.13, 8.74)
Tomy Starck, San Antonio, Texas (10.132)
Walter Stark, Baltimore, Maryland (20.56)
Alfred O Steldt, Minneapolis, Minnesota (15.57)
Alan Sugar, Ann Arbor, Michigan (10.89, 10.90)
Joel Sugar, Chicago, Illinois (8.103, 8.104, 8.105, 8.106, 14.23)
C. Gail Summers, Minneapolis, Minnesota (8.7, 8.16)
Survey of Ophthalmology 38:229, 1993 (8.102)
Hugh Taylor, East Melbourne, Australia (8.107, 8.108, 8.109)
Mark Terry, Portland, Oregon (20.69, 20.70)
Thieme, New York, 1998 (21.10, 21.11)
Keith Thompson, Atlanta, Georgia (10.44, 22.1, 22.2)
Gregory L Thorgaard, Ottumwa, Iowa (13.20, 13.21)
Elias Traboulsi, Cleveland, Ohio (8.40)
David T Tse, Miami, Florida (1.15, 1.16)
Gary Varley, Cincinnati, Ohio (4.14, 11.19)
Arthur W Walsh, Lebanon, New Hampshire (8.129)
Keith Walter, Winston Salem, North Carolina (6.8, 6.9, 21.31, 21.32)
Juanhua Wang, Rochester, New York (20.73)
George O Waring, III, Atlanta, Georgia (5.21, 5.29, 7.10, 10.150, 21.38)
Michael Warner, Hermiston, Oregon (5.1, 5.6, 5.39, 5.41, 5.42, 5.55)
Robert Weisenthal, Dewitt, NY (10.86)
John Wells III, Columbia, South Carolina (8.44, 8.45)
Theodore Werblin, Princeton, West Virginia (22.4)
Jonathan Wirtschafter, Deceased (8.60, 8.61)
Ted H Wojno, Atlanta, Georgia (1.1, 1.2, 1.3, 1.5, 1.8, 1.11, 1.12, 1.14, 2.13, 2.15, 2.19, 2.20, 2.21, 2.22, 2.23, 2.24, 2.27, 2.28, 2.30, 2.31, 2.33, 5.46, 5.56, 5.57, 6.3, 15.23)
Tom Wood, Memphis, Tennessee (5.10, 5.11, 5.12, 14.30, 14.31, 14.32)
Martha Wright, Minneapolis, Minnesota (10.131, 10.148, 10.149)

We would like to thank the staff at Elsevier/Mosby for their wonderful support. It was a pleasure working with them. Although many individuals were involved, it was Paul Fam who went to bat for us when we had ideas which might cost the publisher extra money but in the end would definitely be value-added. An example is the image search capabilities of this book. If our Elsevier publications are judged to be of high quality, a major reason is the support of people like Paul Fam.

Dedication

*With great love and appreciation, I dedicate this book to
my wife, Kathryn, our children, Edward, Kara, and Jill,
our parents, Paul and Rebecca Krachmer
and Louis and Gertrude Maraist*

JAY H. KRACHMER

*To my wife Debra, my children Sarah and Matthew,
and my parents Sandra and Bernard.
Without their love and support this would not have been possible.*

DAVID A. PALAY

Chapter 1

Diseases of the Lid
Anatomic Abnormalities

The eyelids protect the eyes and redistribute the tear film over the ocular surface. Anatomic abnormalities of the eyelids are often associated with corneal exposure and, in severe cases, corneal ulceration.

Ectropion

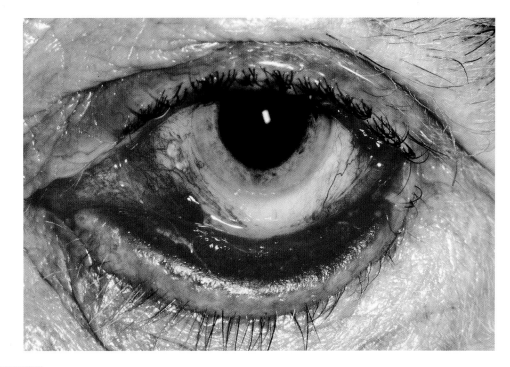

Fig. 1.1 Involutional ectropion. This disorder is caused by laxity of the lid tissue associated with aging. It is almost always seen in the lower lids. The laxity specifically affects the lower lid retractors and/or canthal tendons.

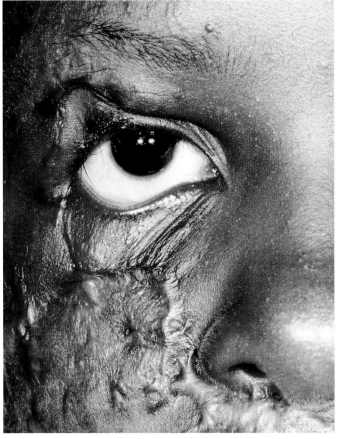

Fig. 1.2 Cicatricial ectropion. This disorder is caused by scarring of the lid tissue or periocular skin. Eversion of the lid results from traction caused by the scar. In this case a burn injury to the skin resulted in lower lid ectropion.

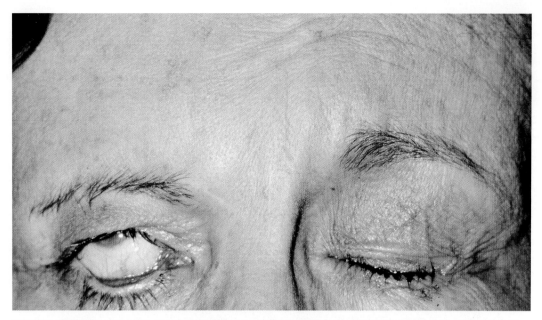

Fig. 1.3 Paralytic ectropion. This disorder is caused by damage to the seventh cranial nerve. Weakness of the orbicularis muscle leads to an out-turning of the lower eyelid. This patient exhibits a paralytic ectropion and a poor Bell's phenomenon caused by a seventh nerve palsy. Normal furrowing of the brow is absent. Exposure keratitis may occur, and these patients require aggressive topical lubrication and, occasionally, a tarsorrhaphy.

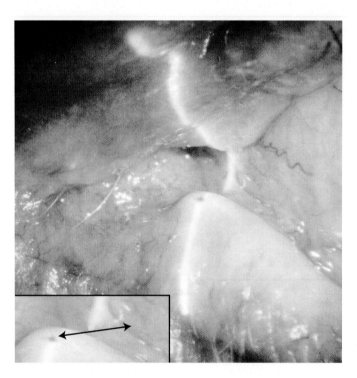

Fig. 1.4 Punctal ectropion. This disorder may occur in an otherwise normally positioned lid. The arrow indicates an abnormal space between the lid and the eye (inset). Repair may be needed in patients with epiphora.

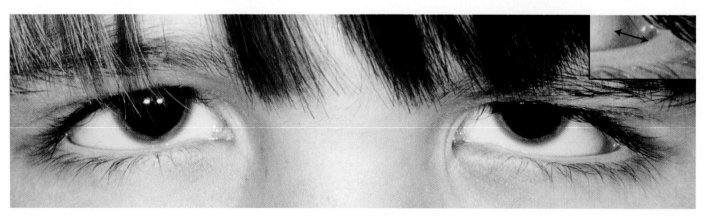

Fig. 1.5 Congenital ectropion. The arrow indicates the malposition of the lower eyelid (inset). This patient also has features of blepharophimosis syndrome, including telecanthus, epicanthus, ptosis, and a poorly developed nasal bridge.

Entropion

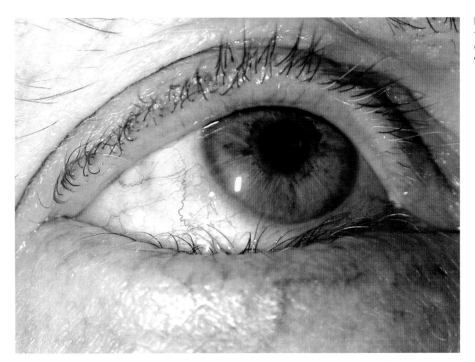

Fig. 1.6 Involutional entropion. The lower eyelid is turned in and the eyelashes rub on the conjunctiva and cornea. This condition occurs with aging and is a result of laxity of the lower lid combined with weakness of the retraction complex.

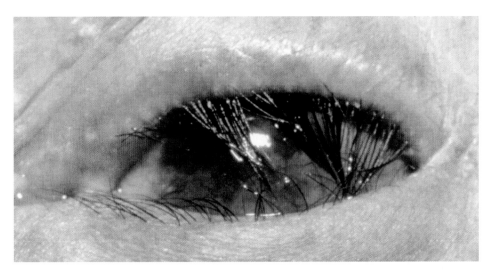

Fig. 1.7 Cicatricial entropion. This disorder is caused by scarring of the palpebral conjunctiva, with resultant in-turning of the lid margins. In this case the conjunctival scarring resulted from trachoma. Other conditions in which cicatricial entropion is seen are Stevens–Johnson syndrome, ocular cicatricial pemphigoid, herpes zoster ophthalmicus, and severe burns.

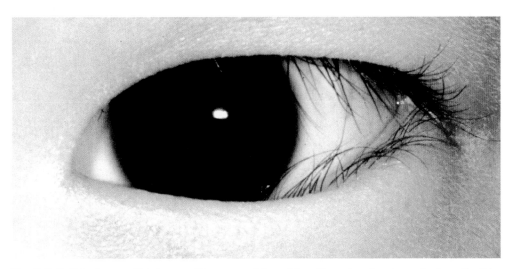

Fig. 1.8 Epiblepharon. This is caused by an overriding of the skin and pretarsal muscle above the lid margin, which causes an in-turning of the lid margin and lashes. Epiblepharon usually resolves with aging and rarely requires treatment.

Trichiasis

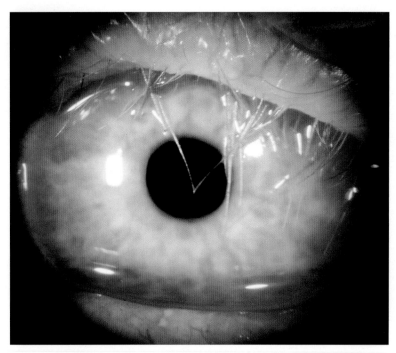

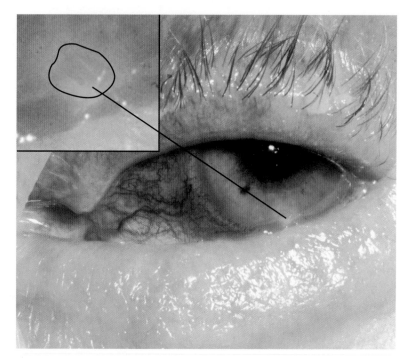

Fig. 1.9 Trichiasis. This is an acquired malposition of the eyelashes. In this patient the eyelashes rub on the superior cornea.

Fig. 1.10 Spastic entropion. This can be caused by acute ocular inflammation or irritation in a patient with a previously unrecognized involutional entropion. Here the lashes rub on the lower cornea and have caused a corneal erosion (inset).

Distichiasis

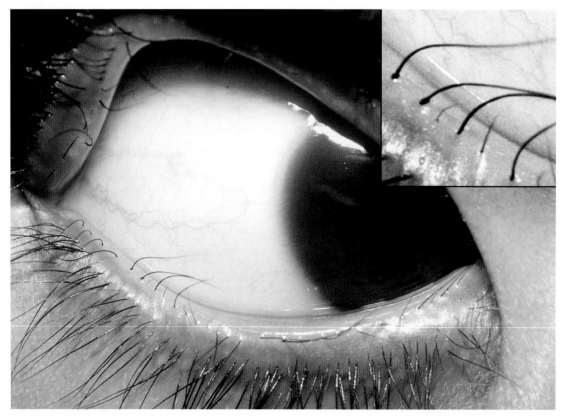

Fig. 1.11 Distichiasis. In this rare condition an extra row of eyelashes exits from the meibomian orifices (inset). The eyelashes may rub on the conjunctiva or cornea.

Lagophthalmos

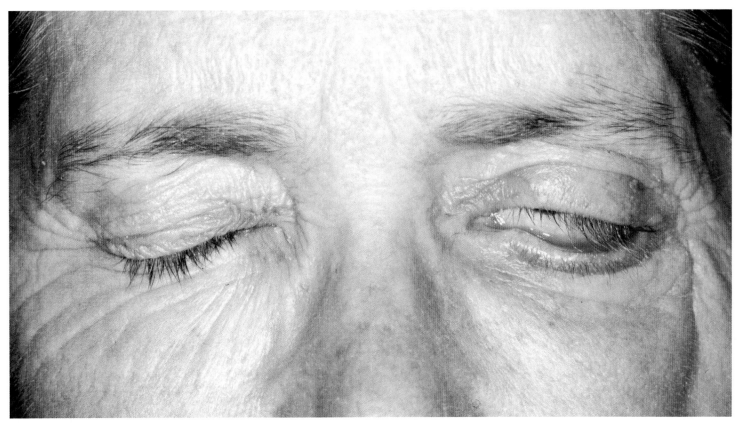

Fig. 1.12 Lagophthalmos. This is the inability to appose the eyelids on attempted eyelid closure. In this case a left seventh nerve palsy has caused a lower lid paralytic ectropion and lagophthalmos.

Ptosis

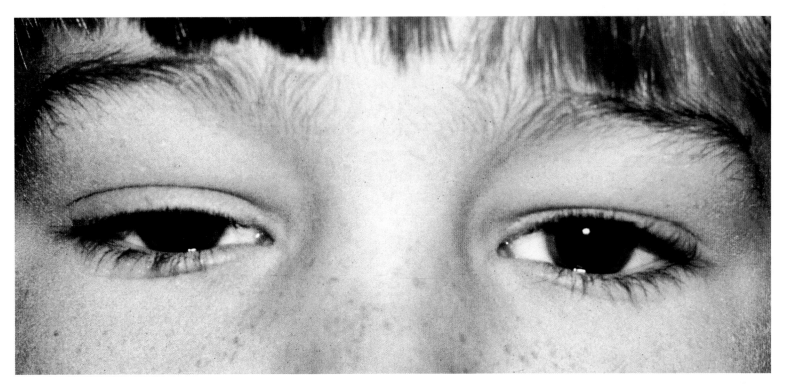

Fig. 1.13 Ptosis. This patient has ptosis of the right upper eyelid with narrowing of the palpebral fissure. The right brow is elevated in an attempt to raise the abnormally low right upper eyelid. The abnormal lid position has induced astigmatism in the right eye. Results of keratometry in the right eye are 47.00 × 87/42.25 × 174; in the left eye, results are nearly spherical.

Floppy Eyelid Syndrome

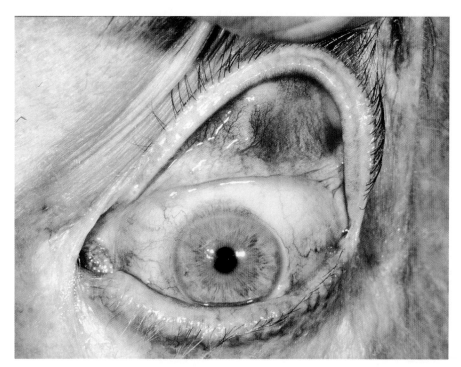

Fig. 1.14 Floppy eyelid syndrome. This syndrome is associated with excessive laxity of the upper eyelid. The eyelid is easily everted with superior traction. Patients often complain of redness, irritation, and mucoid discharge. The symptoms are worse in the morning and may be related to nocturnal eversion of the eyelids leading to corneal exposure.

Lower Lid Imbrication

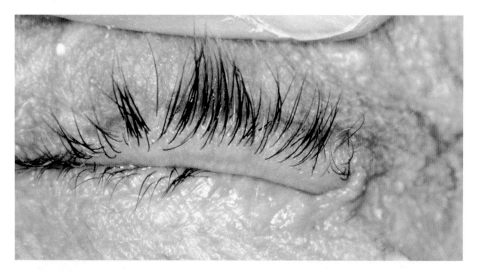

Fig. 1.15 Eyelid imbrication syndrome. The upper eyelid rides over the lower eyelid. This syndrome shares many features with floppy eyelid syndrome, including redness, irritation, and a mucoid discharge. Nocturnal eversion of the eyelids may also occur.

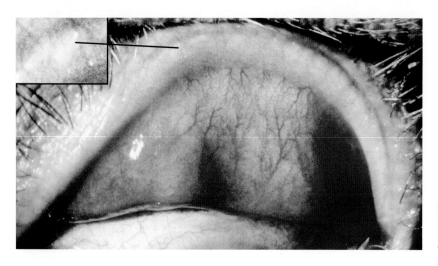

Fig. 1.16 Eyelid imbrication syndrome. Keratinization of the upper palpebral conjunctiva (inset) and papillary conjunctivitis occur with lower lid imbrication. The keratinization is caused by chronic rubbing of the upper lid over the lower lid.

Chapter 2

Diseases of the Lid
Tumors

Patients with abnormal growths on their eyelids are often initially seen by the general practitioner. It is important to differentiate benign lid tumors from malignant lid tumors. Occasionally, a biopsy is needed to establish the diagnosis.

Benign Lid Tumors

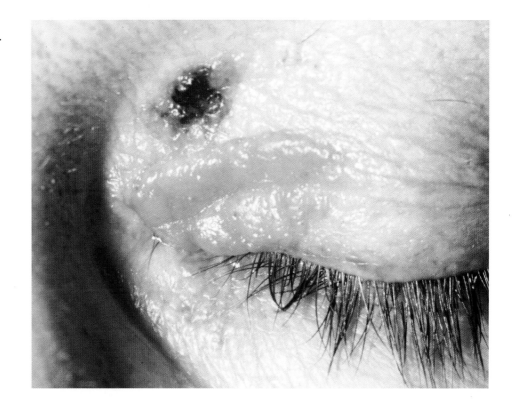

Fig. 2.1 Amyloid deposits from systemic amyloidosis.
These appear as elevated, waxy, yellow deposits in the skin. The deposits are usually bilateral and symmetric. They are occasionally associated with a superficial hemorrhage, as seen in this case.

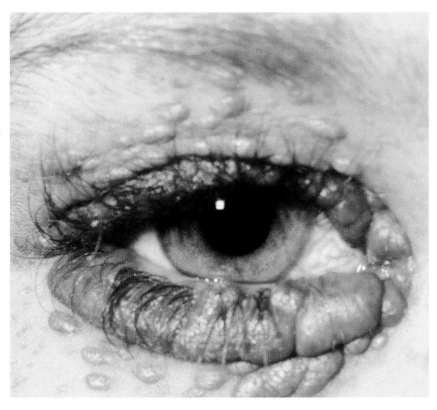

Fig. 2.2 Xanthogranuloma deposits in the eyelid of an 8-year-old boy. Xanthogranuloma is a non-Langerhans histiocytic cell proliferation of unknown etiology. It usually occurs in childhood and is more common in males. The skin lesions usually resolve spontaneously in 3–6 years. Xanthogranulomas can also occur on the cornea (see Fig. 5.53) and iris. Children with iris xanthogranulomas may initially present to the ophthalmologist with visual problems related to spontaneous hyphemas.

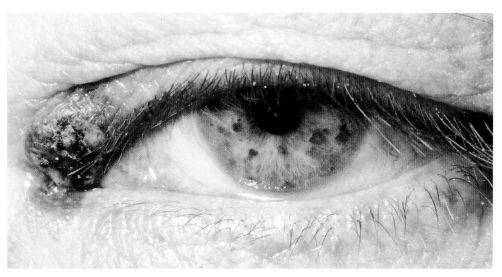

Fig. 2.3 Nevus of the lids. Nevi may be congenital or acquired, and pigmented or nonpigmented. This split nevus or "kissing nevus" occurs when the tumor involves both upper and lower eyelids.

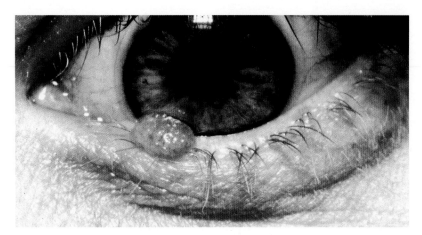

Fig. 2.4 Intradermal nevus. The nevus cells are located exclusively within the dermis, as seen on the lower eyelid in this patient. These nevi are often nonpigmented and elevated.

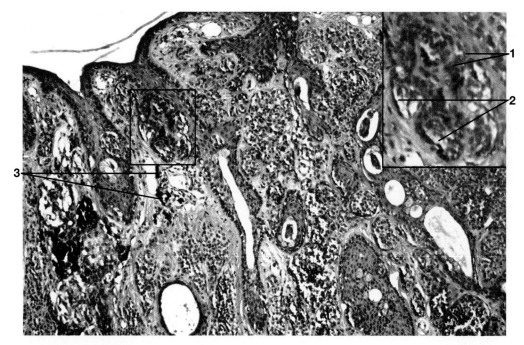

Fig. 2.5 Histopathology of a compound nevus. Nests of nevus cells (1) are lined by clear melanocytes (2). Melanophages (3) are at the junction of the epidermis and dermis and in the dermis.

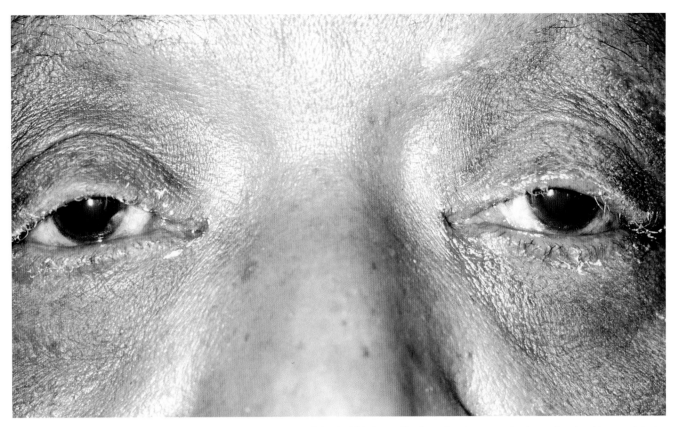

Fig. 2.6 Congenital oculodermal melanocytosis (nevus of Ota). This is a collection of melanocytes in the periocular skin associated with melanosis oculi (see Fig. 2.7). It most commonly occurs in Asian and African-American patients.

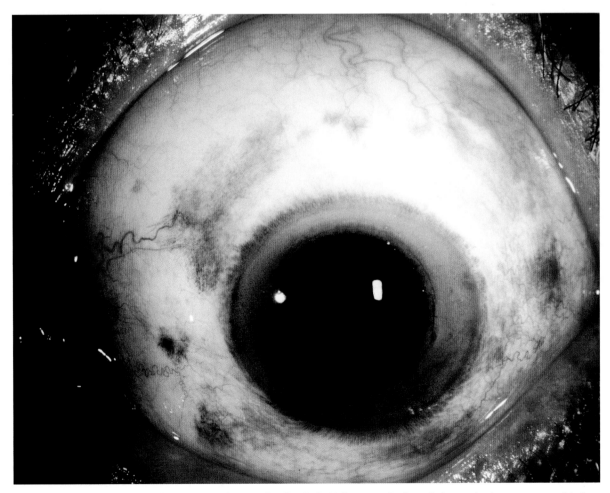

Fig. 2.7 Melanosis oculi in the same patient as in Fig. 2.6. Melanocytes in the episclera and sclera are responsible for the slate-blue discoloration. The conjunctiva over these lesions is mobile. The risk of uveal malignant melanomas is increased in Caucasian patients with this lesion.

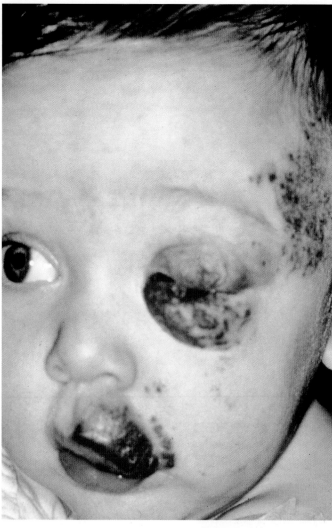

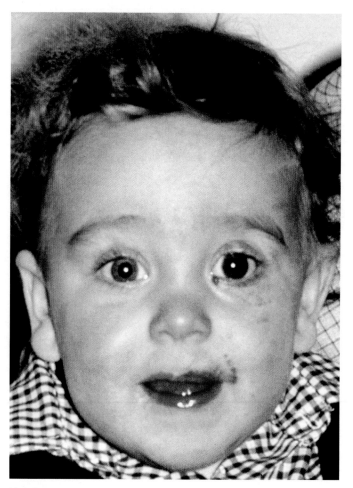

Fig. 2.9 Same patient as in Fig. 2.8, after treatment with intralesional corticosteroids.

Fig. 2.8 Capillary hemangiomas of the lids, mouth, and temporal skin. These tumors are first seen several weeks after birth and grow rapidly during the first year of life. They often resolve spontaneously, but treatment is needed when severe disfigurement, anisometropia, strabismus, or amblyopia occurs.

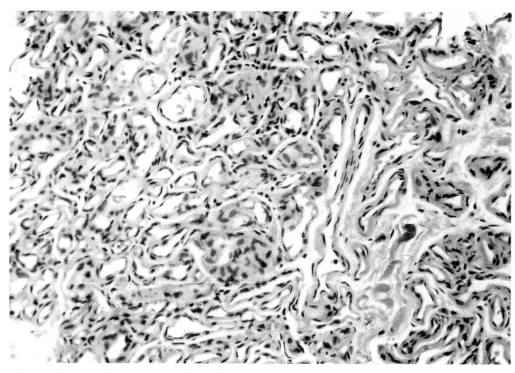

Fig. 2.10 Histopathology of a capillary hemangioma. Multiple small capillary channels lined with endothelial cells are seen.

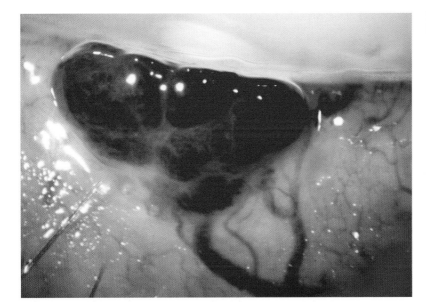

Fig. 2.11 Capillary hemangioma of the lid. This is an isolated capillary hemagioma involving the eyelid margin in an adult.

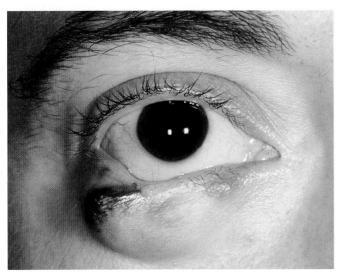

Fig. 2.12 Cavernous hemangioma of the lid. Cavernous hemangiomas are more commonly found in the orbit and are rarely seen in the eyelid. When found on the skin, they are elevated lesions that are compressible with palpation.

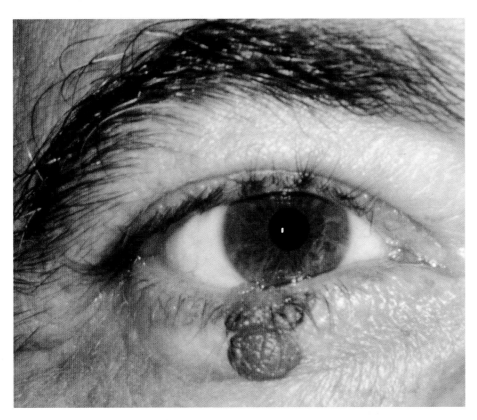

Fig. 2.13 Seborrheic keratosis. This elevated, oily, crusted lesion appears to be stuck onto the surrounding skin. The lesion is common in older persons and is not premalignant.

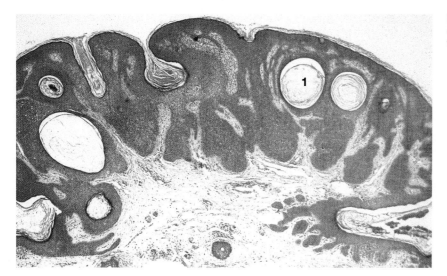

Fig. 2.14 Histopathology of a seborrheic keratosis. A nodule of elevated epithelium is seen. Pseudocysts with keratin (1) are found within the lesion.

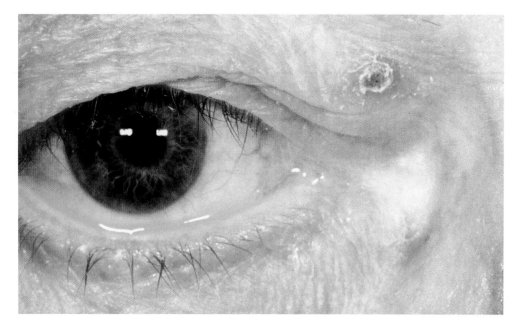

Fig. 2.15 Actinic keratoses. These flat, scaly lesions arise in sun-exposed areas. They are premalignant and may develop into basal or squamous cell carcinoma.

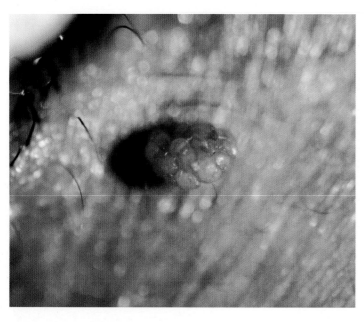

Fig. 2.16 Acrochordon (skin tag). Acrochordons are small skin-colored or lightly pigmented lesions that develop in areas of the body with multiple skin folds such as the eyelids. They are benign lesions that are usually asymptomatic, but occasionally may be associated with itching or discomfort. Simple excision is curative.

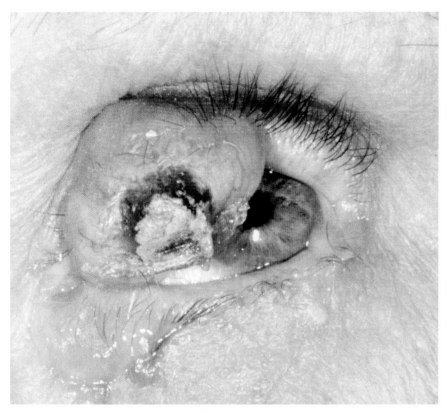

Fig. 2.17 Keratoacanthoma. This rapidly enlarging growth may be seen on the eyelids. There is a central crater filled with keratin. These lesions may involute spontaneously, but are often excised for cosmetic concerns and to exclude the possibility of a malignant lesion.

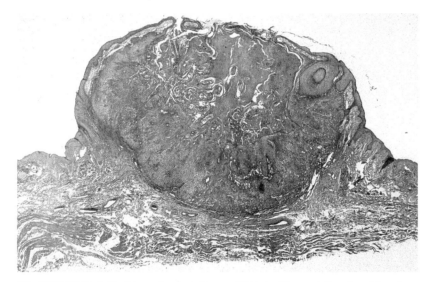

Fig. 2.18 Histopathology of a keratoacanthoma. The central crater of keratin is buttressed by normal epithelium on both sides.

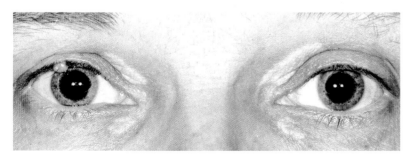

Fig. 2.19 Xanthelasma. These bilateral yellow plaques usually occur in the medial canthal regions. These lesions may be associated with hypercholesterolemia, particularly when they occur in a young patient. In addition, this patient has a probable intradermal nevus on the right upper eyelid margin.

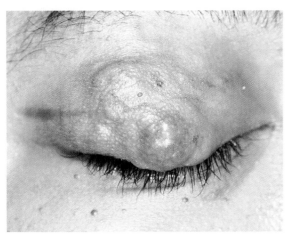

Fig. 2.20 Varices. Varices composed of dilated venous channels are seen in the upper eyelid, giving a blue discoloration to the overlying skin.

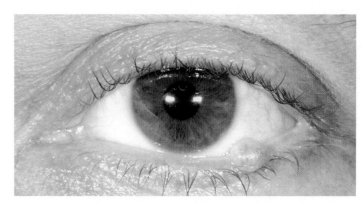

Fig. 2.21 Neurofibromas. Composed of proliferating Schwann cells, they may be seen as elevated nodules and found on the skin anywhere in the body. Here the neurofibroma is on the lower lid margin.

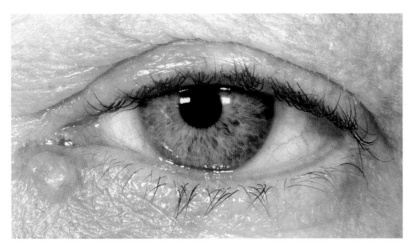

Fig. 2.22 Cysts of Moll's gland. These slow-growing tumors are usually found on the lower lid near the puncta.

Malignant Lid Tumors

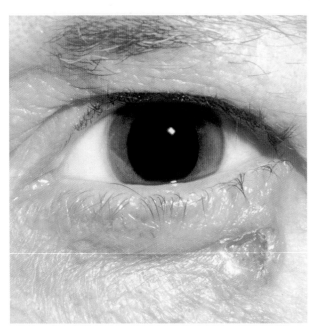

Fig. 2.23 Basal cell carcinomas. These slow-growing tumors are found in sun-exposed areas. They are the most common eyelid malignancy and are usually located on the lower eyelid.

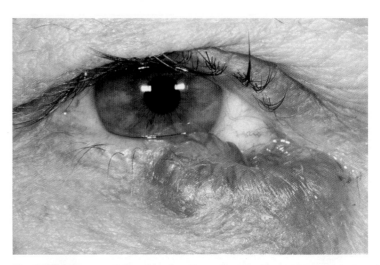

Fig. 2.24 Large, nodular, basal cell carcinoma. The edges are raised and pearly, with a central ulceration.

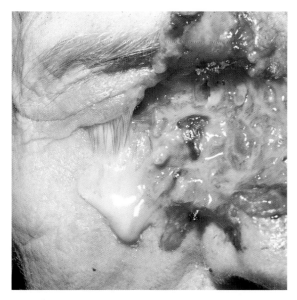

Fig. 2.25 Large basal cell carcinoma. This lesion has invaded deep into the periorbital tissue. Basal cell carcinomas rarely metastasize but may exhibit extensive local invasion if neglected.

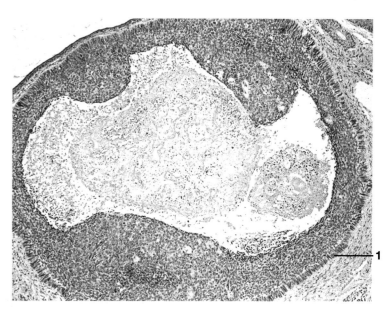

Fig. 2.26 Histopathology of a basal cell carcinoma. Basophilic nests of cells with peripheral palisading (1) are seen.

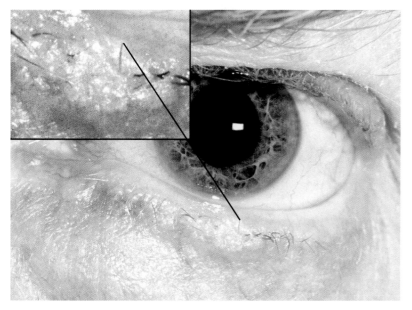

Fig. 2.27 Squamous cell carcinoma. This is a rare malignancy of the eyelids. It commonly arises in sun-exposed areas and may resemble other lesions of the eyelid, such as keratoacanthoma, basal cell carcinoma, and seborrheic keratosis. The inset shows pearly raised margins of a small squamous cell carcinoma.

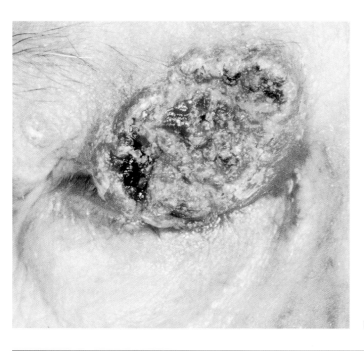

Fig. 2.28 Extensive squamous cell carcinoma of the upper eyelid.

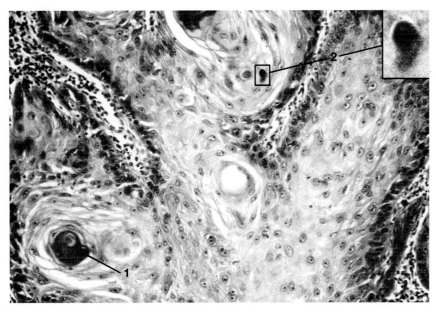

Fig. 2.29 Histopathology of squamous cell carcinoma. Eosinophilic cells with large cytoplasms are shown. Keratin pearls (1) and dyskeratotic cells (2) are seen within the lesion. Dyskeratotic cells have small, dark nuclei and produce keratin.

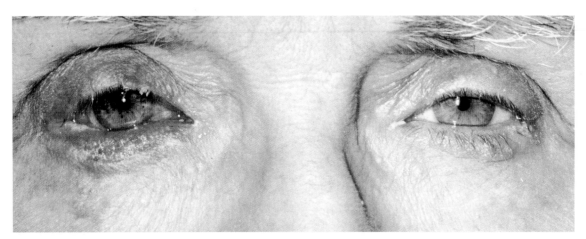

Fig. 2.30 Sebaceous cell carcinoma of the right eyelids. A unilateral or asymmetric chronic blepharitis in an older patient should always raise the suspicion of sebaceous cell carcinoma. This tumor is more common in women and usually located on the upper eyelid, but can be found on both eyelids as seen here.

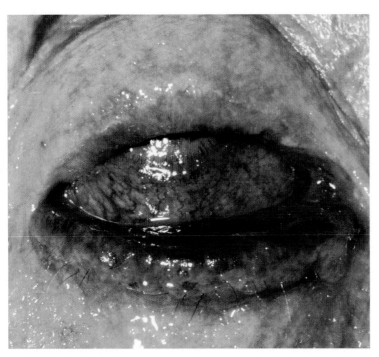

Fig. 2.31 Lid margin in sebaceous cell carcinoma. The lid is thickened and erythematous, and there is extensive lash loss. This tumor is highly malignant and may spread by direct extension, lymphatics, or blood vessels. The mortality rate is as high as 28%.

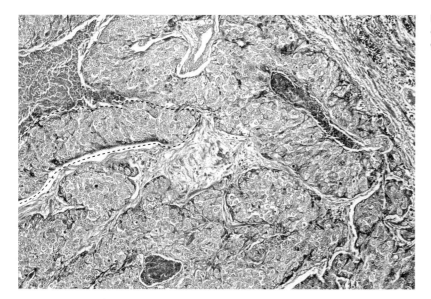

Fig. 2.32 Histopathology of sebaceous cell carcinoma. Cells in nests and cords (outline) with vacuolated, foamy cytoplasms are shown. When the diagnosis is suspected, a full-thickness lid biopsy should be performed.

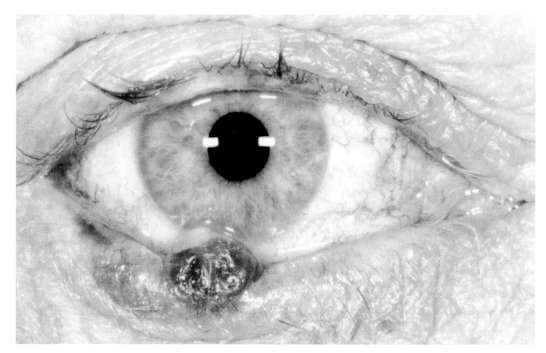

Fig. 2.33 Nodular malignant melanoma of the lower eyelid. This extremely rare malignancy of the eyelid may arise de novo or from preexisting nevi. The prognosis depends on the depth of tumor invasion. This tumor can spread hematogenously and through lymphatic channels.

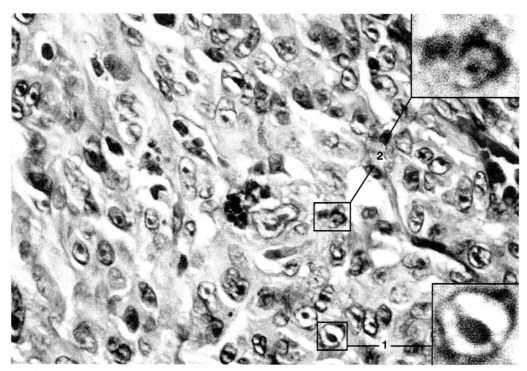

Fig. 2.34 Histopathology of a malignant melanoma of the eyelid. Epithelioid cells with pleomorphic nuclei and eosinophilic nucleoli (1) are shown. Clumps of melanin are seen within the cytoplasm (2).

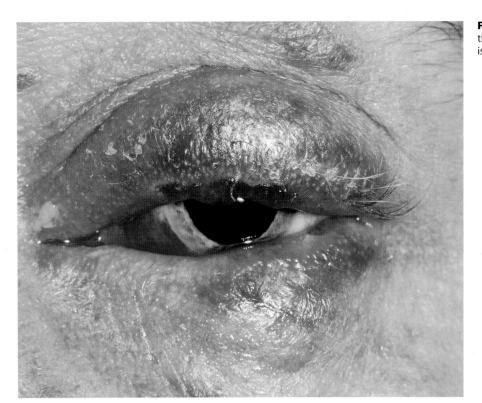

Fig. 2.35 Kaposi's sarcoma of the eyelids. This lesion infiltrates the lid diffusely and has a reddish or purple discoloration. This tumor is found almost exclusively in immunocompromised patients.

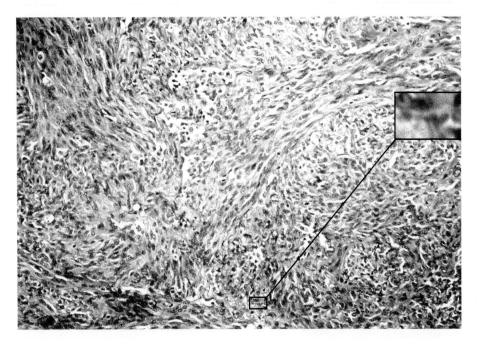

Fig. 2.36 Histopathology of Kaposi's sarcoma. There is proliferation of spindle cells with slit-like spaces between the cells. Erythrocytes (inset) can be seen within the slit-like spaces.

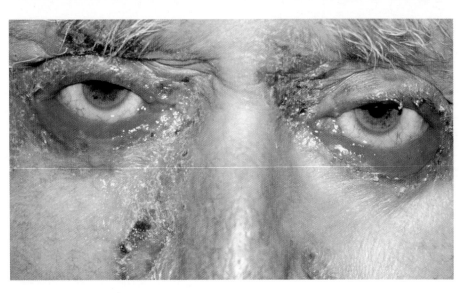

Fig. 2.37 Mycosis fungoides. This is a cutaneous T-cell lymphoma that occasionally involves the periocular skin. Early in the disease process the lesions are eczematoid; they later progress to indurated plaques.

Chapter 3

Diseases of the Lid
Immunologic, Infectious, and Traumatic

Infectious and inflammatory diseases of the eyelids are often associated with conjunctivitis and symptoms of ocular discomfort. These patients are commonly seen in clinical practice.

Blepharitis

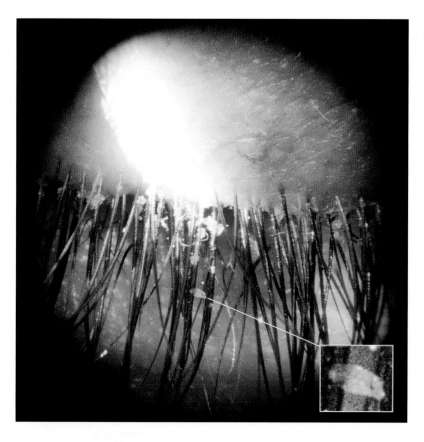

Fig. 3.1 Seborrheic blepharitis. This disorder is often associated with seborrheic dermatitis. Patients complain of redness, burning, and mattering of the eyelids. The condition is usually bilateral and often associated with meibomian gland dysfunction. The lashes are covered with greasy yellow scales. The scales are translucent and easily removed (inset).

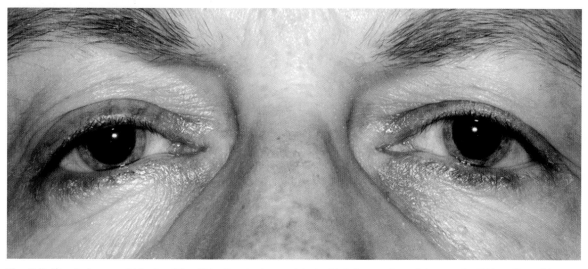

Fig. 3.2 Staphylococcal blepharitis. This disorder is associated with inflammation of the anterior lid lamella and is usually not seen with meibomian gland dysfunction. Erythema of the anterior lid margin, lash loss, misdirected lashes, and ocular discharge are common findings.

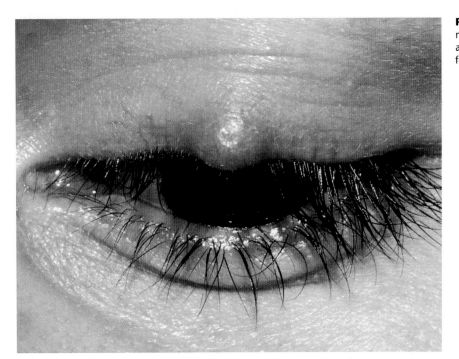

Fig. 3.3 Hordeolum (stye). This is an acute inflammation of the lid margin. An internal hordeolum originates in the meibomian glands, and an external hordeolum originates in Moll's glands, Zeis' glands, or lash follicles. This external hordeolum is on the upper eyelid.

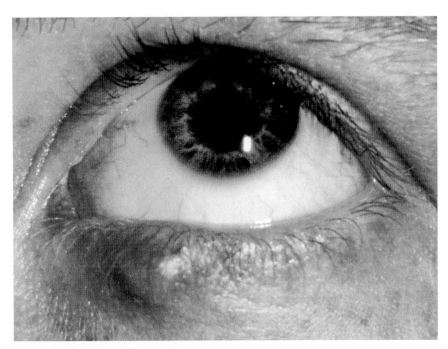

Fig. 3.4 Chalazion. This is an acute inflammation of the eyelid caused by a localized obstruction of meibomian glands. The histopathology shows sebaceous secretions surrounded by a granulomatous reaction.

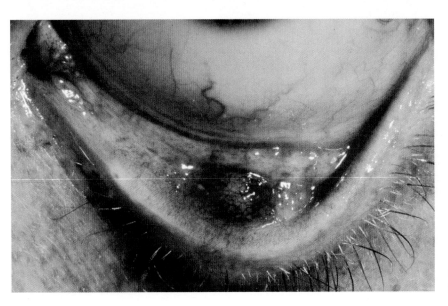

Fig. 3.5 Same patient as in Fig. 3.4. The lower lid is everted, and a focal nodular conjunctivitis is seen overlying the chalazion.

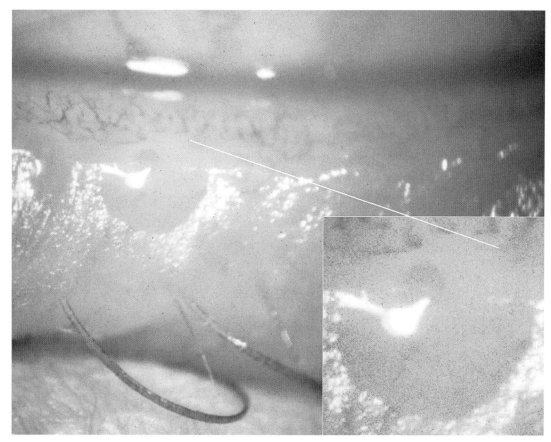

Fig. 3.6 Meibomitis. The lid margin is erythematous, and a loose, oily discharge is easily expressed from the meibomian orifices (inset). This condition is often associated with seborrheic blepharitis.

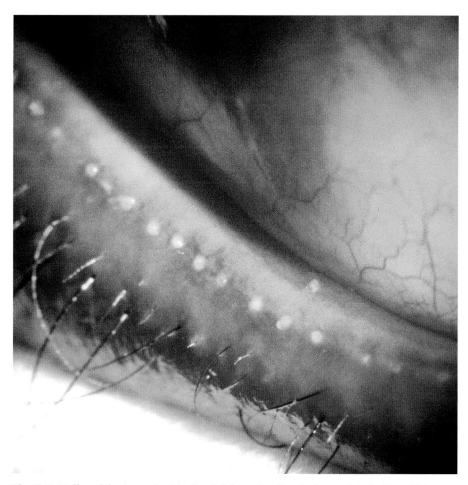

Fig. 3.7 Meibomitis. In contrast to Fig. 3.6, here the disorder is associated with a thick, toothpaste-like secretion. The glands are plugged, and the secretions can be expressed with moderate pressure on the lid margin.

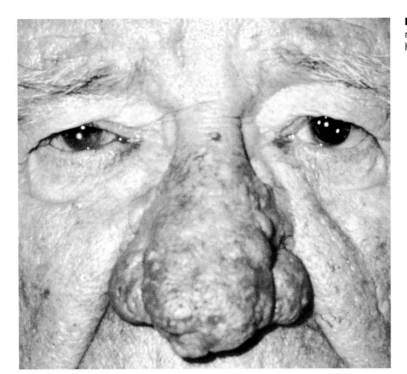

Fig. 3.8 Rosacea. This is a chronic sebaceous gland dysfunction of the skin. This man exhibits rhinophyma, an enlargement of the nose secondary to sebaceous gland hypertrophy.

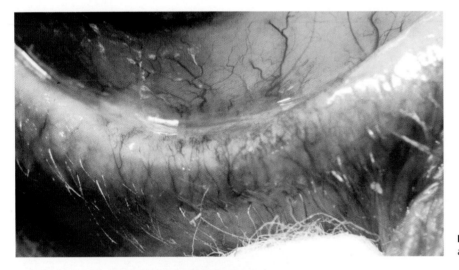

Fig. 3.9 Rosacea. This condition is often associated with blepharitis and meibomian gland dysfunction.

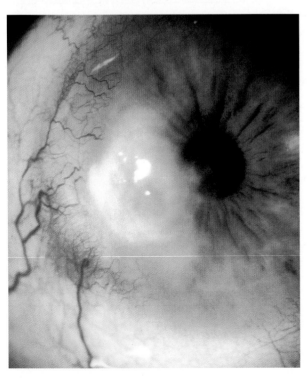

Fig. 3.10 Chronic rosacea. Corneal vascularization and scarring can result.

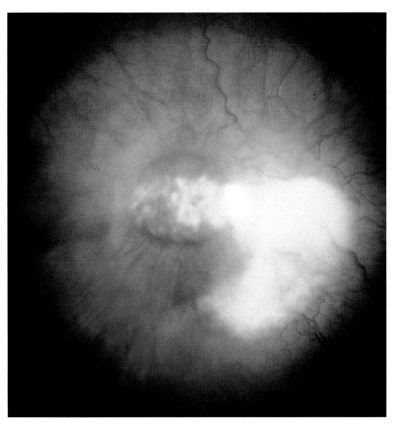

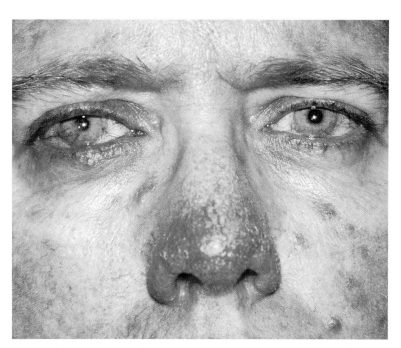

Fig. 3.12 Rosacea. Occurring with greater frequency in females, as in this patient, rosacea often involves erythema, telangiectasia, and acne as common skin findings.

Fig. 3.11 Chronic rosacea keratitis. This patient has severe corneal scarring, vascularization, and lipid degeneration.

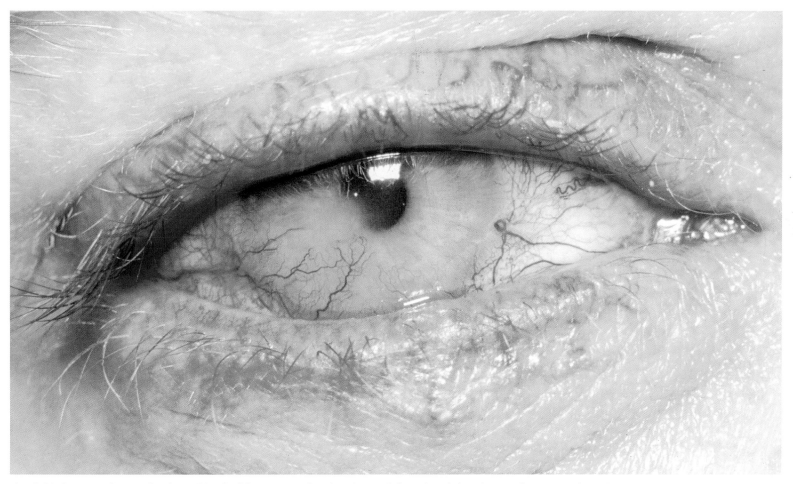

Fig. 3.13 Same patient as in Fig. 3.12. The lid margins and conjunctiva are inflamed, and there is corneal pannus and scarring.

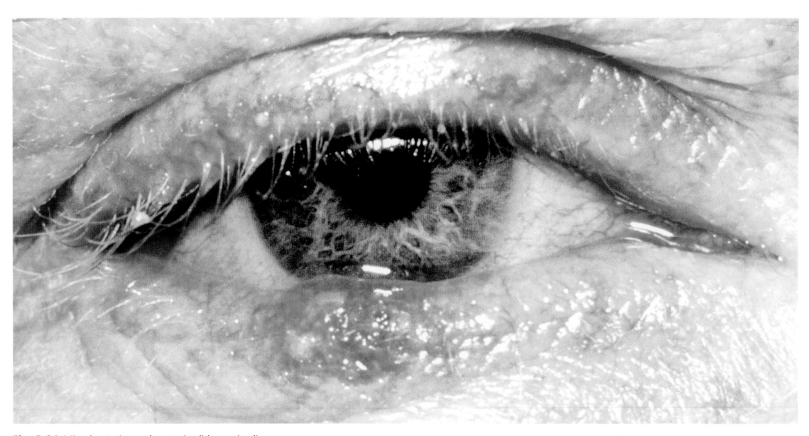

Fig. 3.14 Mixed anterior and posterior lid margin disease.

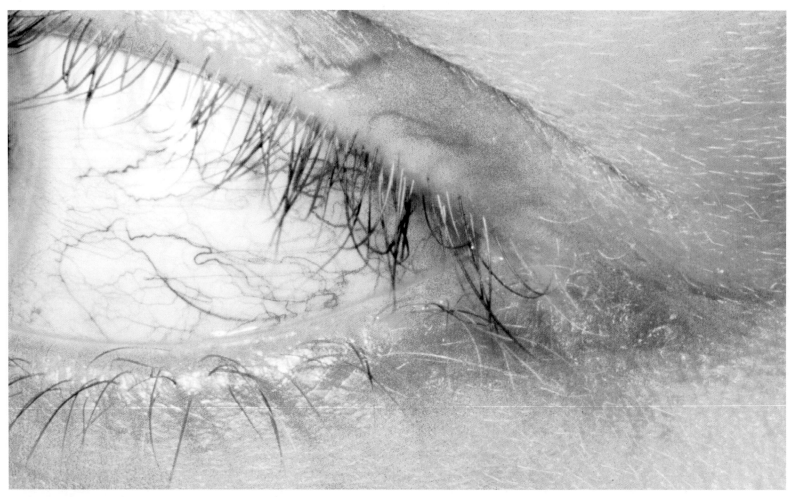

Fig. 3.15 Angular blepharitis. This is an inflammation of the lateral lid margins and canthal region. When infectious, it is often associated with bacterial infection by *Moraxella* or *Staphylococcus* species.

Bacterial Infections

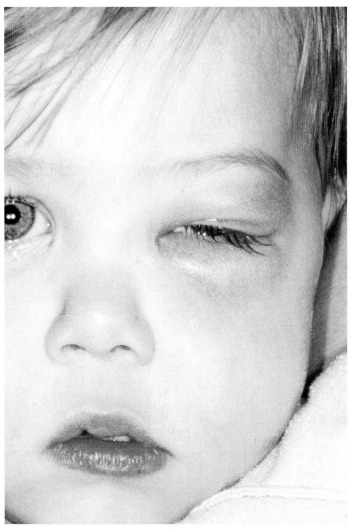

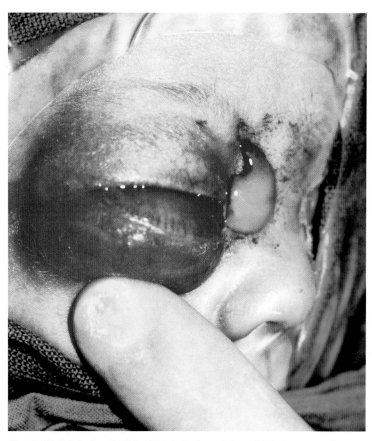

Fig. 3.17 Orbital cellulitis. This infection of the orbital tissues usually extends from an infection in the paranasal sinuses. Here an ethmoid sinusitis has extended into the orbital tissues. Clinical features that distinguish an orbital cellulitis from a preseptal cellulitis include fever, proptosis, severe chemosis, ocular motility disturbances, pupillary abnormalities, and decreased vision.

Fig. 3.16 Preseptal cellulitis. This is an infection of the periorbital tissue anterior to the orbital septum. Visual acuity, pupil reactivity, and ocular motility are normal.

Viral Infections

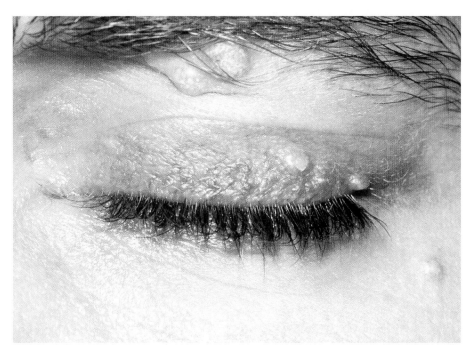

Fig. 3.18 Multiple molluscum contagiosum lesions on the periocular lid in a patient with AIDS. The small elevated lesions with a central umbilicated core are caused by a pox virus.

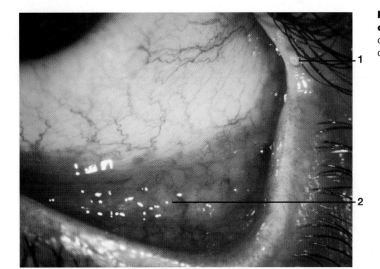

Fig. 3.19 Chronic follicular conjunctivitis from mucocutaneous molluscum contagiosum lesion. A small molluscum lesion (1) is the cause of a chronic follicular conjunctivitis (2). The lesion is small and solitary, and could easily have been missed as the cause of this patient's chronic follicular conjunctivitis.

Parasitic Infections

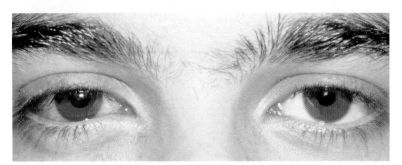

Fig. 3.20 Lid infestation with the crab louse (Phthirus pubis). Chronic conjunctivitis is seen in this patient's right eye. Symptoms include itching, redness, and irritation.

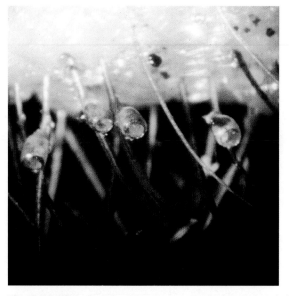

Fig. 3.22 Nits. Ovoid eggs are seen attached to the eyelashes. They hatch 1–2 weeks after they are laid. The reddish-brown granular material on the lid seen here and in Fig. 3.21 is feces from the lice.

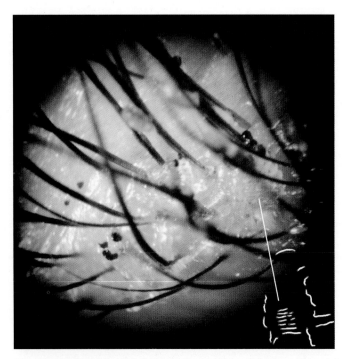

Fig. 3.21 Phthirus pubis infestation of the eyelashes. The adult louse has six legs and appears transparent with direct illumination. The schematic (lower right) shows the outline of a louse.

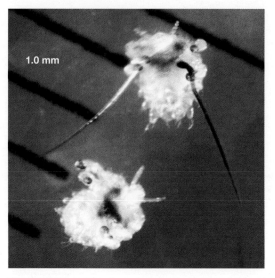

Fig. 3.23 Lice. Two lice are seen after removal from the eyelid. The upper louse is clinging to cilia. Crab lice usually measure 2 mm or less, whereas head and body lice are usually 2–4 mm long.

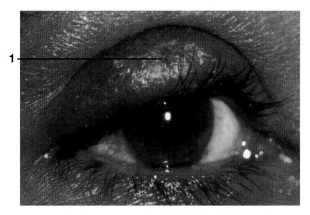

Fig. 3.24 Leishmaniasis of the lid. A healing pustule (1) is seen on the upper eyelid. Leishmaniasis is caused by protozoa transmitted between infected hosts (humans, rodents, and canines) by the bite of the sandfly. The eyelid is an uncommon site of involvement owing to the blinking action of the lid, which makes it more difficult for the sandfly to bite in this area. Most lesions are self-limiting, healing within 3–24 months.

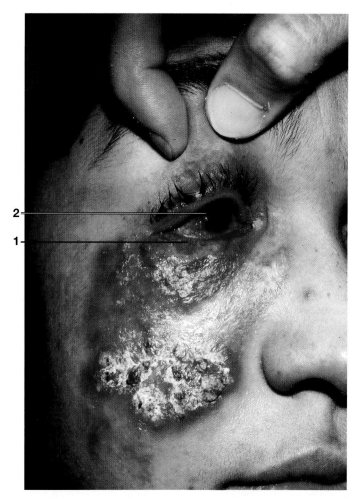

Fig. 3.25 Leishmaniasis of face, lids, conjunctiva, and cornea. A chronic form of leishmaniasis may cause psoriaform plaques on the skin. This form is often resistant to therapy and may result in disfiguring scars on the face. Lid involvement (1) can result in cicatricial ectropion. Conjunctival and corneal involvement (2) can result in ulceration and scarring.

Allergic Inflammations

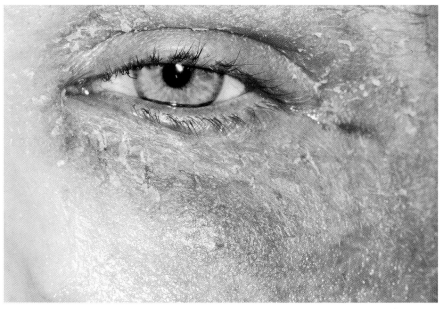

Fig. 3.26 Contact dermatitis. This may develop after prolonged use of a topical medication. Clinically, an eczematous reaction of the lid margin and redness of the periocular skin occur. Symptoms include itching and irritation. This patient developed a reaction to tape after several days of pressure patching of a corneal abrasion.

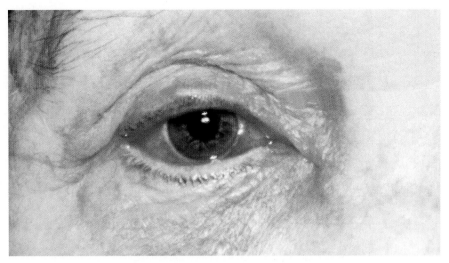

Fig. 3.27 Hypersensitivity reaction. Thimerosal is believed to cause a type IV hypersensitivity reaction of the conjunctiva. Here the thimerosal was a preservative in a contact lens solution. It is now used less frequently in a contact lens solution because of this type of reaction.

Alopecia

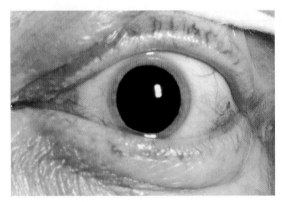

Fig. 3.28 Alopecia. There is complete loss of all of the eyelashes. The underlying skin is hypopigmented and slightly erythematous.

Trauma

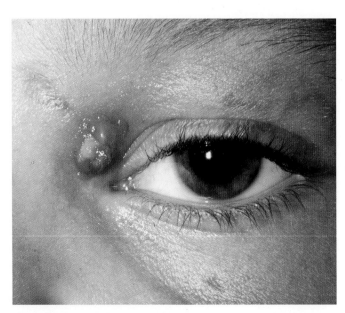

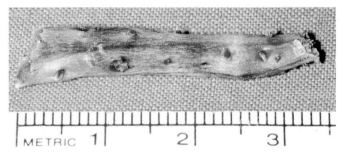

Fig. 3.30 Foreign body. The wooden foreign body was approximately 3.5 cm long.

Fig. 3.29 Foreign body reaction. A retained foreign body may present as a localized area of eyelid inflammation. Here an occult wooden foreign body was removed surgically.

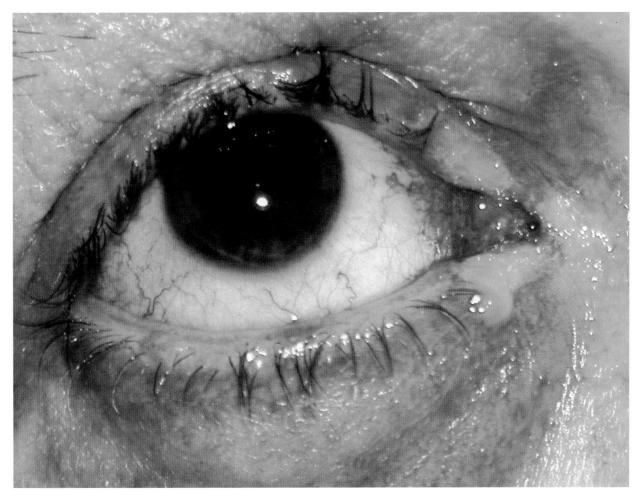

Fig. 3.31 Thermal burns to right upper and lower lids.

Chapter 4

Disorders of Tear Production and the Lacrimal System

The tear film is composed of three layers: the mucous layer, the aqueous layer, and the lipid layer. The mucous layer is produced by conjunctival goblet cells and is in direct contact with the corneal epithelium. The aqueous layer is produced by the main lacrimal gland and the accessory lacrimal glands. The most anterior layer is the lipid layer, which is produced by the meibomian glands.

Dry Eye

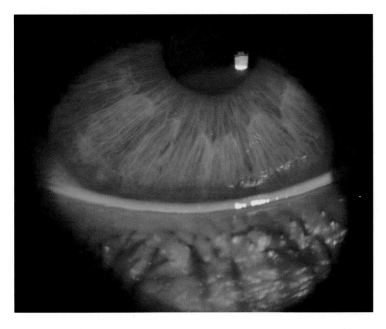

Fig. 4.1 Normal tear film. In this example of a normal tear film, there is an adequate tear lake between the lower lid and the cornea. The cornea is clear and there are no staining irregularities of the corneal epithelium.

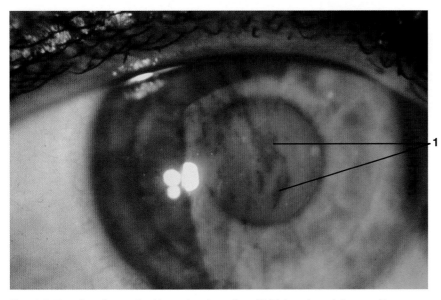

Fig. 4.2 Tear break-up. Rapid tear break-up time (BUT) is a sign of dry eye. To measure tear break-up time, the patient is asked to blink; this distributes the tear film evenly across the cornea. As the tear film thins, dry spots (1) develop on the surface of the cornea. The time taken for this to occur is measured. Tear break-up times of 10 seconds or less are considered abnormal.

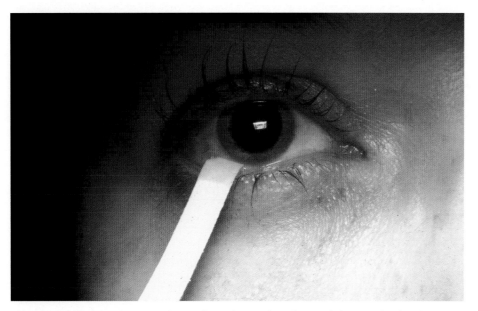

Fig. 4.3 Schirmer strip. To perform Schirmer's test, the inferior cul-de-sac is dried with a cotton swab. A standardized strip of filter paper is placed over the lateral third of the lower lid. This test can be performed with or without anesthesia. Schirmer's test without anesthesia measures basal tear secretion and reflex tear secretion. Schirmer's test with anesthesia measures only basal tear secretion by eliminating the irritation from the filter paper that causes reflex tearing. With anesthesia, the interpretation is as follows: 0–5 mm of wetting, severe dry eyes; 5–10 mm of wetting, moderately dry eyes; 10–15 mm of wetting, mildly dry eyes, and more than 15 mm of wetting, normal tear function. Without anesthesia, wetting of less than 15 mm indicates dry eyes, and less than 5 mm indicates very severe dry eyes.

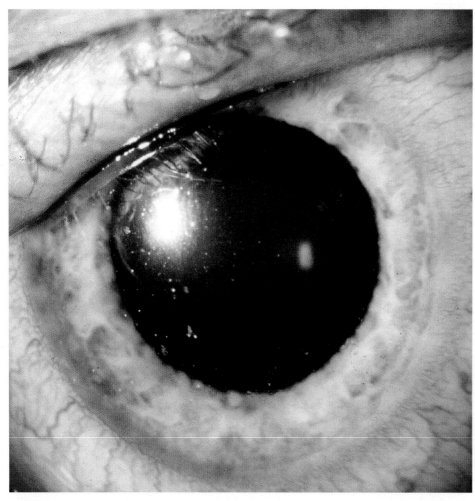

Fig. 4.4 Dry eye syndrome. This is often associated with lid margin disease. Dry eyes can occur as both quantitative and qualitative disorder of tear production. In this example, the upper lid margin is inflamed and shows lash loss. The corneal surface is dry, and there is an irregular light reflex. Mucus is evident on the corneal surface.

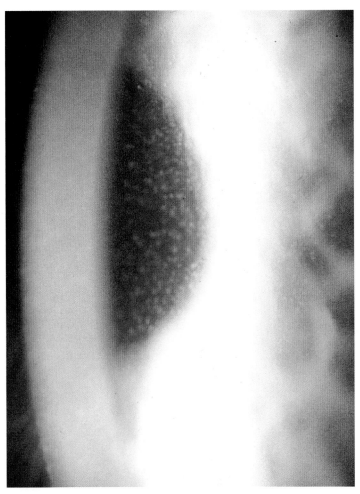

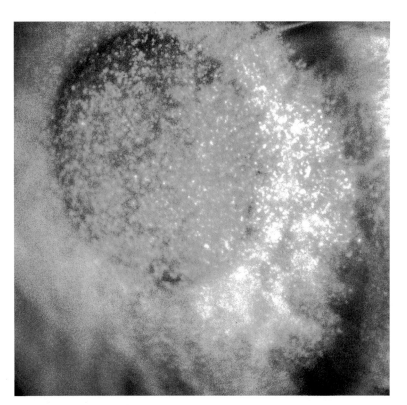

Fig. 4.6 Fluorescein staining in the same patient as in Fig. 4.5. Fluorescein is a water-soluble dye that stains in areas of missing epithelium.

Fig. 4.5 Superficial punctate keratopathy. This is a common finding in patients with dry eye syndrome. The irregular epithelial surface can be appreciated without special stains.

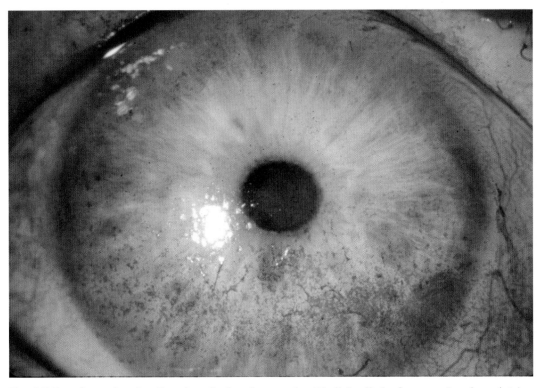

Fig. 4.7 Rose bengal stain of conjunctival and corneal epithelial cells in dry eyes. Rose bengal stains conjunctival and corneal epithelial cells with a disruption to the overlying mucin layer or damage to the epithelial cell wall.

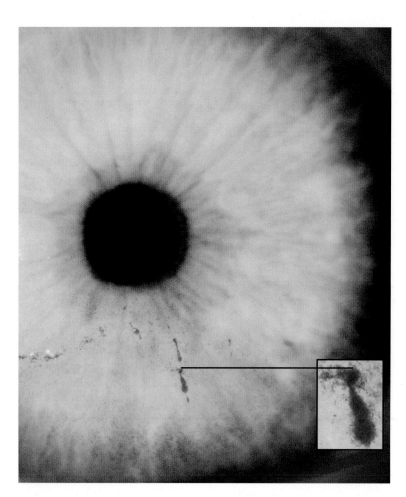

Fig. 4.8 Dry eye syndrome. In addition to epithelial cells, rose bengal also stains mucous filaments (inset). Mucus does not stain well with fluorescein.

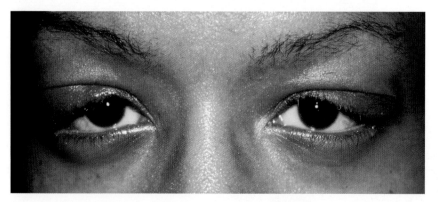

Fig. 4.9 Bilateral lacrimal gland enlargement from sarcoidosis. Enlargement of the lacrimal gland from sarcoidosis has caused inferior displacement of the lateral lid margins. The lid margins assume a characteristic **S** shape.

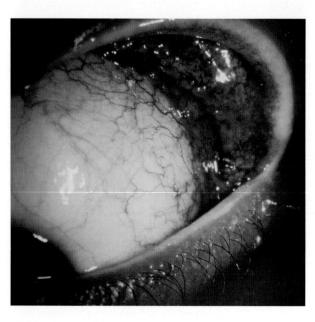

Fig. 4.10 Sarcoidosis; same patient as in Fig. 4.9. The lacrimal gland is inflamed and enlarged.

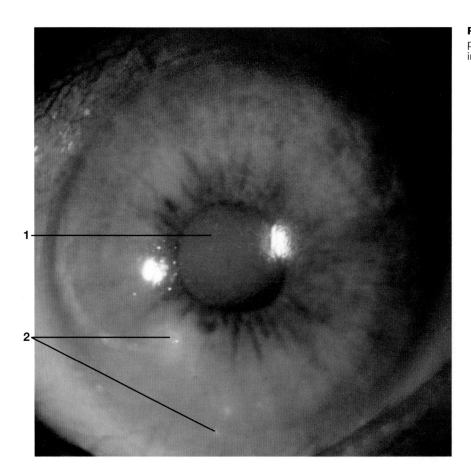

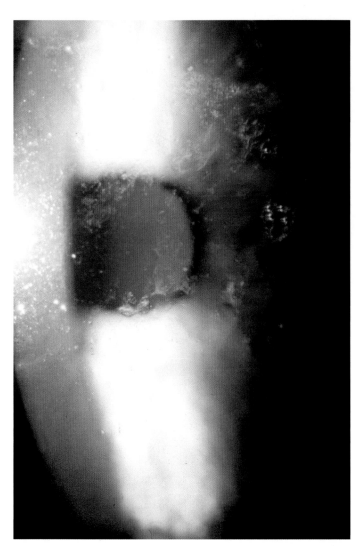

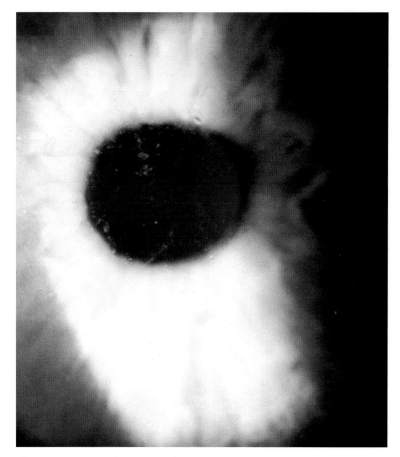

Fig. 4.11 Lacrimal gland tumor resulting in a dry eye. In this patient with pseudotumor of the lacrimal gland, the corneal surface is irregular (1) and there are mucous filaments (2).

1

2

Fig. 4.13 Same patient as in Fig. 4.12. Several minutes after administration of 10% acetylcysteine (Mucomyst), this was the appearance of the eye. Acetylcysteine is a mucolytic agent that is effective in the treatment of excessive mucus.

Fig. 4.12 Dry eye syndrome. Mucous debris is stuck on the epithelium.

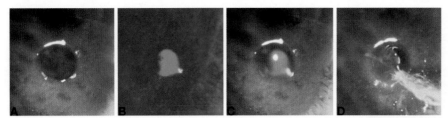

Fig. 4.14 Dry eye with an epithelialized ulcer. A, White light without fluorescein suggests an ulcer (stromal tissue loss with an overlying epithelial defect). **B,** Colbalt blue light with fluorescein apparently confirms an overlying epithelial defect. **C,** White light with fluorescein apparently further confirms an overlying epithelial defect. **D,** Clearing the pool of fluorescein with a cotton applicator reveals that there was pooling of the fluorescein simulating an active corneal ulcer. Active corneal ulcers with stromal thinning show fluorescein staining of the overlying epithelial defects, whereas stromal thinning without ulceration may show pooling of fluorescein dye that simulates an active corneal ulcer.

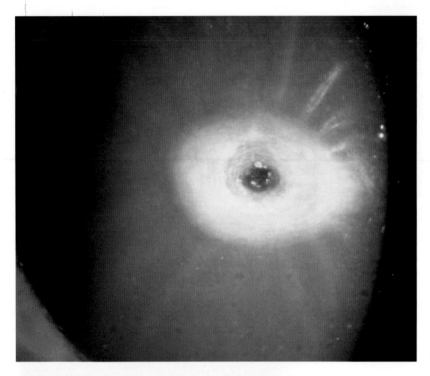

Fig. 4.15 Severe dry eyes. Sterile ulceration can result.

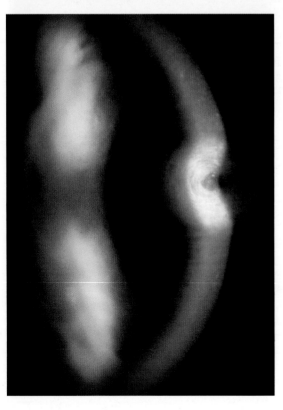

Fig. 4.16 Dry eye syndrome. Slit-beam examination of this patient's cornea shows extensive tissue loss with a descemetocele.

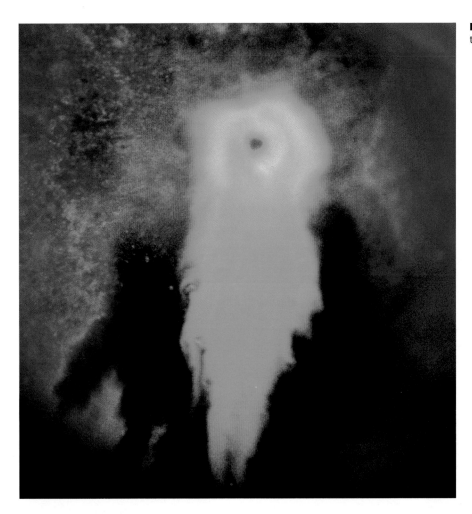

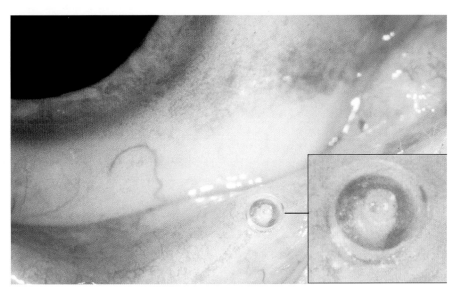

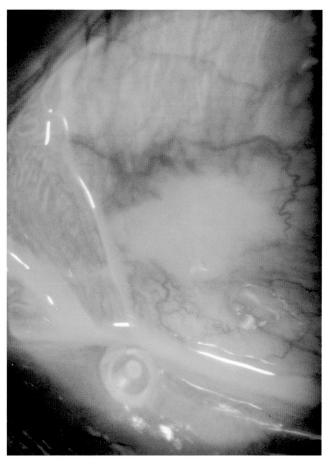

Fig. 4.18 Dry eye syndrome. A silicone punctal plug (inset) has been placed in the right inferior punctum. The plug increases the volume of the tear film by decreasing tear outflow.

Fig. 4.19 Dry eye syndrome. Silicone plugs can rub on the conjunctiva. Fluorescein stains an area of conjunctival erosion.

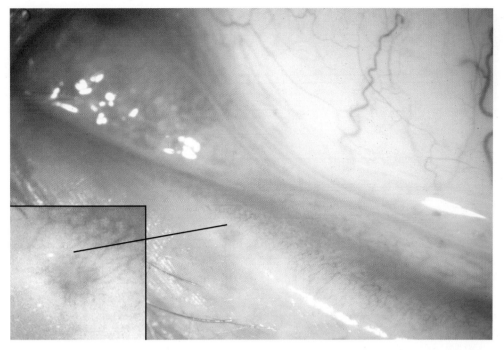

Fig. 4.20 Dry eye syndrome. Permanent punctal occlusion can be performed with cautery. The left lower punctum has been occluded, and fluorescein pools in the occluded area (inset).

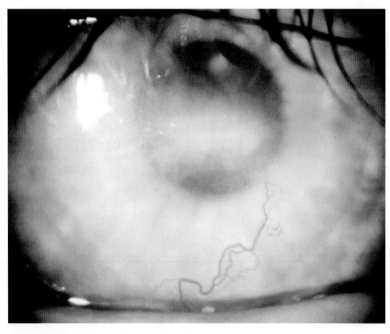

Fig. 4.21 Dry eye syndrome. Familial dysautonomia (Riley–Day syndrome) causes systemic autonomic instability. Here the cornea is scarred from a previous corneal ulcer. These patients have corneal hypesthesia and dry eyes.

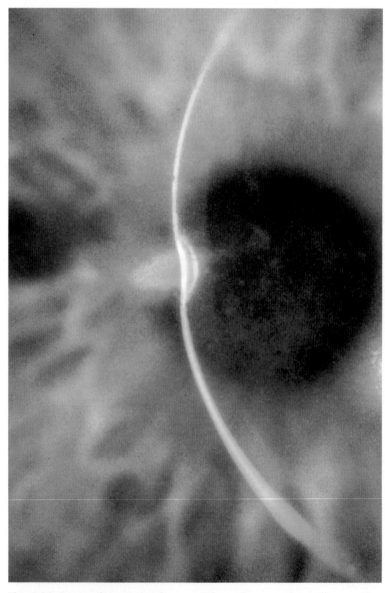

Fig. 4.22 Severe dry eye syndrome with graft-versus-host disease. Here a sterile corneal ulceration is seen.

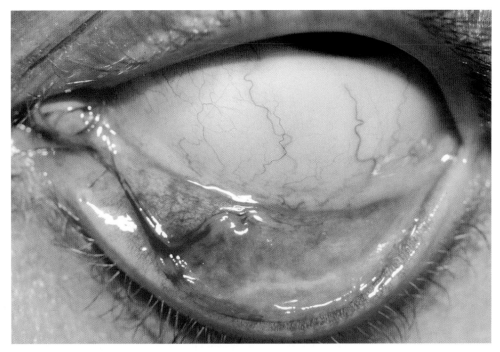

Fig. 4.23 Dry eye syndrome with graft-versus-host disease. This patient has a severe dry eye and membranous conjunctivitis.

Dacryoadenitis, Dacryocystitis, and Canaliculitis

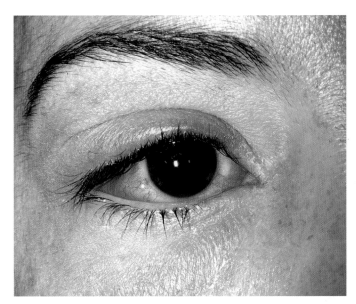

Fig. 4.24 Dacryoadenitis. This is an inflammation of the lacrimal gland. The superior temporal lid is erythematous, and the lid margin is **S**-shaped as a result of the underlying enlargement of the lacrimal gland.

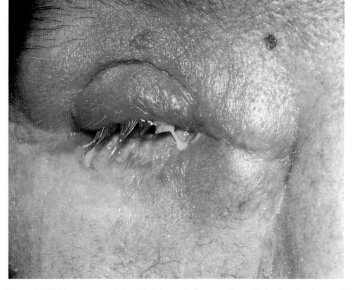

Fig. 4.25 Dacryocystitis. This is an inflammation of the lacrimal sac. Here an acute infection is seen, with erythema and enlargement lateral to the nasal bridge. Mucopurulent conjunctivitis is also present.

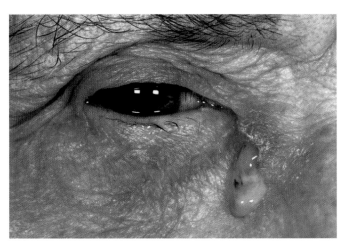

Fig. 4.26 Dacryocystitis. In this case, a fistulous tract has developed from the lacrimal sac to the overlying skin. Purulent material is seen exiting the fistula.

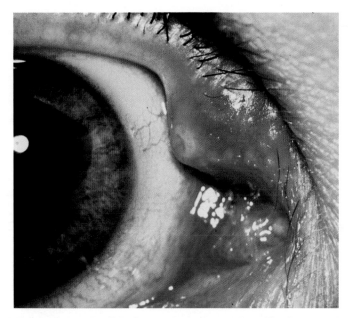

Fig. 4.27 Canaliculitis due to Actinomyces israelii. The signs of canaliculitis include a chronic conjunctivitis and an inflamed pouting punctum. Canaliculitis and low-grade dacryocystitis are often overlooked as causes of chronic conjunctivitis.

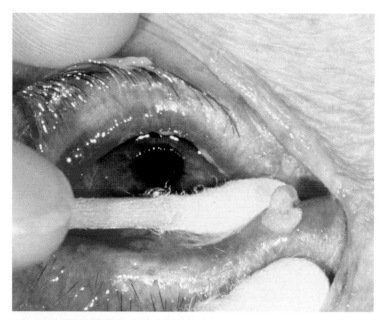

Fig. 4.28 Canaliculitis due to Actinomyces israelii. When external pressure is placed on the puncta, a thick concretion with sulfur granules is expressed. The *Actinomyces* organism is often sequestered in diverticula within the canaliculus, and treatment involves surgical opening and irrigation of the canaliculus.

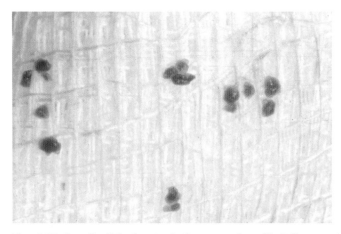

Fig. 4.29 Canaliculitis due to Actinomyces israelii. Sulfur granules composed of branching filaments are found within the discharge. This organism was once thought to be a fungus due to the morphology of the branching filaments, but it is now known to be an anaerobic bacteria with variable Gram-positive and acid-fast staining characteristics.

Chapter 5

Conjunctival Disease
Tumors

Conjunctival tumors can be divided into squamous neoplasms, melanocytic neoplasms, and subepithelial neoplasms. It is often possible to differentiate benign lesions from malignant lesions based on the appearance of the lesion; however, in some cases a biopsy is necessary.

Squamous Neoplasms of the Conjunctiva

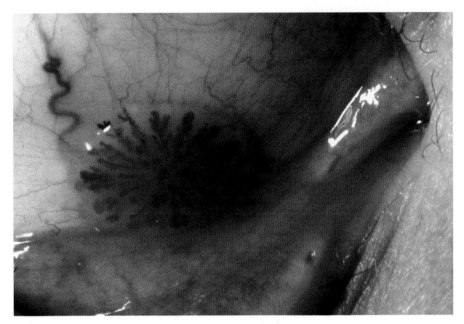

Fig. 5.1 Sessile papilloma. This benign lesion of the conjunctiva consists of multiple fibrovascular connective tissue cores with an overlying epithelium. Lesions may be sessile or pedunculated. They are caused by human papillomavirus (subtypes 6, 11, 16, and 18); in older adults these lesions can be premalignant.

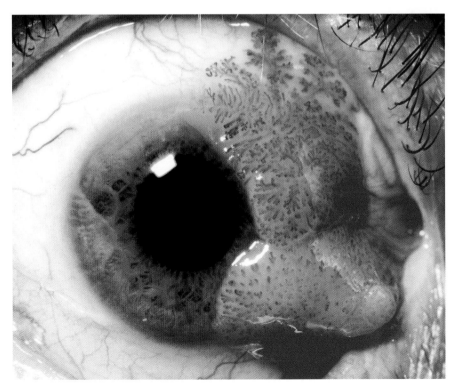

Fig. 5.2 Large papilloma. This papilloma extends onto the corneal surface.

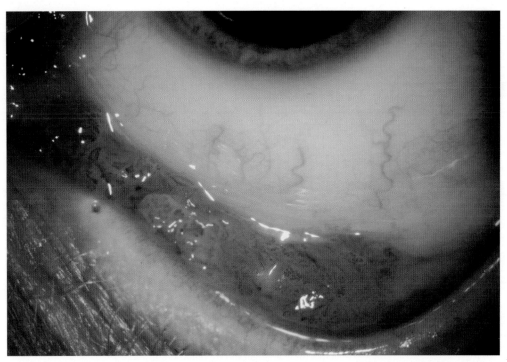

Fig. 5.3 Condyloma acuminatum of the conjunctiva. Clinically, this squamous papilloma extends from the caruncle deep into the inferior and superior fornix of both eyes. In this case, molecular diagnostic polymerase chain reaction studies confirmed human papilloma virus (HPV) subtype 11. Commonly, HPV 6 and 11 are benign strains associated with genital cervical warts. HPV 16, 18, and 31 can be associated with premalignant cervical lesions. When exuberant bilateral squamous papillomas are derived from a sexually transmitted HPV infection, they can be referred to as condyloma acuminatum of the conjunctiva.

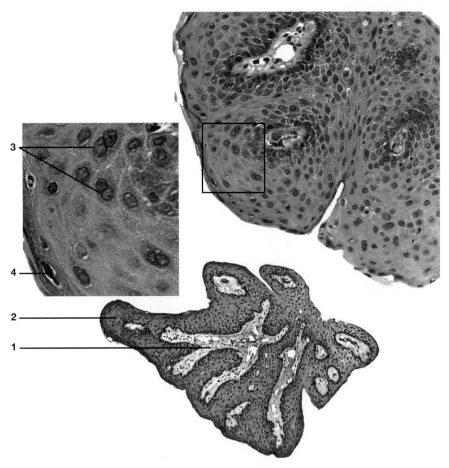

Fig. 5.4 Condyloma acuminatum of the conjunctiva; pathology of patient in Fig. 5.3. The low-power specimen below demonstrates a frond composed of a fibrovascular core (1) and thickened epithelium (2). The higher-magnification specimen above this HPV-induced squamous papilloma demonstrates binucleate cells (3) and perinuclear cytoplasmic clearing (4), also known as koilocytosis.

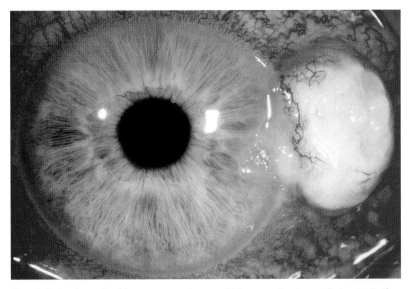

Fig. 5.5 Conjunctival keratoacanthoma. This exceedingly rare lesion is similar to keratoacanthoma on the skin. The lesions arise rapidly, are elevated, and contain a central keratin core.

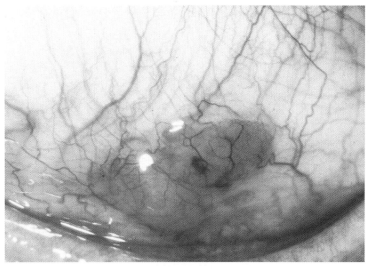

Fig. 5.6 Conjunctival dacryoadenoma. Clinically, this is a soft, pink, mobile mass. Histologically, it is composed of lacrimal secretory cells arising from the conjunctival epithelium. It is a benign tumor. The lacrimal gland is embryologically derived from the conjunctiva.

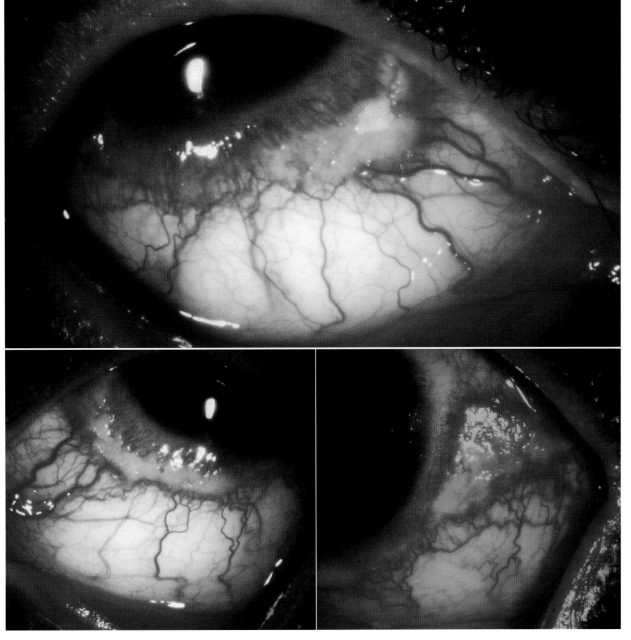

Fig. 5.7 Hereditary benign intraepithelial dyskeratosis. This autosomal dominant condition is seen primarily in the Haliwa Indians (an inbred triracial isolate of white, American Indian, and black origin) of northeastern North Carolina. The primary feature is white dyskeratotic plaques on the peri-limbal bulbar conjunctiva. Corneal and buccal mucosal plaques have been described. The lesions tend to wax and wane, and most patients can be treated with conservative measures. Rarely, large lesions require surgical resection.

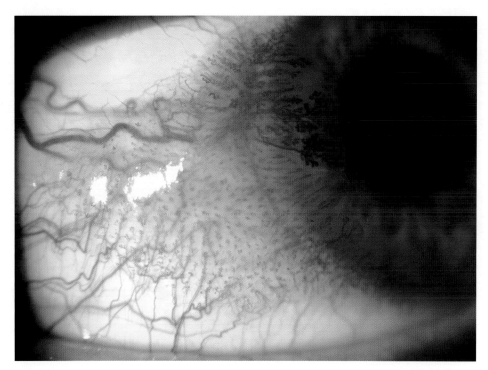

Fig. 5.8 Conjunctival and corneal intraepithelial neoplasia. This occurs predominantly in older Caucasians. When it is seen in a younger patient, as in this case, a thorough search for systemic immunodeficiency syndromes should be undertaken. The condition usually begins at the limbus in the interpalpebral region and often extends onto the cornea. It is associated with chronic sun exposure. The lesions are characteristically elevated and have a gelatinous appearance. The conjunctiva is diffusely injected around the lesion, and within the lesion there are loops of vessels. The lesion may resemble a papilloma.

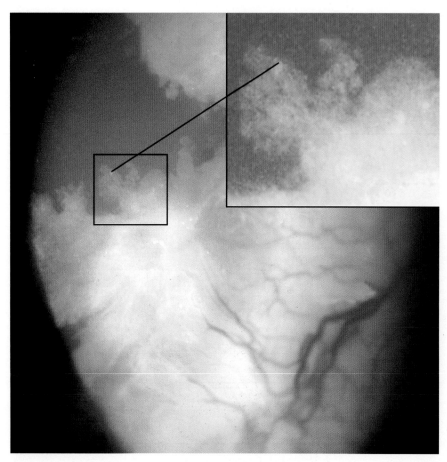

Fig. 5.9 Conjunctival intraepithelial neoplasia. In many cases, the lesion extends onto the cornea and has waxy, scalloped extensions (inset).

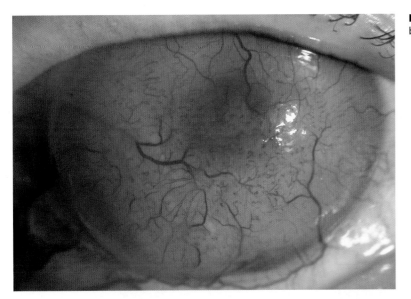

Fig. 5.10 Corneal intraepithelial neoplasia. This is the appearance of the eye before treatment with topical mitomycin.

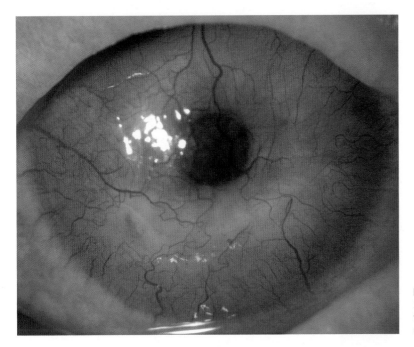

Fig. 5.11 Corneal intraepithelial neoplasia; same patient as in Fig. 5.10. Six weeks after treatment with topical mitomycin the cornea is less opacified. At that time, because of burning, the concentration of mitomycin was reduced and used for two more weeks.

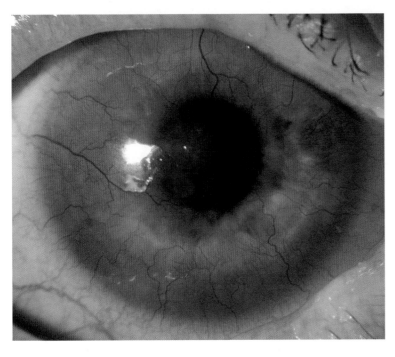

Fig. 5.12 Corneal intraepithelial neoplasia; same patient as in Figs 5.10 and 5.11. This is the appearance of the eye 7 months later. The vision has improved from hand motions to 20/200.

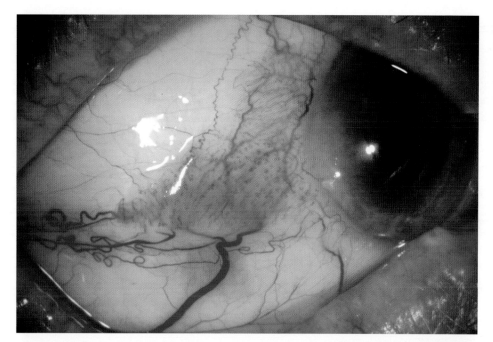

Fig. 5.13 Conjunctival intraepithelial neoplasia before treatment with interferon alpha-2b. This 68-year-old man had noted a lesion in his right eye for several months. Impression cytology confirmed the diagnosis of conjunctival intraepithelial neoplasia. The patient was started on topical interferon alpha-2b four times daily.

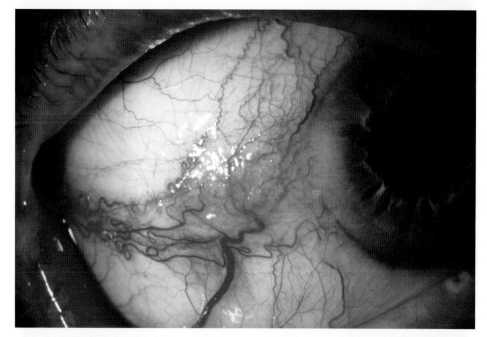

Fig. 5.14 Conjunctival intraepithelial neoplasia; same patient as in Fig. 5.13. Two months after treatment with interferon alpha-2b, there is partial resolution of the lesion.

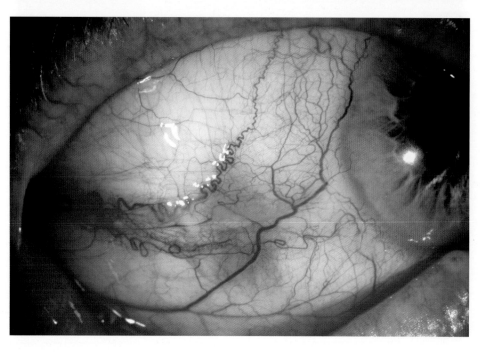

Fig. 5.15 Conjunctival intraepithelial neoplasia; same patient as in Figs 5.13 and 5.14. Three months after treatment with interferon alpha-2b, the lesion has resolved completely.

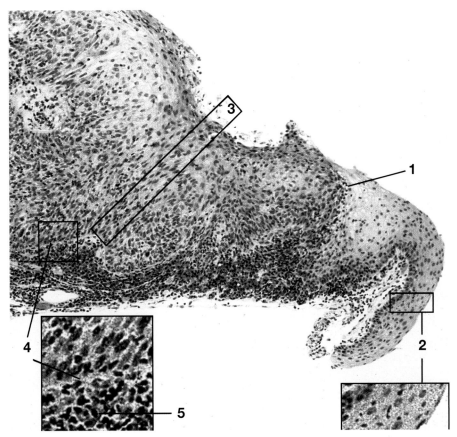

Fig. 5.16 Conjunctival intraepithelial neoplasia. There is a junction between normal epithelium on the right and neoplastic epithelium on the left (1). Normal cells show a maturation continuum from immature cells in the basal layer to mature anterior cells (2). In contrast, on the neoplastic side, immature cells extend through the full thickness of the epithelial layers (3). The basement membrane underlying the neoplastic cells is intact (4). Beneath it are chronic inflammatory cells (5).

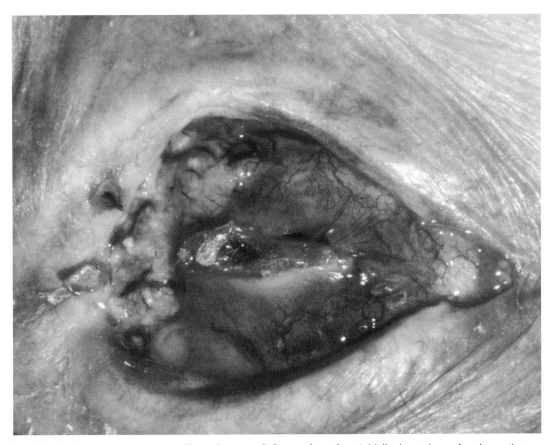

Fig. 5.17 Extensive squamous cell carcinoma of the conjunctiva. Initially the patient refused resection and then returned with this advanced lesion.

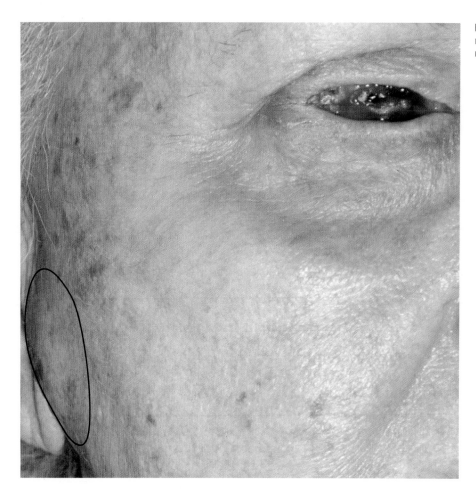

Fig. 5.18 Same patient as in Fig. 5.17. The lesion has metastasized to the preauricular nodes (circled). The nodes are firm, raised, and immobile.

Melanocytic Neoplasms and Other Pigmented Lesions of the Conjunctiva

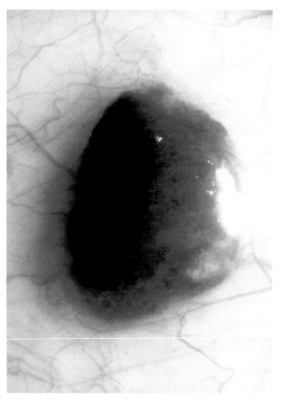

Fig. 5.19 Nevi. These are benign pigmented lesions of the conjunctiva. They usually occur on the bulbar conjunctiva and are freely mobile over the sclera. This is an elevated conjunctival nevus.

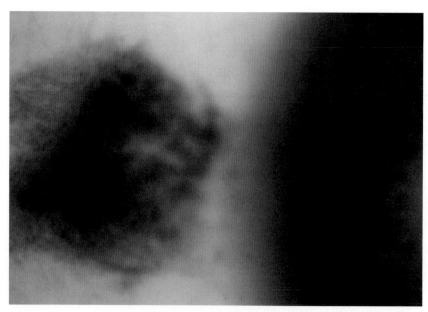

Fig. 5.20 Nevus. This is an example of a flat conjunctival nevus.

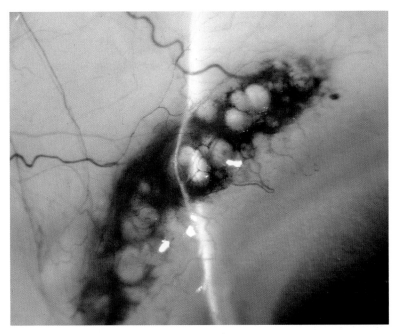

Fig. 5.21 Nevi. Occasionally, nevi develop clear cystic spaces.

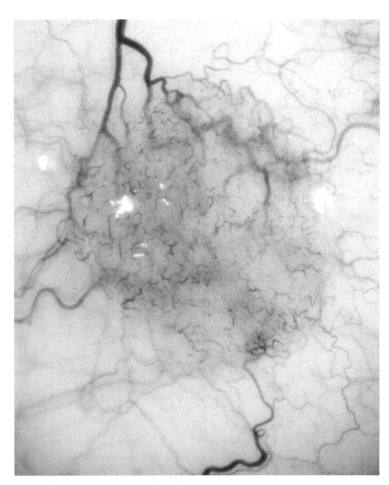

Fig. 5.22 Nevi. Some are lightly pigmented or nonpigmented.

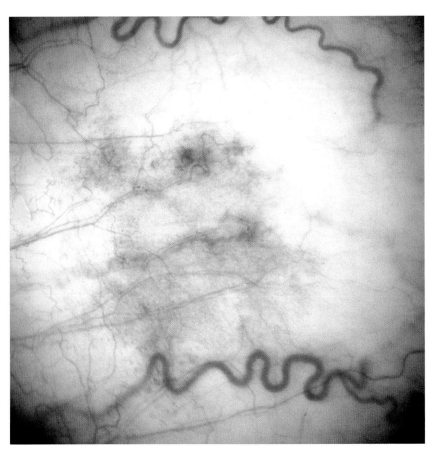

Fig. 5.23 Primary acquired melanosis (PAM). This is a flat, golden-brown or tan pigmentation of the conjunctiva; its appearance may change with time. This acquired lesion usually occurs in the fourth decade of life or later, primarily in Caucasians. PAM with atypia may progress to malignant melanoma.

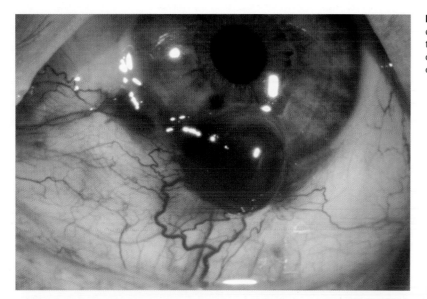

Fig. 5.24 Malignant melanoma of the conjunctiva. This lesion can arise de novo, from a preexisting nevus, or from preexisting PAM with atypia. This tumor may appear on the palpebral conjunctiva or the bulbar conjunctiva, and commonly occurs at the limbus. It is elevated and highly vascular and is occasionally accompanied by a hemorrhagic component, as in this case.

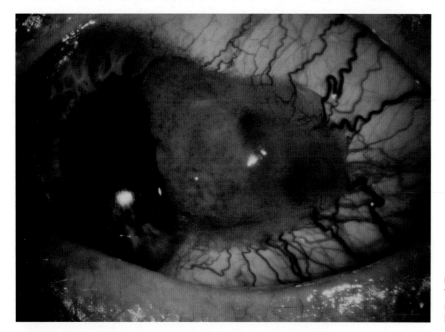

Fig. 5.25 Malignant melanoma of the conjunctiva and cornea. This is a large conjunctival melanoma arising from the limbal region. The most common sites of metastasis are ipsilateral facial lymph nodes, brain, lung, and liver.

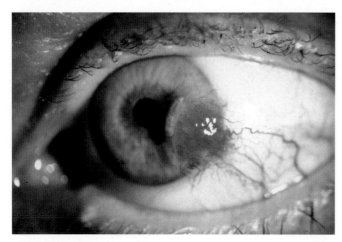

Fig. 5.26 Malignant melanoma of the conjunctiva and cornea. This is another example of a conjunctival and corneal melanoma that is located primarily on the cornea.

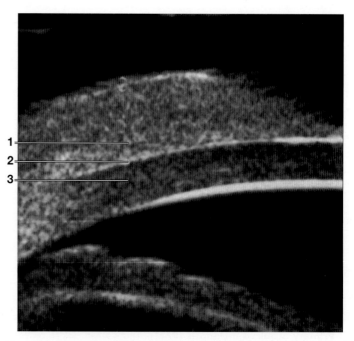

Fig. 5.27 Ultrasonography of the patient in Fig. 5.26. Ultrasound biomicroscopy shows that the lesion (1) is superficial to Bowman's membrane (2) with an underlying cornea (3) of normal thickness.

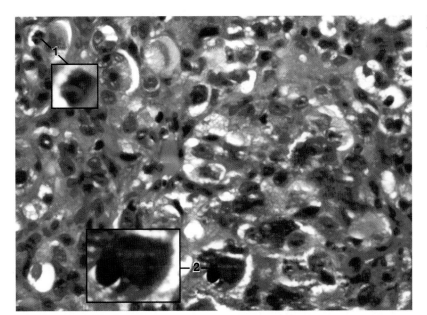

Fig. 5.28 Histopathology of a conjunctival malignant melanoma. There is invasion of the substantia propria with pleomorphic melanocytes (1) and melanophages (2) with pigment.

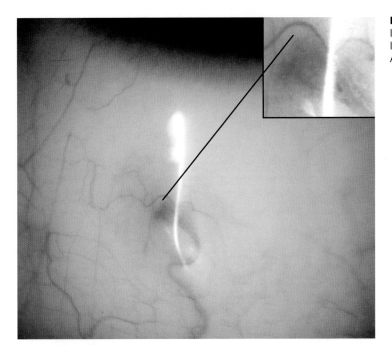

Fig. 5.29 Melanosis. Pigmentation can occur around an Axenfeld's intrascleral nerve loop. The pigmentation is found near the limbus and is benign and nonmobile, as it is located within the sclera. These areas of pigmentation are more common in African-American patients.

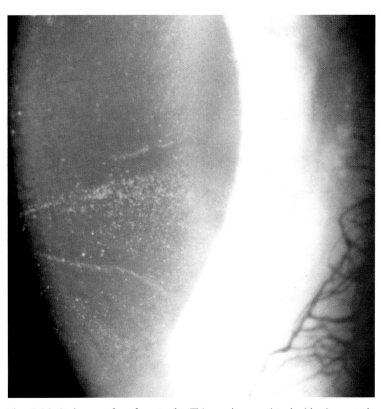

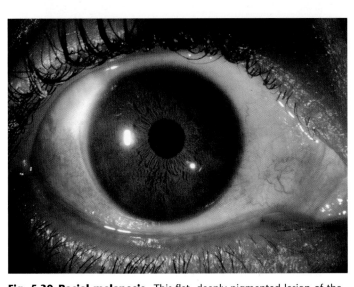

Fig. 5.30 Racial melanosis. This flat, deeply pigmented lesion of the conjunctiva is commonly found near the limbus and in the interpalpebral area. It develops early in life, is uninflamed, and rarely changes in appearance. It occurs primarily in darkly pigmented patients and has no malignant potential.

Fig. 5.31 Striate melanokeratosis. This can be associated with pigmented limbal lesions, such as racial melanosis. Chronic irritation of the corneal epithelium results in migration of pigmented stem cells from the limbus onto the cornea. The corneal lesion appears whorl-like, indicating the path of epithelial cell migration.

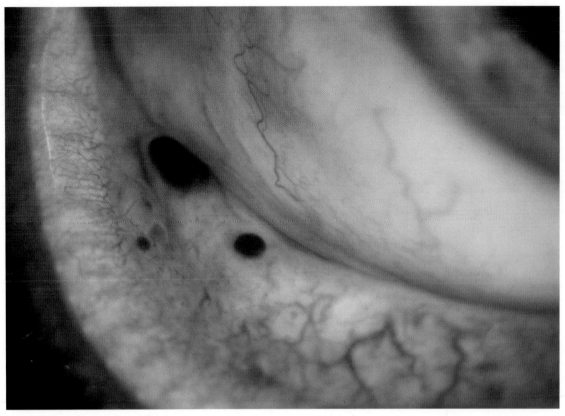

Fig. 5.32 Paraneoplastic syndrome. This 45-year-old woman presented with a 3-month onset of multiple, well circumscribed, bilateral bulbar and palpebral conjunctival lesions. One week before presentation she was diagnosed with an ovarian tumor. A rare paraneoplastic disorder, bilateral conjunctival pigment proliferation can be the initial presenting sign of occult malignancy. This clinical diagnosis is a variant of bilateral diffuse uveal melanocytic proliferation (BDUMP), a recognized uveal pigment response to a primary gynecologic carcinoma.

Subepithelial Neoplasms and Other Lesions

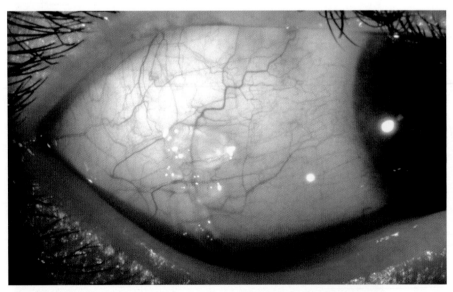

Fig. 5.33 Lymphangiectasis. There is a collection of dilated lymphatic channels within the conjunctiva. They are clear, elevated, and cystic.

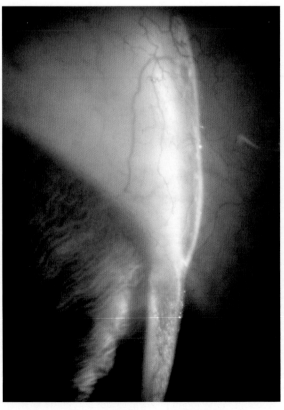

Fig. 5.34 Lymphangiectasis. A thin slit-beam view shows the lymphatic channels to be cystic and elevated.

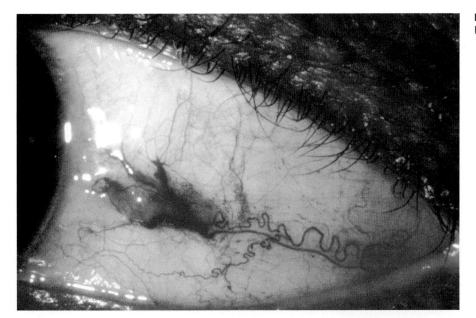

Fig. 5.35 Lymphangiectasis. Occasionally, this disorder has a hemorrhagic component.

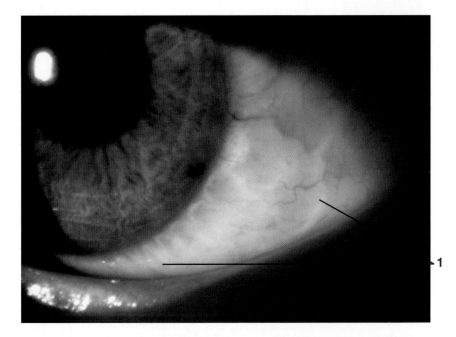

Fig. 5.36 Lymphangiectasis in Turner's syndrome. Congenital lymphoedema is common in Turner's syndrome. Lymphangiectasis of the conjunctiva (1) may also be seen with this syndrome.

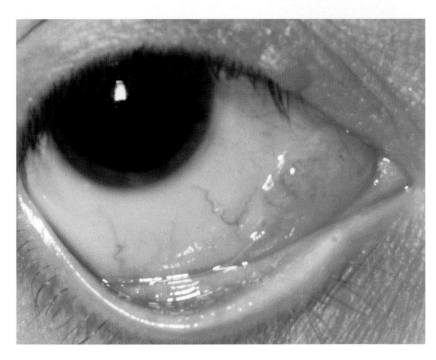

Fig. 5.37 Lymphangioma within the conjunctiva. These rare tumors usually occur during the first decade of life and often enlarge with upper respiratory tract infections. In contrast to lymphangiectasis, these lesions are composed of a proliferation of lymphatic channels and lymphoid tissue.

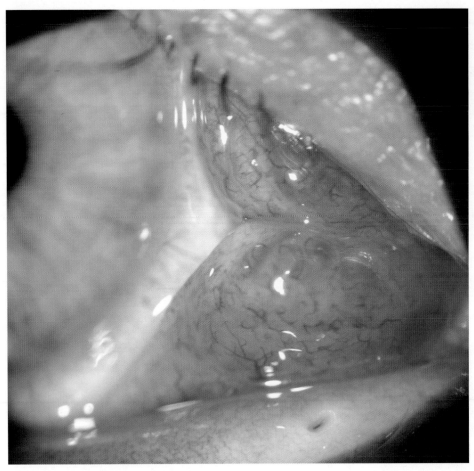

Fig. 5.38 Lymphangioma within the conjunctiva. This is another example of a lymphangioma within the conjunctiva. These lesions are characteristically multiloculated and contain cystic channels.

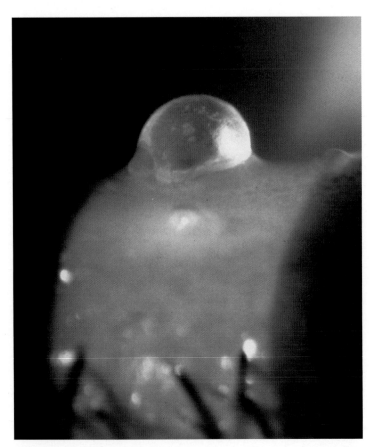

Fig. 5.39 Lymphangioma involving the lid. This patient has lid and orbital involvement.

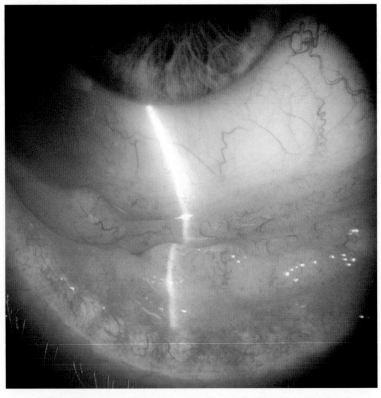

Fig. 5.40 Benign lymphoid hyperplasia. Lymphoid lesions of the conjunctiva are typically elevated and salmon-colored. The surrounding tissue is uninflamed. A local biopsy is necessary to establish the diagnosis.

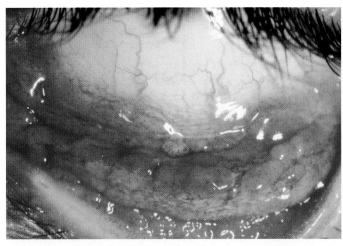

Fig. 5.41 Subconjunctival lymphoma. This lesion is salmon-colored and has a nodular or follicular appearance. All patients with biopsy-proven subconjunctival lymphoma need an extensive systemic work-up at the time of diagnosis and frequently thereafter. The risk of developing systemic lymphoma is 10–15% within 5 years of diagnosis and 28% within 10 years of diagnosis.

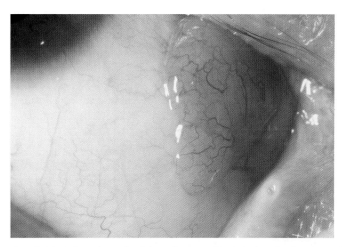

Fig. 5.42 Subconjunctival lymphoma. This is a sharply demarcated, salmon-colored, subconjunctival lymphoma. The mass is freely mobile and the surrounding tissue in uninflamed.

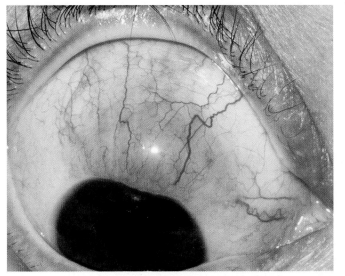

Fig. 5.43 Conjunctival lesion in a patient with systemic lymphoma. Similar to the lesions already noted, this is elevated and salmon-colored; the surrounding tissue is uninflamed.

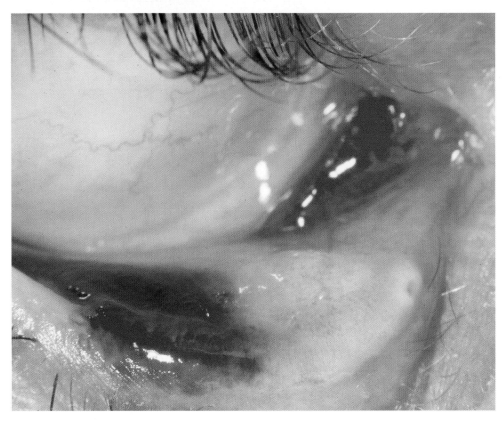

Fig. 5.44 Kaposi's sarcoma of the conjunctiva and lower lid in a patient with AIDS. The lesion is elevated and highly vascular.

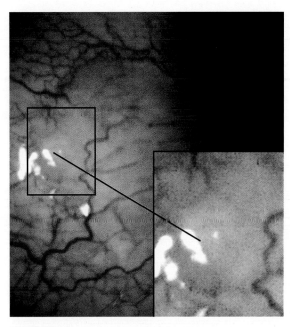

Fig. 5.45 Limbal sarcoid nodule (inset).

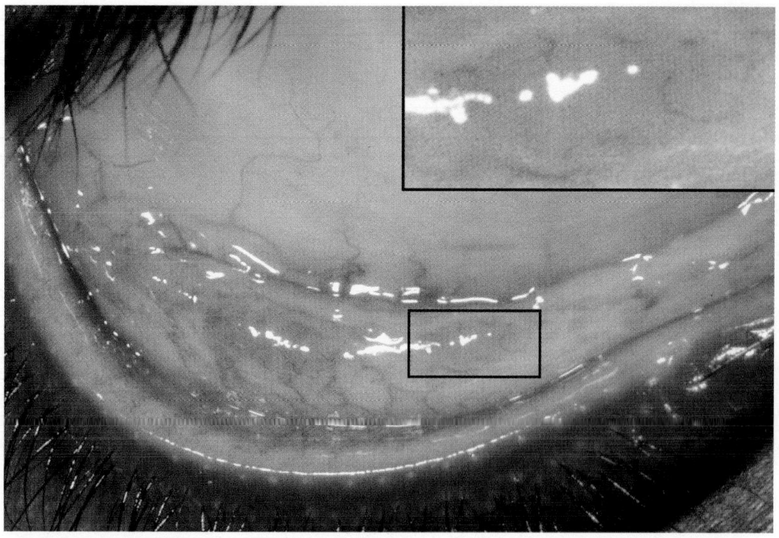

Fig. 5.46 Multiple sarcoid nodules in the inferior fornix. These solid, raised lesions (insert) may resemble follicles.

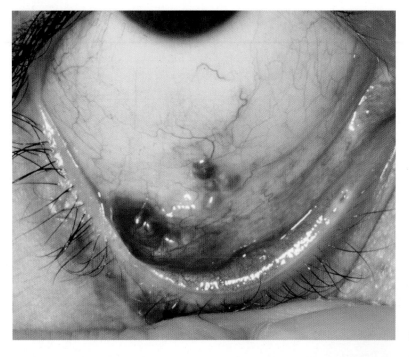

Fig. 5.47 Hemangiomas. These lesions rarely occur in the conjunctiva.

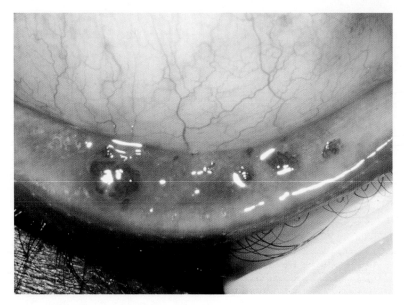

Fig. 5.48 Conjunctival hemangiomas in a patient with Osler–Weber–Rendu disease.

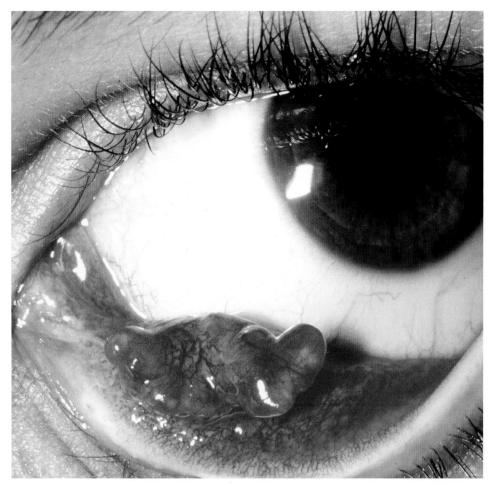

Fig. 5.49 Pyogenic granuloma. This lesion arises after inflammation of the conjunctiva and is often seen after a surgical procedure. It is composed of granulation tissue, fibroblasts, and capillaries, and does not contain granulomas.

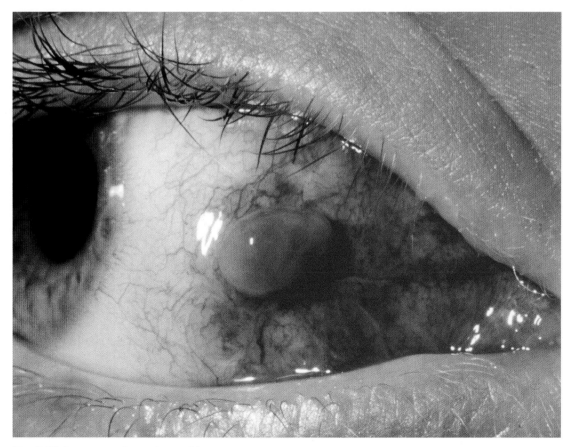

Fig. 5.50 Suture granuloma after strabismus surgery.

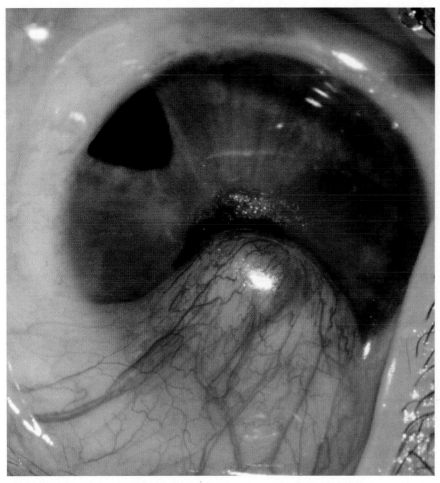

Fig. 5.51 Recurrent keloid on the left cornea in a patient with Lowe's syndrome. Unlike a pterygium, this lesion extends from the inferior limbus onto the cornea and deep into the corneal stroma.

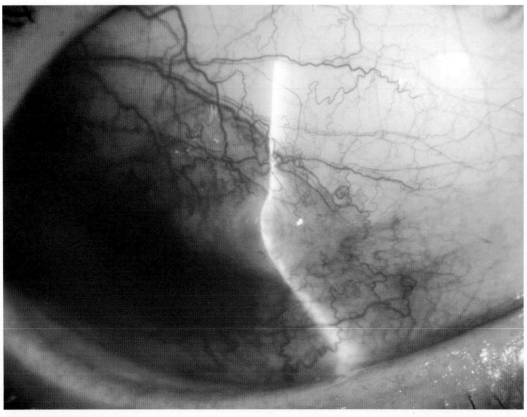

Fig. 5.52 Nodular fasciitis. This lesion is an acute proliferation of sheets of immature fibroblasts. It occurred in response to multiple self-inflicted needle punctures to the conjunctiva.

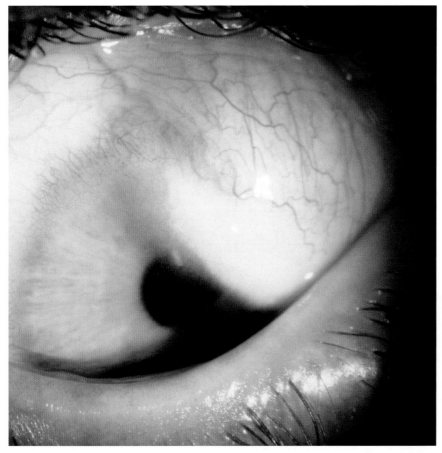

Fig. 5.53 Xanthogranuloma on the cornea of an 8-year-old boy.
Xanthogranulomas can also occur on the skin (see Fig. 2.2) and the iris. Children with iris xanthogranulomas may initially present to the ophthalmologist with visual problems related to spontaneous hyphemas.

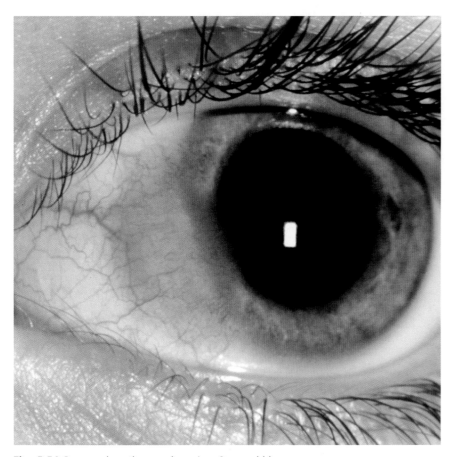

Fig. 5.54 Presumed xanthogranuloma in a 9-year-old boy.

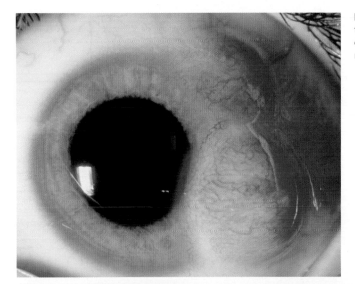

Fig. 5.55 Conjunctival ectopic lacrimal gland tumor. This bilobed, fleshy, choristoma tumor arose from ectopic lacrimal tissue in the conjunctiva. The lacrimal gland is derived embryologically from the conjunctiva. This lesion extends deep into the sclera and cornea making complete resection difficult.

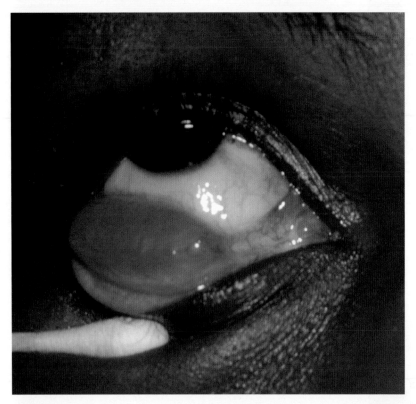

Fig. 5.56 Large conjunctival cyst arising from the palpebral conjunctiva. The central cyst is clear, and the margins of the cyst are easily seen.

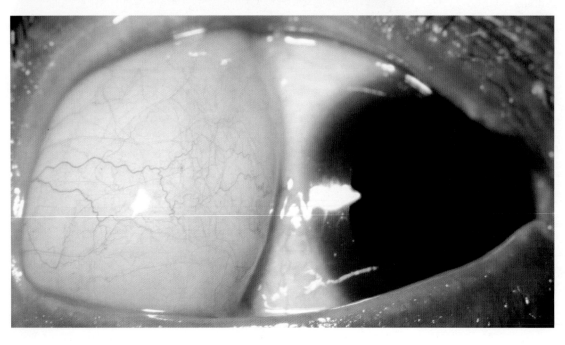

Fig. 5.57 Prolapsed orbital fat mistaken for a conjunctival cyst. In contrast to the conjunctival cyst in Fig. 5.56, this lesion is not clear and the margins cannot be easily seen. With digital pressure, the prolapsed fat can be pushed back into the orbit, but it returns when the pressure is removed.

Chapter 6

Conjunctivitis

Conjunctivitis is one of the more common conditions seen in general practice. Certain signs of conjunctival inflammation, such as follicles, giant papillae, membranes, and symblepharon, may be helpful in establishing a definitive diagnosis.

Clinical Features

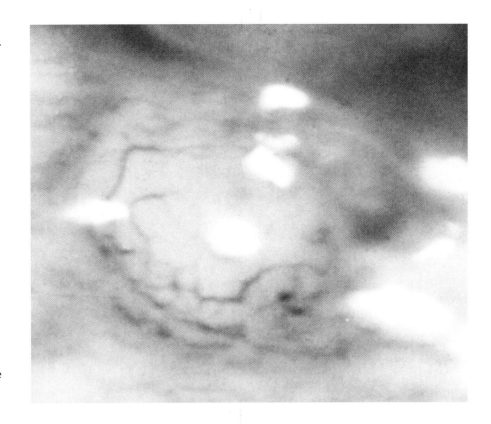

Fig. 6.1 Conjunctival follicle. This is a lymphocytic response in the conjunctiva. Vessels are on the surface and especially around the base of the follicle, but they lack the central vascular core seen in a papilla. Follicles are more rounded and deeper than papillae.

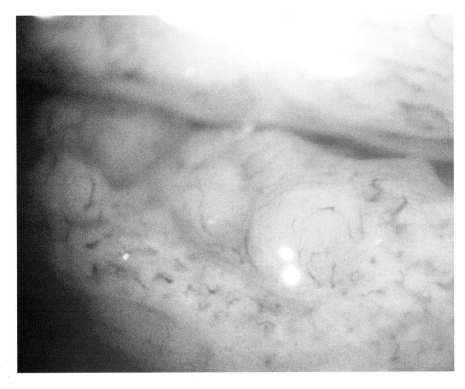

Fig. 6.2 Conjunctival follicles in the inferior palpebral conjunctiva. Causes of acute follicular conjunctivitis include adenoviral keratoconjunctivitis, adult inclusion conjunctivitis, and primary herpes simplex keratoconjunctivitis. Causes of chronic follicular conjunctivitis include adult inclusion conjunctivitis, trachoma, toxic response to medications or molluscum contagiosum lesions, and Parinaud's oculoglandular syndrome.

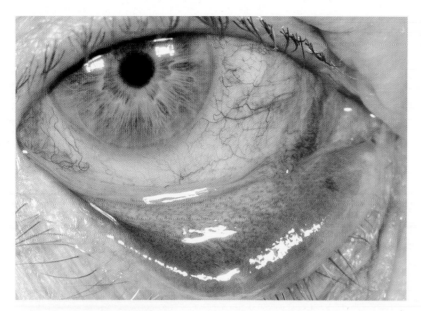

Fig. 6.3 Chronic conjunctival inflammation. A papillary response is a nonspecific response to chronic conjunctival inflammation and can occur along with a follicular response. In contrast to follicles, papillae are smaller and contain a central fibrovascular core.

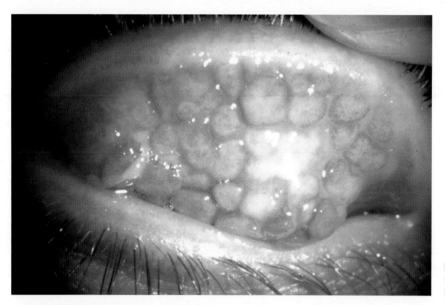

Fig. 6.4 Giant papillary conjunctivitis. This is seen in vernal keratoconjunctivitis or as a response to chronic irritation from a contact lens, an ocular prosthesis, or an exposed suture.

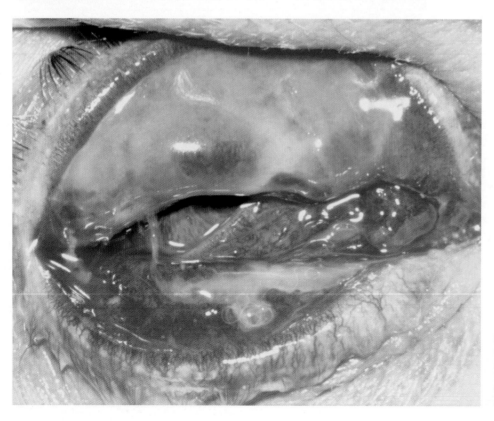

Fig. 6.5 Membranous conjunctivitis. A transudation of protein and fibrin from the conjunctiva can cause a membranous or pseudomembranous conjunctivitis. Pseudomembranes can be easily stripped from the conjunctiva, whereas membranes are more adherent to the underlying conjunctiva.

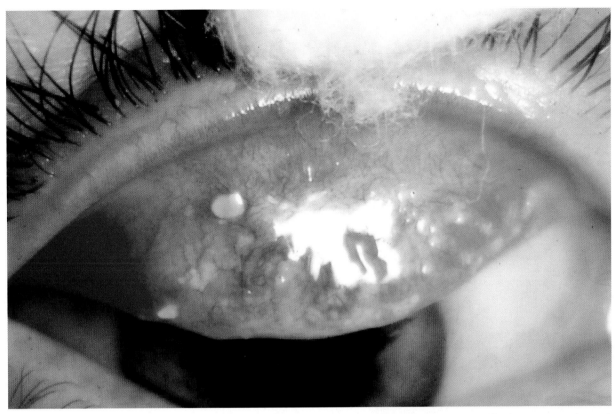

Fig. 6.6 Conjunctival concretions. These are benign lesions of the palpebral conjunctiva. Occasionally, they are extensive and can cause ocular irritation. Surgical excision is usually curative.

Bacterial Conjunctivitis

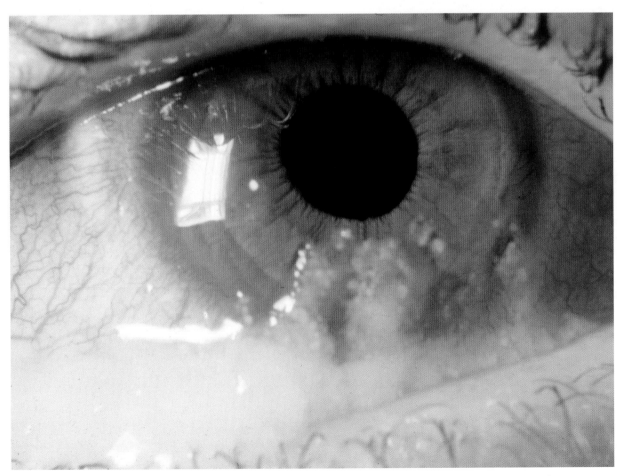

Fig. 6.7 Bacterial conjunctivitis. There may be a prominent purulent or mucopurulent discharge.

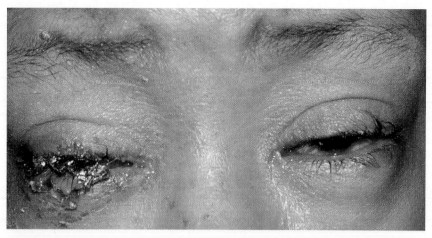

Fig. 6.8 Hyperacute conjunctivitis. This disorder is characterized by a rapidly progressing conjunctivitis. Chemosis and conjunctival membranes are often present. This type of conjunctivitis can be unilateral or bilateral and is often associated with a prominent preauricular node. Here the right eye is infected by *Neisseria gonorrhoeae*. *N. meningitidis* may produce a similar clinical picture.

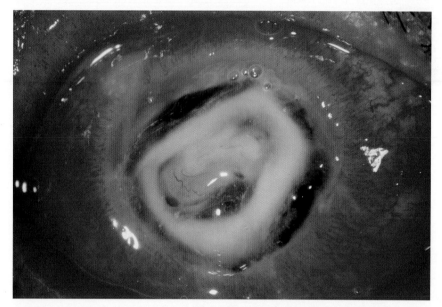

Fig. 6.9 Extensive corneal ulcer with perforation of the right eye of the patient in Fig. 6.8. The patient experienced an expulsive hemorrhage, and retina plugs the perforation site.

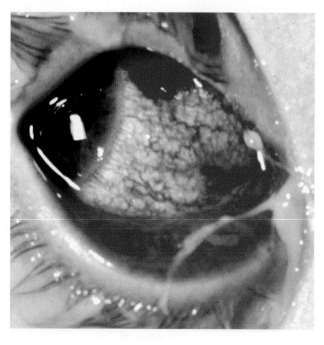

Fig. 6.10 Gonococcal conjunctivitis. There is a prominent mucopurulent discharge.

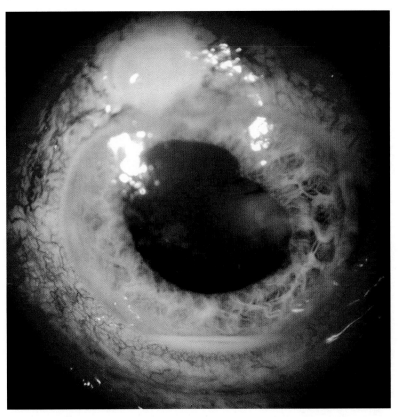

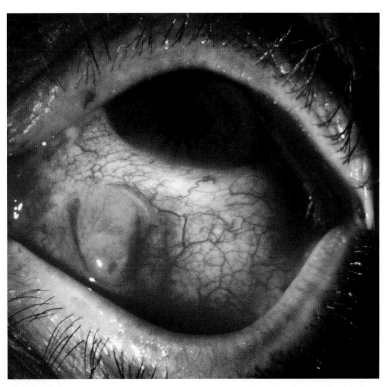

Fig. 6.12 Chronic conjunctivitis caused by an extruding scleral buckle.

Fig. 6.11 Infection in a filtering bleb leading to endophthalmitis. The bleb is white compared with the surrounding conjunctiva. A hypopyon is present.

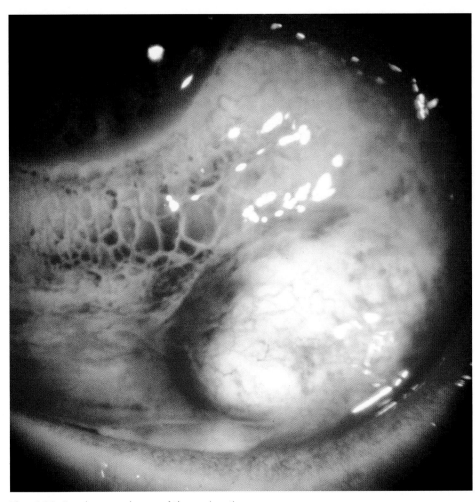

Fig. 6.13 *Pseudomonas* abscess of the conjunctiva.

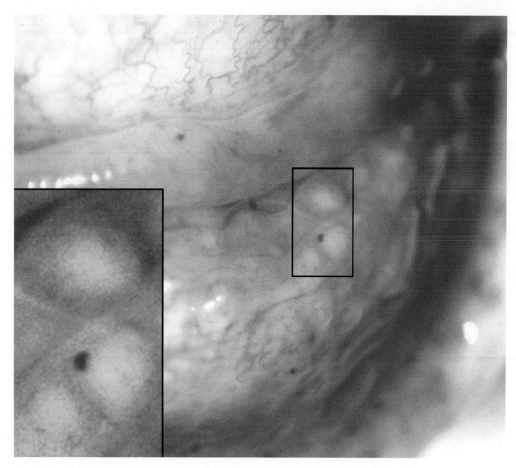

Fig. 6.14 Epidemic keratoconjunctivitis (EKC). Extremely contagious, EKC is usually associated with adenoviral serotypes 8 and 19, although many other serotypes can cause conjunctivitis. EKC is usually bilateral, with the second eye infected 3–7 days after the first. It causes a follicular conjunctivitis, as seen here. Often, small petechial hemorrhages are present (inset).

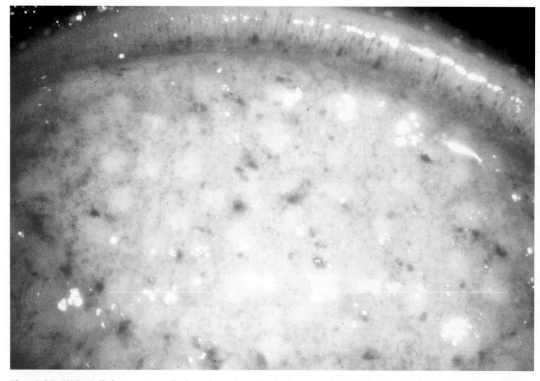

Fig. 6.15 EKC. Follicles are typically found on the palpebral conjunctiva of both the upper and lower lids. Small petechial hemorrhages are often present.

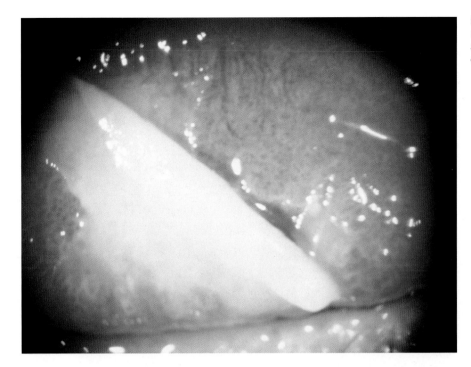

Fig. 6.16 EKC. In severe cases, transudation of protein and fibrin can result in a pseudomembrane. As noted in Fig. 6.5, a pseudomembrane, as opposed to a membrane, can be easily stripped from the underlying conjunctiva.

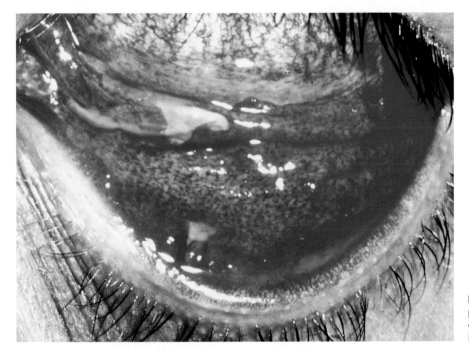

Fig. 6.17 Same patient as in Fig. 6.16, after removal of the pseudomembrane. There is a diffuse papillary response in the conjunctiva and a small residual piece of the pseudomembrane in the inferior fornix.

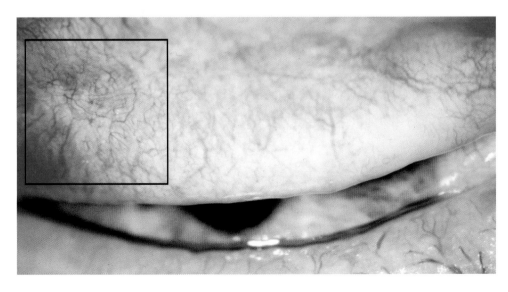

Fig. 6.18 EKC. After the lesion has resolved, an unusual complication can be scarring of the conjunctiva (box).

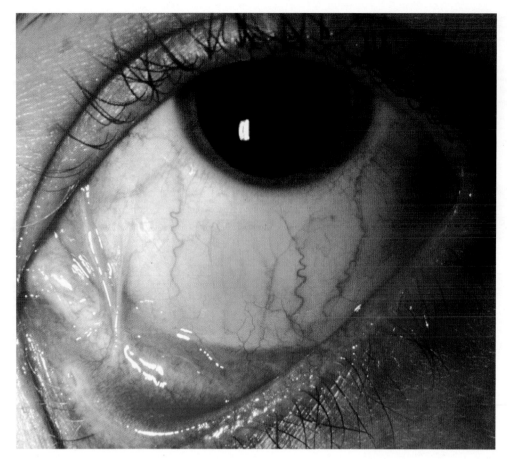

Fig. 6.19 EKC. Rarely, symblepharon develop after a severe case of EKC.

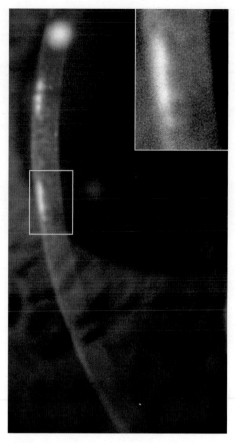

Fig. 6.21 EKC. A thin slit-beam view demonstrates that subepithelial infiltrates are located in the anterior stroma (inset).

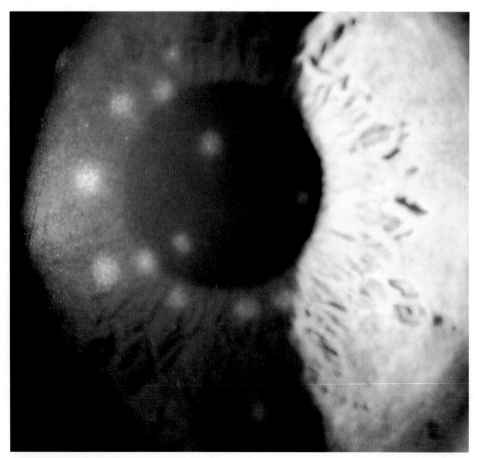

Fig. 6.20 EKC. Subepithelial infiltrates may develop 10–14 days after the acute infection. Histologically, they are composed of lymphocytes and may be an immunologic reaction to viral proteins in the cornea.

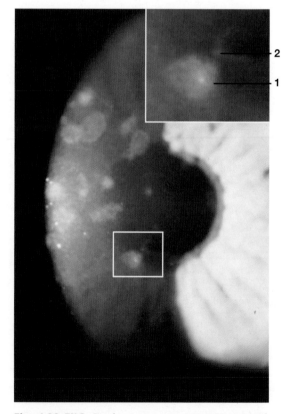

Fig. 6.22 EKC. Rarely, severe cases can cause corneal scarring (1). A change in the tear distribution over the corneal surface has resulted in iron deposition (2) in the corneal epithelium.

Chlamydial Infections—Adult Inclusion Conjunctivitis

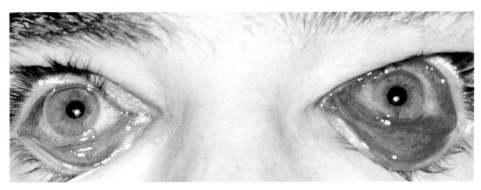

Fig. 6.23 Adult inclusion conjunctivitis. This chlamydial infection is associated with serotypes D through K. The source of infection is usually the genitalia. This is a bilateral case, but unilateral cases are more prevalent. Enlarged preauricular nodes are often present in acute cases.

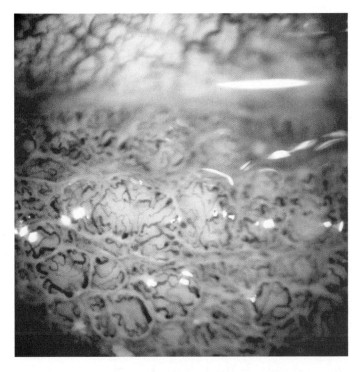

Fig. 6.24 Adult inclusion conjunctivitis. During an acute infection, prominent follicular conjunctivitis and moderate injection of the conjunctiva occur.

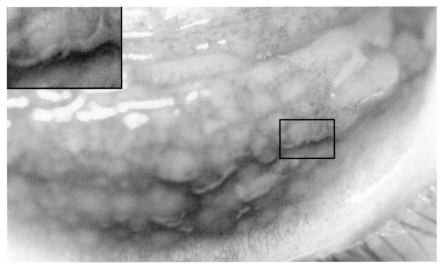

Fig. 6.25 Chronic adult inclusion conjunctivitis. The follicles remain but are associated with less injection of the conjunctiva. Scant mucopurulent discharge is present (inset).

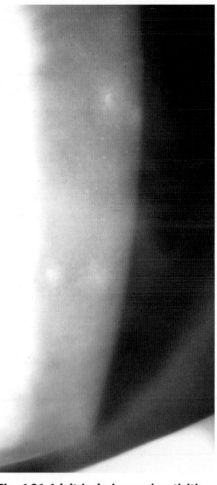

Fig. 6.27 Adult inclusion conjunctivitis. Subepithelial infiltrate (1) and superficial vascularization (2) in the peripheral cornea.

Fig. 6.26 Adult inclusion conjunctivitis. Peripheral subepithelial infiltrates can occur 2–3 weeks after the initial infection. They are believed to be an immunologic response to chlamydial antigens.

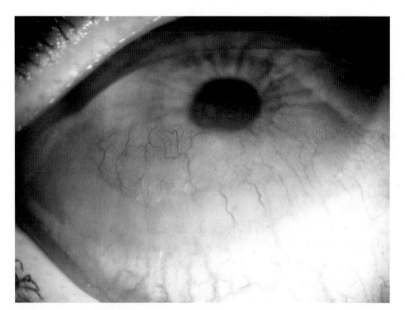

Fig. 6.28 Chronic adult inclusion conjunctivitis. An inferior vascular pannus may develop.

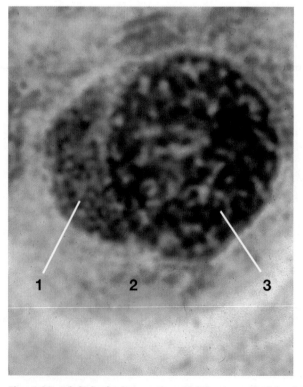

Fig. 6.29 Adult inclusion conjunctivitis. An epithelial cell from a conjunctival scraping shows basophilic inclusion bodies (1), cell cytoplasm (2), and the cell nucleus (3).

Chlamydial Infections—Trachoma

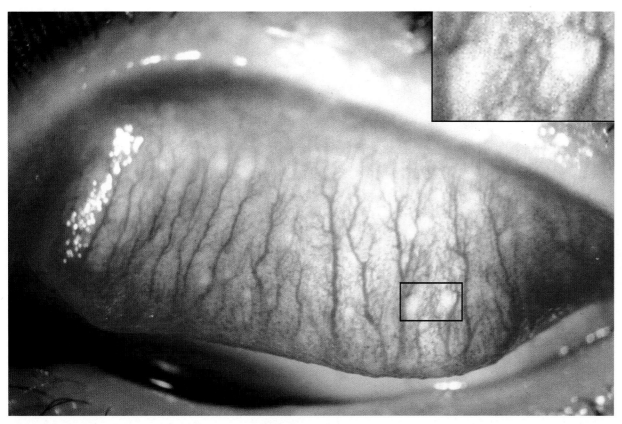

Fig. 6.30 Trachoma. This chlamydial infection is caused by serotypes A through C. The disease is extremely rare in the United States, although it is epidemic in some Native American tribes. In acute trachoma, there is a follicular response of the conjunctiva that is more prominent on the superior tarsal conjunctiva (inset). The World Health Organization classification is as follows: trachomatous inflammation-follicular (TF).

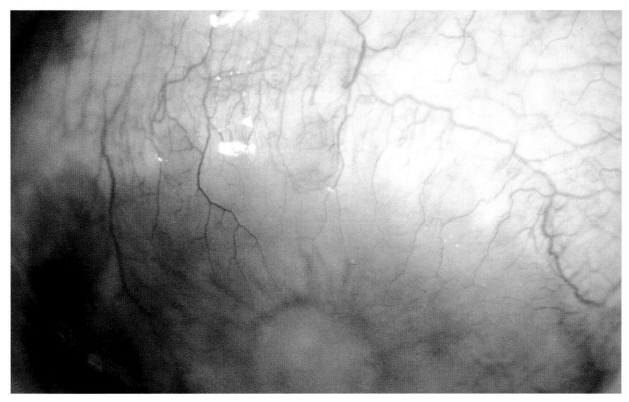

Fig. 6.31 Trachoma. A corneal pannus may be seen in advanced disease. In addition, Herbert's pits are seen at the superior limbus.

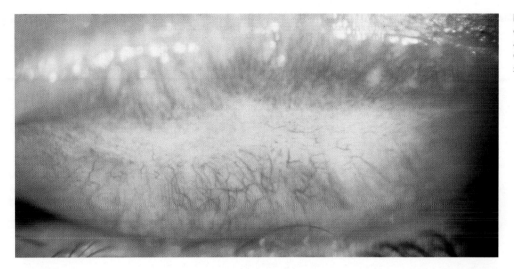

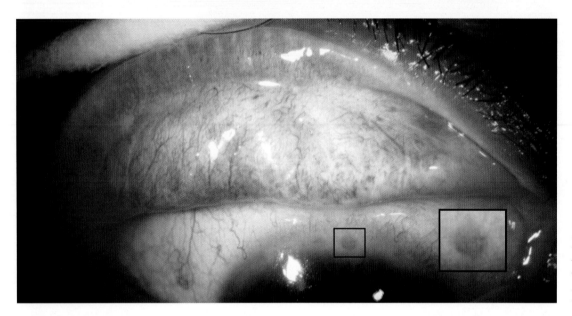

Fig. 6.32 Trachoma. Arlt's lines are horizontal bands of conjunctival scarring on the upper tarsal conjunctiva and are associated with advanced trachoma. The World Health Organization classification is as follows: trachomatous scarring (TS).

Fig. 6.33 Trachoma. Herbert's pits are round, depressed, limbal scars with an overlying thickened epithelium (inset). These pits are formed from limbal follicles that leave a scar when they resolve. This patient also has significant scarring on the upper tarsal conjunctiva.

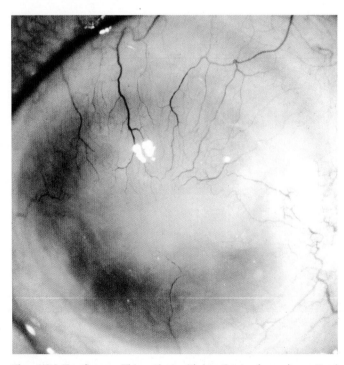

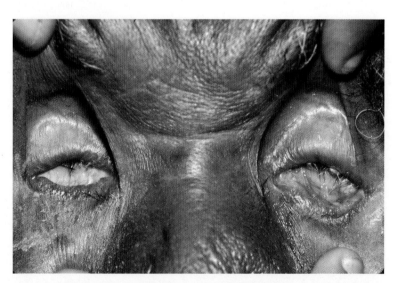

Fig. 6.35 Trachoma. Cicatricial entropion and trichiasis have developed. The World Health Organization classification is as follows: trachomatous trichiasis (TT).

Fig. 6.34 Trachoma. This patient with inactive trachoma has extensive corneal vascularization and scarring. The World Health Organization classification is as follows: corneal opacity (CO). Worldwide it is estimated that 4.9 million people are blind from corneal scarring caused by trachoma.

Ophthalmia Neonatorum

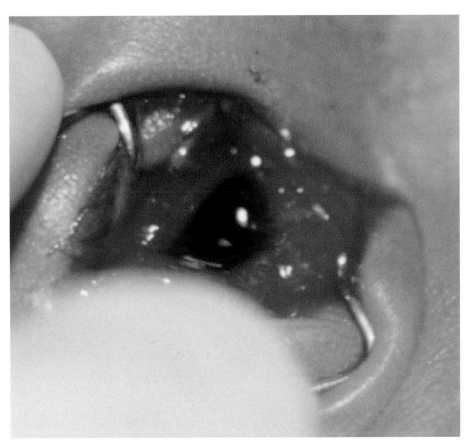

Fig. 6.36 Neonatal inclusion conjunctivitis (inclusion blennorrhea). This is acquired during passage through the birth canal and occurs several days after birth. In contrast to adult inclusion conjunctivitis, the response is papillary rather than follicular. The conjunctivitis is more intense, it may be associated with chemosis or pseudomembranes, and a mucopurulent discharge may be present.

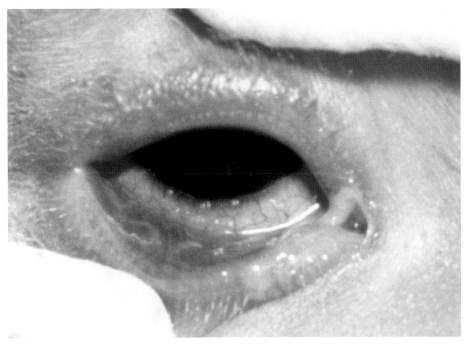

Fig. 6.37 Gonococcal conjunctivitis of the newborn. This is acquired during passage through the birth canal and occurs a few days after birth. A mucopurulent discharge is usually present. Gram staining reveals intraepithelial Gram-negative diplococci. Aggressive treatment with systemic and topical antibiotics is indicated, as severe corneal ulceration can occur.

Parinaud's Syndrome

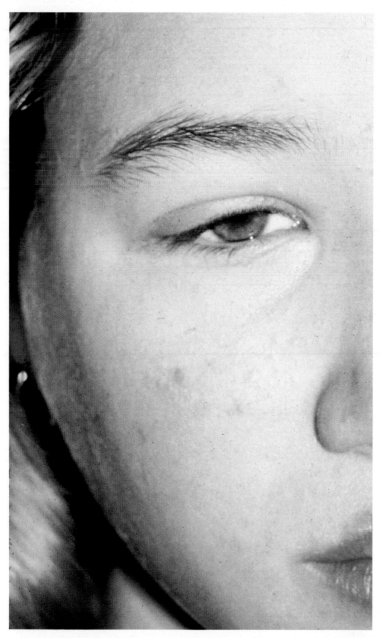

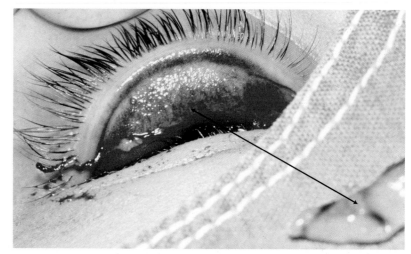

Fig. 6.38 Parinaud's oculoglandular syndrome. This group of diseases is characterized by localized conjunctival granulomas and regional lymphadenopathy. The most common etiology is cat scratch disease, which is attributed to the bacterium *Bartonella henselae*. This patient had a conjunctival granuloma on the palpebral conjunctiva of the upper lid with resultant ptosis. Prominent preauricular adenopathy is present.

Fig. 6.39 Parinaud's oculoglandular syndrome. Same patient as in Fig. 6.38; the granuloma was excised. The arrow points to the site of the excision.

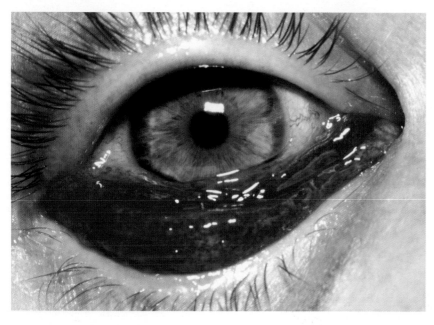

Fig. 6.40 Parinaud's oculoglandular syndrome; cercopithecine herpesvirus 1 (B virus). This is the right eye of a primate center worker 14 days after being splashed in the eye with biologic material (possibly fecal) from a rhesus macaque monkey. A large nodular granuloma with overlying follicles is seen in the inferior fornix. Preauricular lymphadenopathy was present. Despite treatment with systemic antiviral medication, the patient died 42 days after exposure from encephalomyelitis. Herpes B virus can be isolated from at least 70% of adult macaque monkeys, and exposure to blood or biologic material is a serious health risk among primate workers.

Parasitic Conjunctivitis

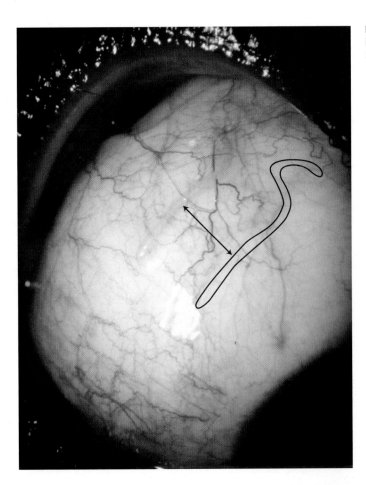

Fig. 6.41 Loiasis. This parasitic infection is confined primarily to Africa. The microfilariae are inoculated into the subcutaneous tissue by the bite of the mango fly. In this patient, the *Loa loa* worm is located beneath the conjunctiva (above and left of the drawn outline).

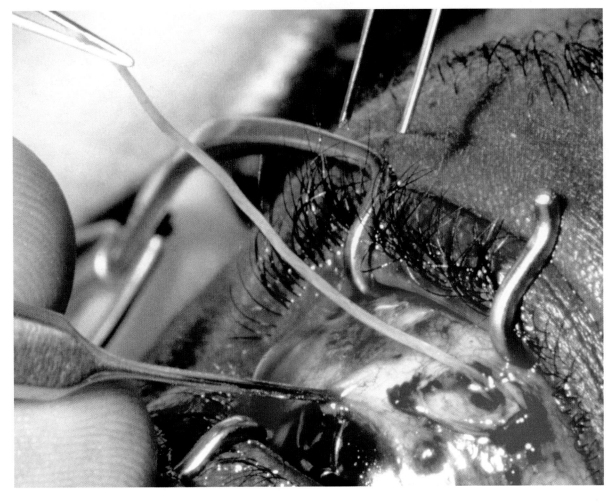

Fig. 6.42 Loiasis. Surgical removal of the worm from the patient in Fig. 6.41.

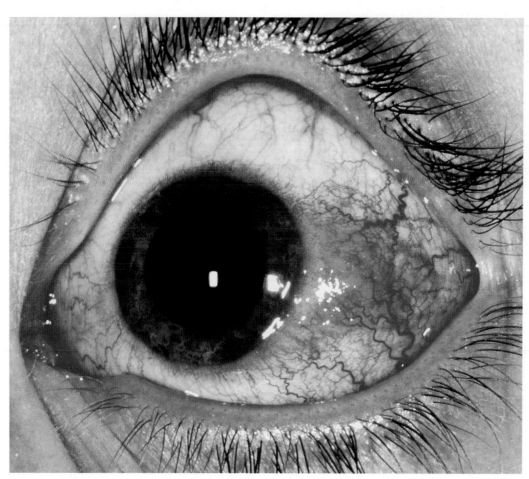

Fig. 6.43 Localized allergic conjunctivitis resulting from poison ivy.

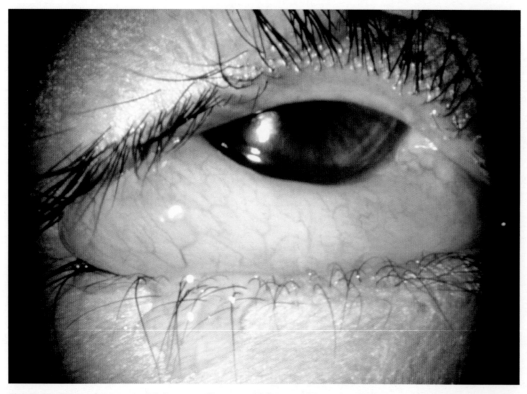

Fig. 6.44 Type I hypersensitivity reaction caused by an airborne allergen. Common inciting agents include animal dander, dust, plant pollens, ragweed, and mold spores. Symptoms of itching and irritation occur shortly after exposure. Ocular signs include a diffuse conjunctivitis accompanied (in this case) by severe chemosis.

Vernal and Atopic Keratoconjunctivitis

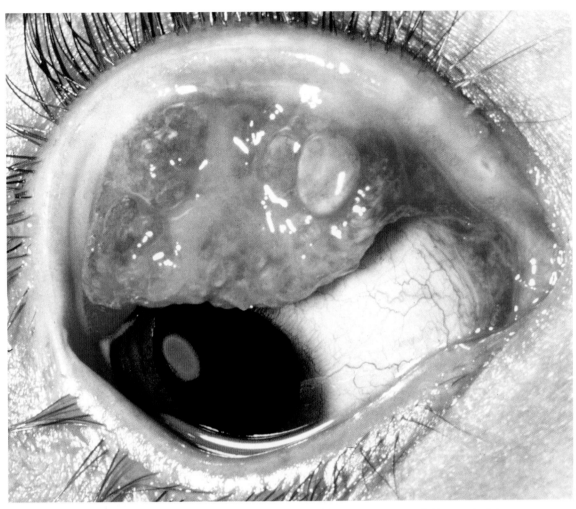

Fig. 6.45 Vernal keratoconjunctivitis. This seasonal conjunctivitis is usually seen in children and adolescents. Symptoms include itching, irritation, and mucoid discharge. Prominent giant papillae with a mucoid discharge are present on the upper palpebral conjunctiva. A shield ulcer is seen on the superior cornea. Mechanical irritation from the giant papillae and eye rubbing may predispose to shield ulcers.

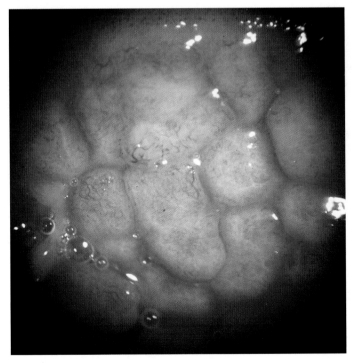

Fig. 6.46 Magnified view of giant papillae in a patient with vernal keratoconjunctivitis.

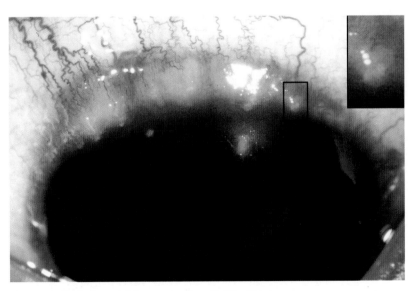

Fig. 6.47 Limbal vernal keratoconjunctivitis. This type is more common in African-Americans and Native Americans, and is characterized by large gelatinous elevations at the corneal limbus. It is often associated with Horner–Trantas' dots (inset). Horner–Trantas' dots are collections of eosinophils usually present for less than 1 week.

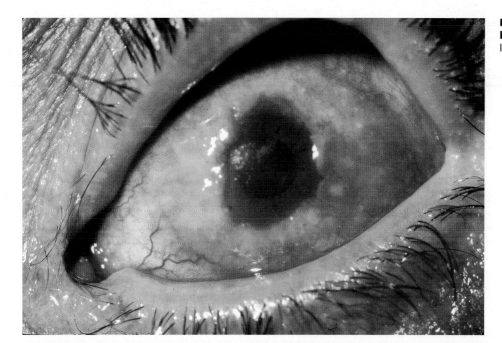

Fig. 6.48 Severe, chronic, limbal vernal keratoconjunctivitis. This is an extreme example of untreated limbal vernal keratoconjunctivitis in an Afghani patient.

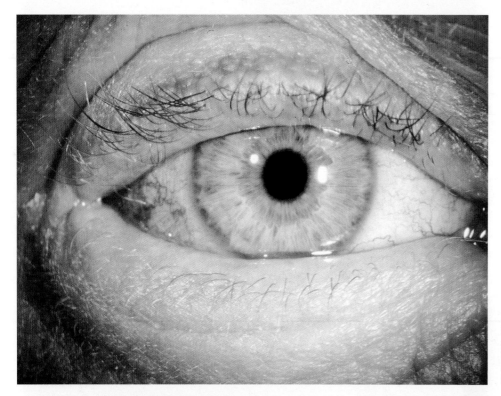

Fig. 6.49 Atopic keratoconjunctivitis. In contrast to vernal keratoconjunctivitis, atopic keratoconjunctivitis occurs in young adults and has no seasonal preference. In its severe form, it is associated with more advanced conjunctival and corneal scarring. This patient has a chronic atopic blepharokeratoconjunctivitis with thickened lid margins.

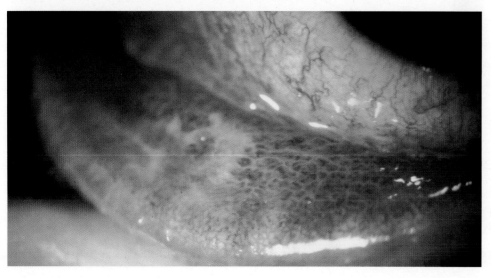

Fig. 6.50 Atopic keratoconjunctivitis. Small to medium-sized papillae and conjunctival scarring are seen on the lower lid.

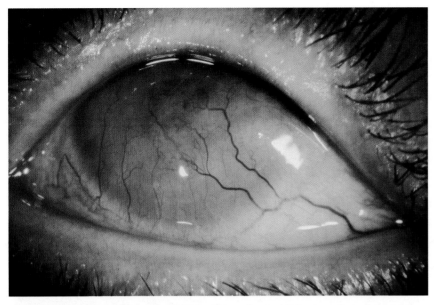

Fig. 6.51 Atopic keratoconjunctivitis. This patient exhibits corneal scarring and vascularization.

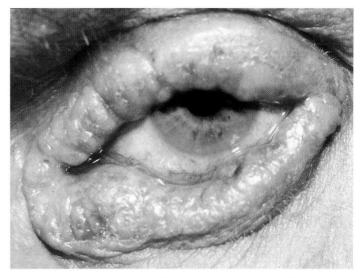

Fig. 6.52 Severe atopic eye disease. Markedly thickened lid margins, chronic conjunctival inflammation, and peripheral corneal scarring are seen.

Giant Papillary Conjunctivitis

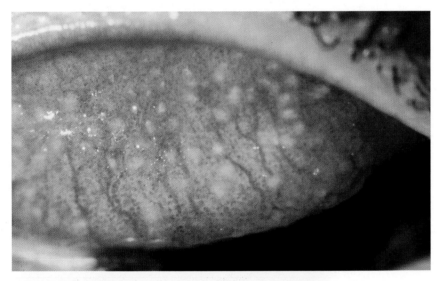

Fig. 6.53 Giant papillary conjunctivitis. This is thought to be a type IV hypersensitivity reaction that is exacerbated by chronic conjunctival irritation. It is most commonly seen in contact lens wearers (see Fig. 16.1). Patients complain of itching, irritation, and a slight mucoid discharge. Giant papillae are seen on the upper palpebral conjunctiva. In this patient, the conjunctivitis was associated with an ocular prosthesis.

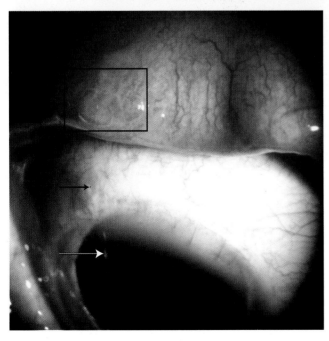

Fig. 6.54 Giant papillary conjunctivitis. An exposed nylon suture (black arrow) has caused a localized area of giant papillary conjunctivitis (box) and filamentary keratitis (white arrow).

Ocular Cicatricial Pemphigoid

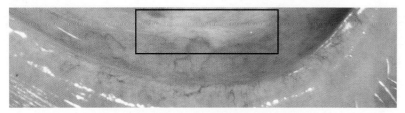

Fig. 6.55 Ocular cicatricial pemphigoid (OCP). This bilateral progressive scarring disease of the conjunctiva is rarely seen before the age of 50 years. It is more common in females. Subepithelial fibrosis is the earliest stage of this disease. Subtle subepithelial fibrotic bands are seen in the inferior fornix (box). This patient had a chronic relapsing blepharoconjunctivitis previously attributed to meibomian gland dysfunction.

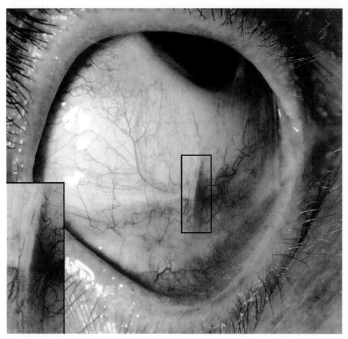

Fig. 6.56 OCP. As the disease progresses, the fornices shorten and there is symblepharon formation (inset).

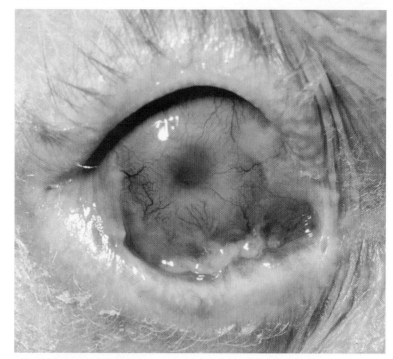

Fig. 6.57 OCP. The fornices are obliterated, and severe vascularization and scarring of the cornea occurs.

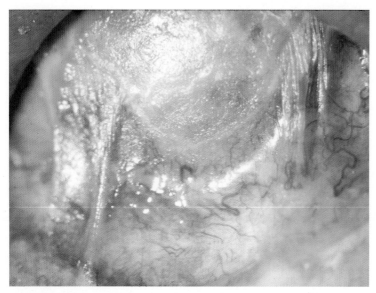

Fig. 6.58 OCP. In the final stages, the conjunctiva and cornea become keratinized.

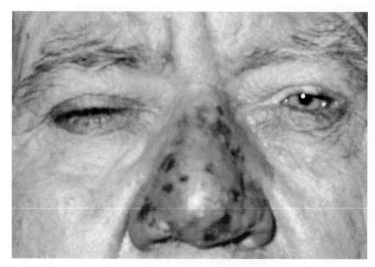

Fig. 6.59 OCP. Approximately 25% of patients have bullous lesions of the skin.

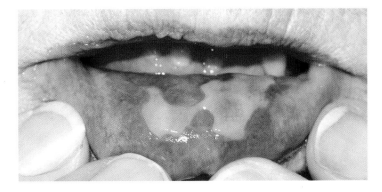

Fig. 6.60 OCP. Approximately 90% of patients have mucosal lesions in the oropharynx.

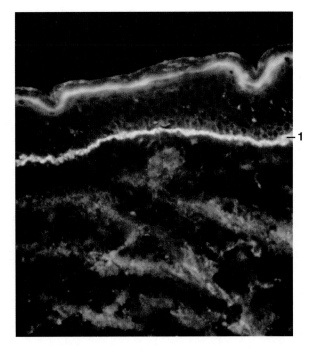

Fig. 6.61 OCP. Immunoglobulin is deposited in the basement membrane tissue (1), as demonstrated by this immunofluorescent stain.

Linear IgA Disease

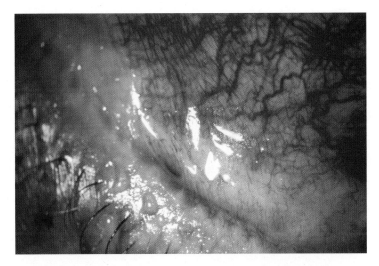

Fig. 6.62 Linear IgA disease. This disorder results in conjunctival scarring and symblepharon formation. The predominant immunoglobulin deposited is IgA, and the prognosis is better than for ocular cicatricial pemphigoid. The IgA antibody deposition is in the epithelial basement membrane.

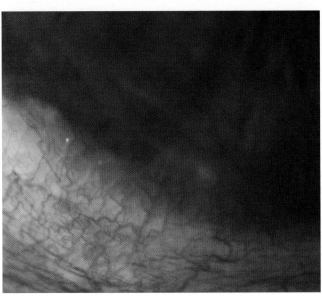

Fig. 6.63 Linear IgA disease. The peripheral cornea shows scarring and vascularization.

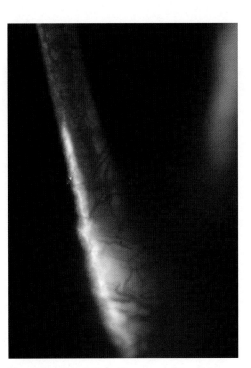

Fig. 6.64 Linear IgA disease. A thin slit-beam view of Fig. 6.63 demonstrates the scarring in the superficial cornea.

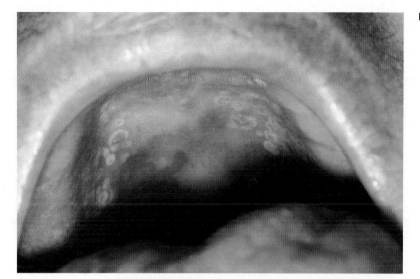

Fig. 6.65 Linear IgA disease. There is ulceration of the oral mucosal.

Pemphigus Vulgaris

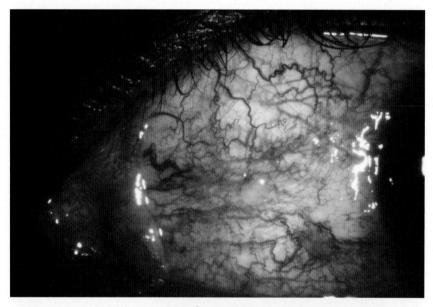

Fig. 6.66 Pemphigus vulgaris. Pemphigus vulgaris is characterized by intraepithelial bullae on the skin and mucous membranes. In this example, there is localized conjunctival inflammation and an active conjunctival epithelial erosion (see fluorescein staining in next figure). Unlike ocular cicatricial pemphigoid and linear IgA disease in which the antibodies deposit in the epithelial basement membrane, the antibodies in pemphigus vulgaris deposit within the epithelium. Conjunctival scarring does not occur.

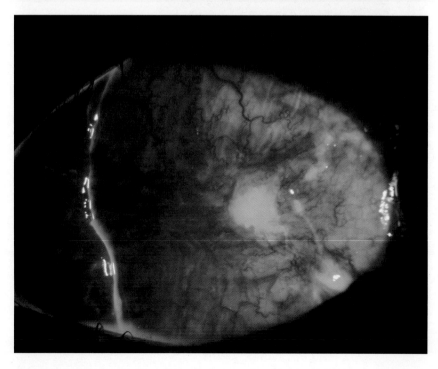

Fig. 6.67 Pemphigus vulgaris. Fluorescein staining of the conjunctiva of the patient in Fig. 6.66 demonstrates a central epithelial erosion.

Stevens–Johnson Syndrome

Stevens–Johnson syndrome is a severe inflammatory disease of the skin and mucous membranes. It can be associated with medications or infectious agents and is believed to be an autoimmune disorder.

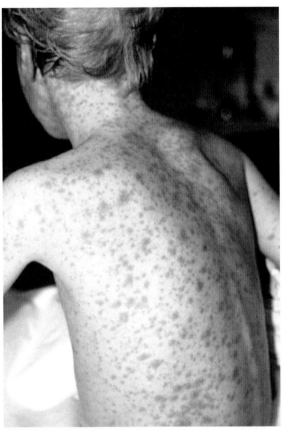

Fig. 6.68 Stevens–Johnson syndrome. This patient has bullous skin lesions on the skin of the back.

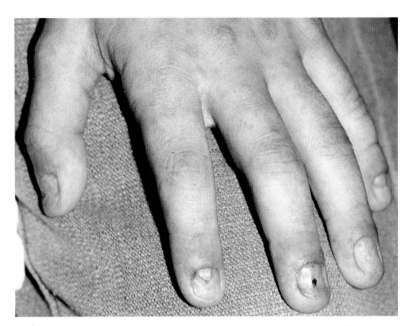

Fig. 6.69 Stevens–Johnson syndrome. Scarring of the hands and fingernails can occur.

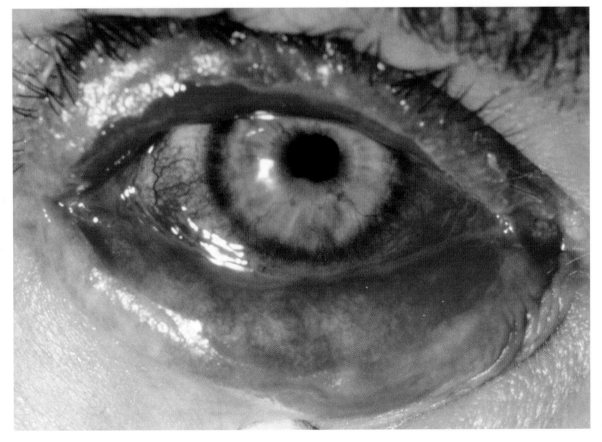

Fig. 6.70 Acute Stevens–Johnson syndrome. The conjunctiva is diffusely injected and thickened. Corneal vascularization occurs in severe cases.

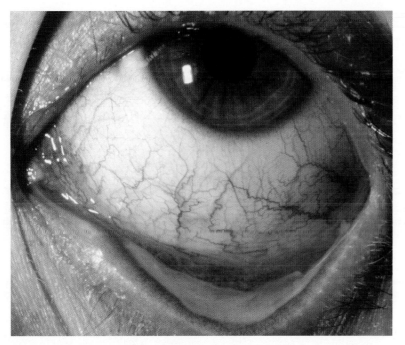

Fig. 6.71 Stevens–Johnson syndrome. Transudation of proteins and fibrin can result in a membranous conjunctivitis.

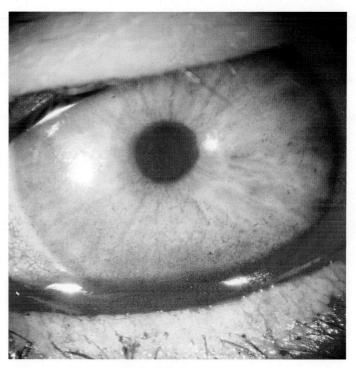

Fig. 6.72 Stevens–Johnson syndrome. Mucin production is altered. This patient has an adequate tear meniscus but demonstrates rose bengal staining of epithelial cells devoid of an overlying mucin layer.

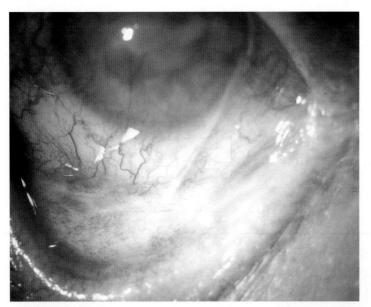

Fig. 6.73 Stevens–Johnson syndrome. Corneal scarring, conjunctival scarring, and symblepharon formation may occur after the acute stage.

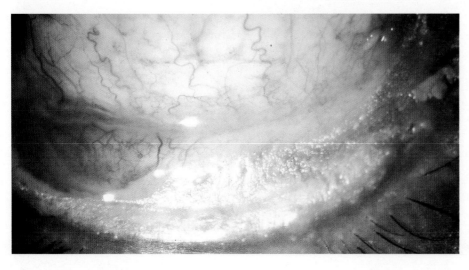

Fig. 6.74 Severe Stevens–Johnson syndrome. There is keratinization of the conjunctiva.

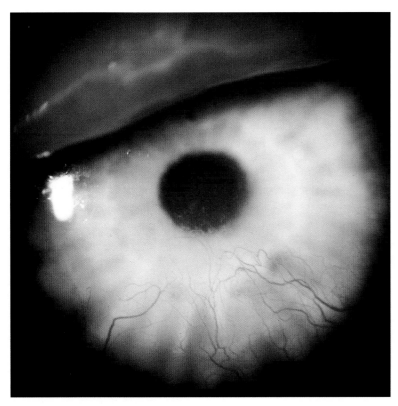

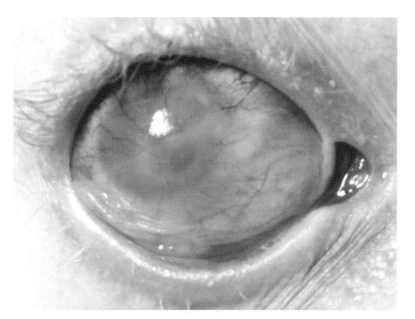

Fig. 6.76 Advanced Stevens–Johnson syndrome. The cornea can become totally vascularized and opaque.

Fig. 6.75 Stevens–Johnson syndrome. There is moderate corneal vascularization and scarring.

Reiter's Syndrome

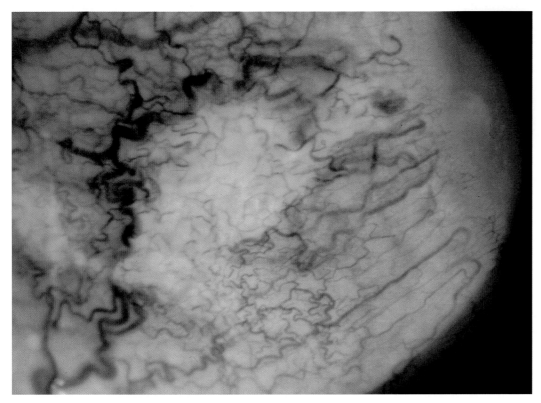

Fig. 6.77 Reiter's syndrome. This syndrome consists of arthritis, urethritis, and conjunctivitis, and occurs primarily in young males. Nonspecific papillary conjunctivitis with a mucopurulent discharge is common. Occasionally, these patients have ulcerations of the conjunctiva (as seen here) or buccal mucosa.

Toxic Conjunctivitis

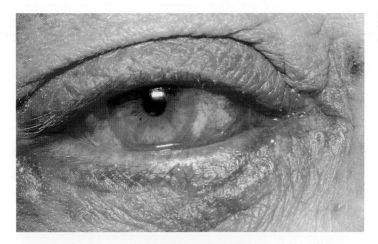

Fig. 6.78 Toxic follicular conjunctivitis. This case occurred after several weeks of Viroptic® (trifluorothymidine) therapy. Other agents causing a toxic follicular conjunctivitis include miotics and atropine.

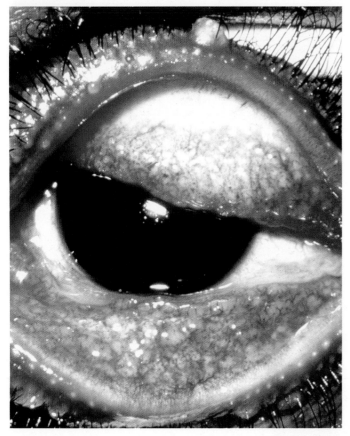

Fig. 6.79 Toxic follicular conjunctivitis. This toxic follicular conjunctivitis was caused by products from a molluscum lesion on the upper eyelid margin.

Theodore's Superior Limbic Keratoconjunctivitis

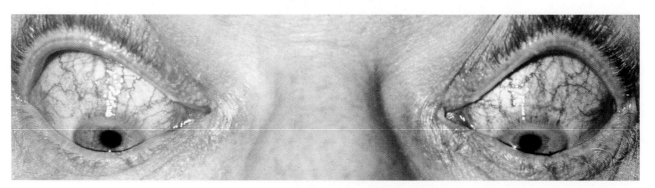

Fig. 6.80 Superior limbic keratoconjunctivitis. This is a bilateral, although often asymmetric, inflammation of the superior bulbar conjunctiva. There is focal injection of the superior conjunctiva, and rose bengal staining or lissamine green staining is often positive in this region. The superior conjunctiva is redundant, and the inflammation may result from chronic rubbing of the superior tarsal conjunctiva with the superior bulbar conjunctiva. Many of these patients have systemic thyroid abnormalities.

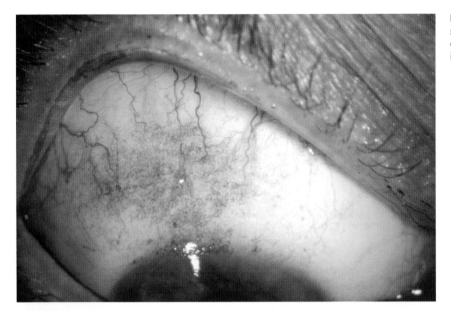

Fig. 6.81 Superior limbic keratoconjunctivitis; lissamine green staining. Lissamine green stains epithelial cells with a disruption to the overlying mucin layer or damage to the epithelial cell wall. It is less irritating to the patient than rose bengal.

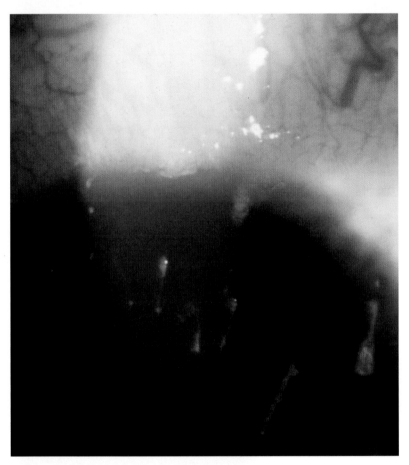

Fig. 6.82 Superior limbic keratoconjunctivitis. This high-power view of superior limbic keratoconjunctivitis shows superior injection of the bulbar conjunctiva, gelatinous hypertrophy of the limbal tissue, and superior filaments on the cornea.

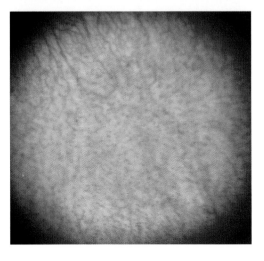

Fig. 6.83 Velvety papillary hypertrophy on the upper tarsal conjunctiva.

Ligneous Conjunctivitis

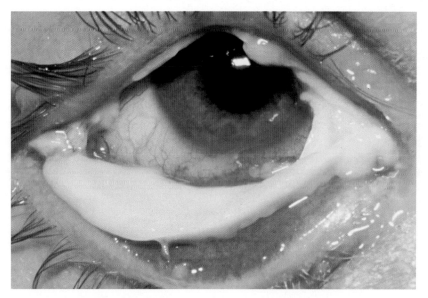

Fig. 6.84 Ligneous conjunctivitis. This is a bilateral chronic conjunctivitis of unknown etiology. The condition usually begins in early childhood and may be precipitated by local injury or a systemic process. It is characterized by exuberant fibrinous conjunctival membranes, which recur despite mechanical removal.

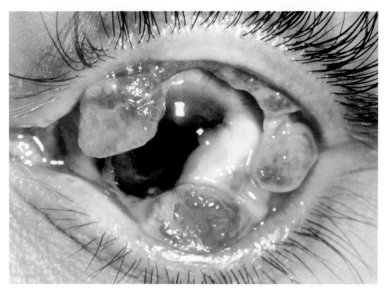

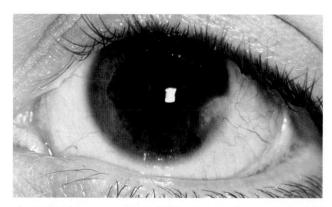

Fig. 6.86 Ligneous conjunctivitis. Same patient as in Fig. 6.85 after treatment with topical cyclosporin A. The conjunctivitis has resolved and there is slight corneal scarring temporally.

Fig. 6.85 Ligneous conjunctivitis. Appearance of the eye before treatment with topical cyclosporin A.

Factitious Conjunctivitis

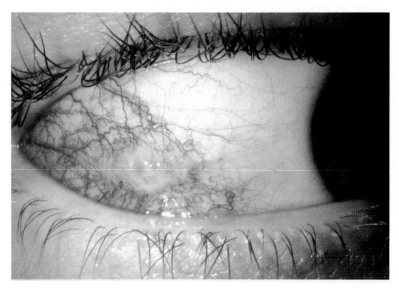

Fig. 6.87 Factitious conjunctivitis. Rarely, conjunctivitis is due to factitious causes. This patient repeatedly stabbed the conjunctiva with a straight pin.

Chapter 7

Normal Anatomy and Developmental Abnormalities of the Cornea

Developmental abnormalities of the cornea result from a complex interaction of genetic and environmental influences. These abnormalities are present at birth, in contrast to other genetic disorders that develop later in life. Many of these disorders develop during the sixth to eighteenth week of gestation, when differentiation of the anterior segment occurs.

Normal Anatomy

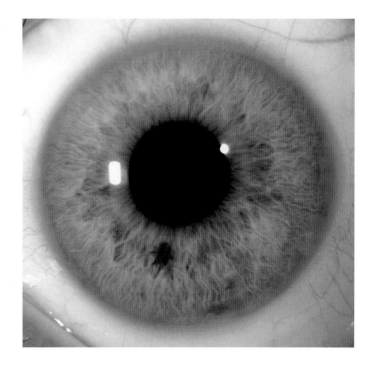

Fig. 7.1 Normal cornea. The normal cornea is transparent and allows an examiner to have a clear view of iris detail. The light reflexes on the cornea are sharply demarcated, indicating that the tear film is evenly distributed over a smooth epithelial surface.

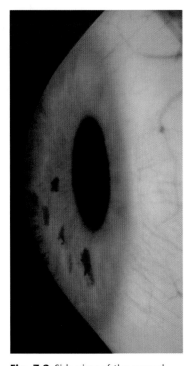

Fig. 7.2 Side view of the normal cornea.

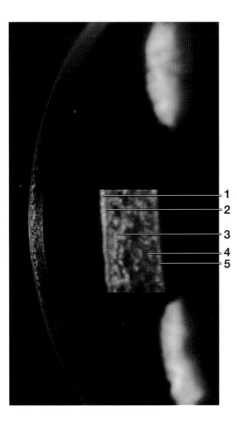

Fig. 7.3 Thin slit-beam view of the normal cornea. The layers seen are: (1) tear film, (2) epithelium, (3) anterior stroma (higher density of keratocytes), (4) posterior stroma (lower density of keratocytes), and (5) posterior layer (Descemet's membrane and endothelium).

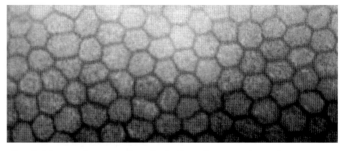

Fig. 7.4 Normal corneal endothelium by specular microscopy. The normal corneal endothelium is an array of hexagonal cells all having nearly the same shape and size.

Method for specular reflection of the central corneal endothelium of the patient's right eye.

1. Position the slit light source (1) so that it is directed from the patient's right side.
2. Position the microscope (2) so that it is directed from the patient's left side. **The examiner will be sitting to the patient's left side. The angle between the light apparatus and the microscope should be 60-70°.**
3. Ask the patient to look straight ahead through the middle of the two devices, as pictured below.
4. Using 16x magnification, put the slit beam on the center of the cornea and focus on the posterior cornea.
5. Change to 40x magnification. **Focus** on the tiny cells with fine black borders (3), the endothelial cells. They are to the right of the dazzling bright reflex (4).

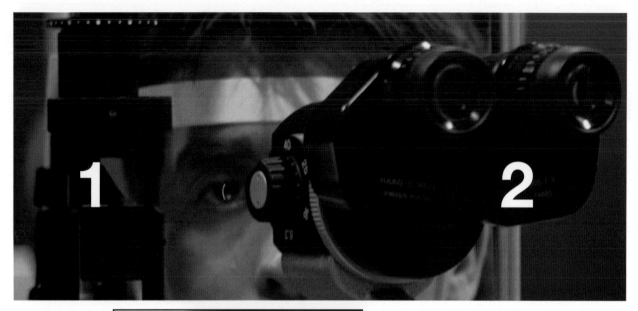

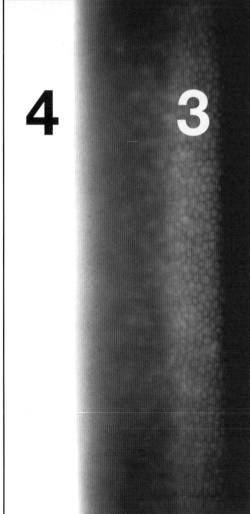

Fig. 7.5

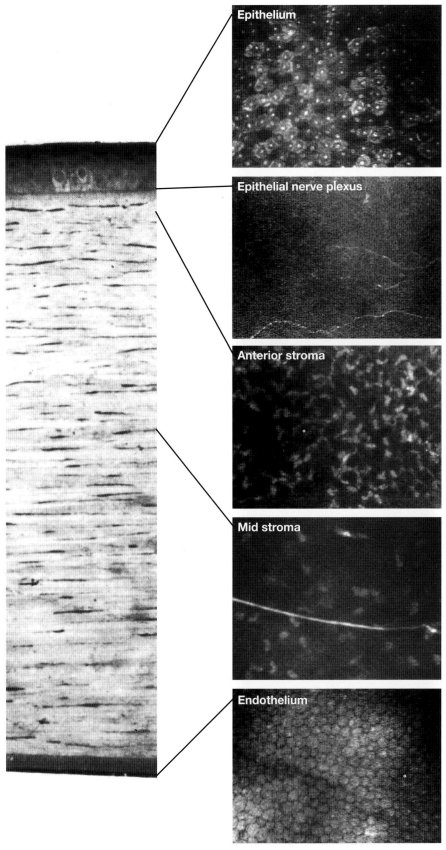

Fig. 7.6 Confocal microscopy of the normal cornea. On the left is a histologic section of the normal cornea in vitro; on the right is the corresponding confocal microscopic images in vivo.

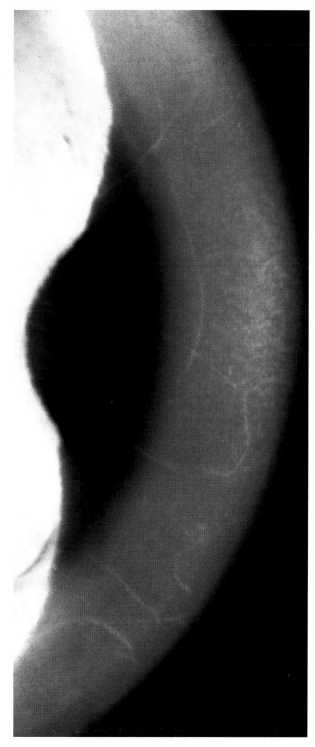

Fig. 7.7 Prominent corneal nerves, a variation of normal. These appear as fine, branching, white lines that originate at the limbus in the mid to anterior stroma. They can also be associated with pathologic states including multiple endocrine neoplasia type IIB, leprosy, Refsum's syndrome, neurofibromatosis, and keratoconus.

Developmental Corneal Opacities and Abnormalities of Size and Shape

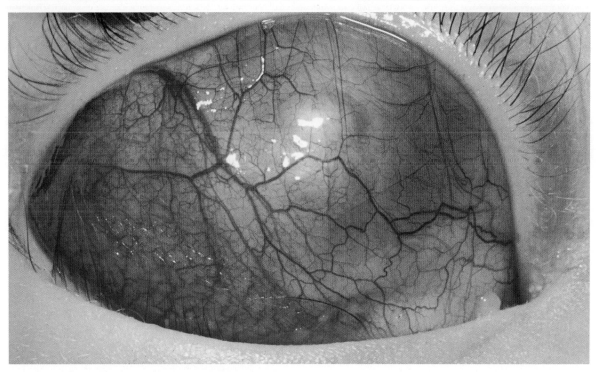

Fig. 7.8 Microphthalmos with cyst. The eye is small and malformed, and a cyst is contiguous with the globe. The cyst is formed from proliferating retina. This abnormality occurs when the embryonic (choroidal) fissure fails to close.

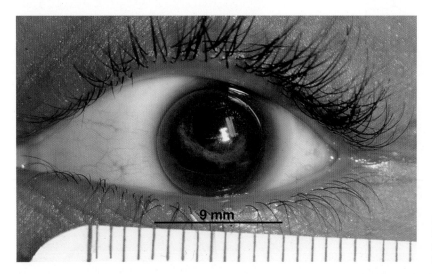

Fig. 7.9 Microcornea. This is defined as a corneal diameter less than 10 mm in an eye of normal size. If the entire eye is small, the condition is termed nanophthalmos. This patient with microcornea had congenital cataracts removed and is wearing an aphakic contact lens.

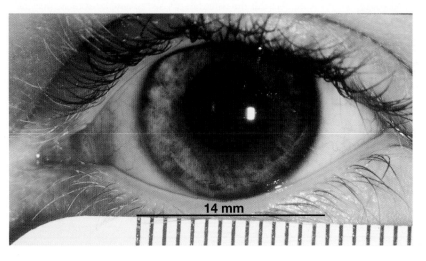

Fig. 7.10 Megalocornea. The corneal diameter is greater than or equal to 13 mm. This condition is transmitted most commonly as an X-linked recessive disorder, and for that reason 90% of affected patients are males. It is associated with numerous ocular and systemic disorders. The relative difference in corneal diameter between Figs 7.9 and 7.10 is the actual difference; the same scale is used for both figures.

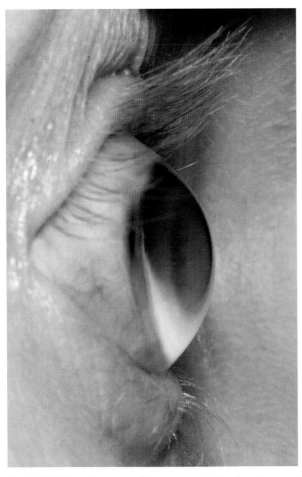

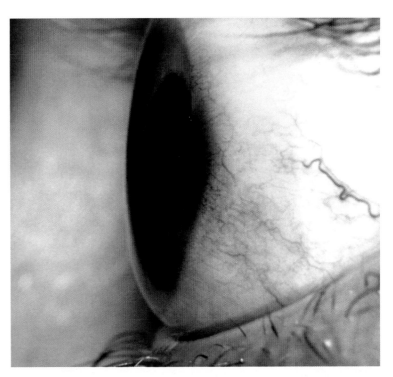

Fig. 7.12 Cornea plana. Both autosomal dominant and recessive cornea plana have been mapped to the long arm of chromosome 12. Clinical features include a greatly reduced corneal dioptric power (37.50–42.75 diopters for the dominant form and 25–35 diopters for the recessive form), hyperopia, slight microcornea, and a marked arcus senilis occurring at a young age.

Fig. 7.11 Megalocornea. The corneas in this disorder are often steep, and the patients are usually myopic.

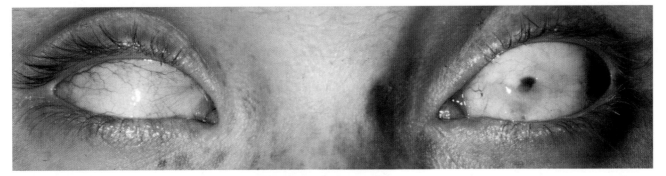

Fig. 7.13 Sclerocornea. There is diffuse whitening or scleralization of the cornea. The cornea may be totally opaque, as in the right eye of this patient, or there may be a central, relatively clearer area, as seen in the left eye. The central cornea is flat because it reflects the curvature of the sclera. There are usually associated ocular abnormalities, and the prognosis for vision with keratoplasty is poor.

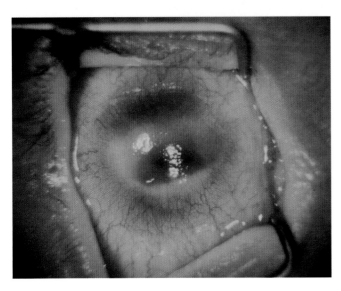

Fig. 7.14 Sclerocornea. In this example of sclerocornea, there is peripheral opacification of the cornea with vascularization.

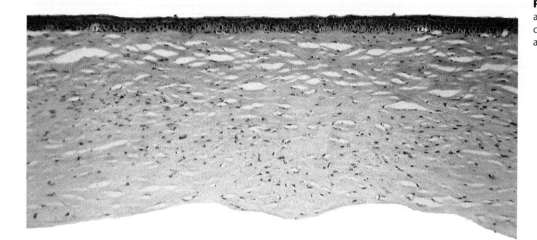

Fig. 7.15 Histopathology of sclerocornea. The absence of Bowman's layer, increased cellularity of the corneal stroma, and loss of the normal collagen lamellar architecture can be seen.

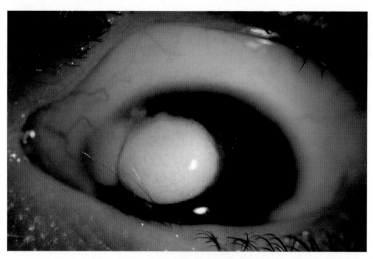

Fig. 7.16 Corneal dermoid. A corneal dermoid is a collection of ectodermal elements such as sweat glands, hair follicles, and sebaceous glands on the corneal surface. These lesions are well circumscribed and elevated. In this case, abnormal lashes from the lower lid are rubbing on the cornea; however, in some cases, lashes are found exiting from the substance of the dermoid.

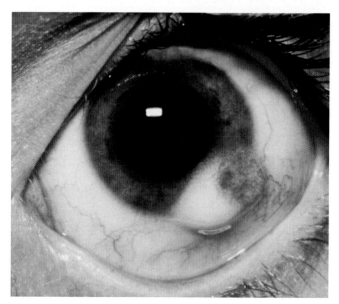

Fig. 7.17 Limbal dermoid. Although this tumor does not extend into the visual axis, it can induce astigmatism and resultant amblyopia.

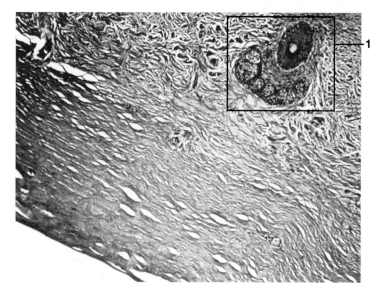

Fig. 7.18 Histopathology of a corneal dermoid. The dermis and dermal-like appendages in the corneal stroma are shown. Pilosebaceous unit (1).

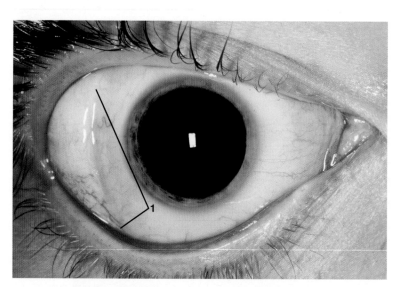

Fig. 7.19 Lipodermoid. These tumors are composed primarily of fatty tissue and are usually located beneath the conjunctiva on the lateral aspect of the globe (1). The posterior aspect of the lesion often extends far posteriorly and cannot be identified in this patient. These tumors can be removed for cosmetic reasons, but it is important to excise only the anterior aspect of the tumor and not to attempt excision of the entire lesion.

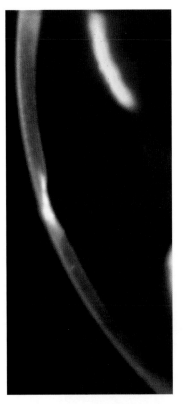

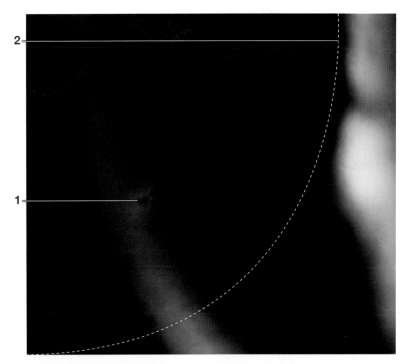

Fig. 7.20 Circumscribed posterior keratoconus. This developmental defect is usually unilateral. There is a focal indentation of the posterior cornea with overlying stromal scarring. The vision is usually not greatly affected.

Fig. 7.21 Posterior corneal vesicles. These are typically noted as an incidental finding. They are unilateral, and vision is not affected. Two vesicular lesions (1) are seen at the level of Descemet's membrane and endothelium. The location of pupil (2) is noted for proportion. These lesions should be distinguished from vesicular lesions in posterior polymorphous dystrophy, which are bilateral and associated with ocular abnormalities in other family members (see Fig. 10.71).

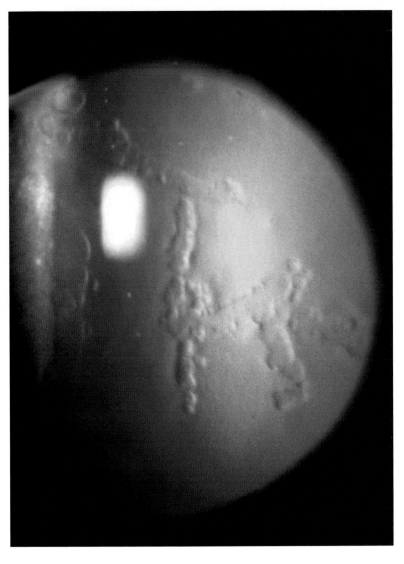

Fig. 7.22 Red reflex view of posterior corneal vesicles. Grouped vesicular lesions are seen throughout the posterior cornea.

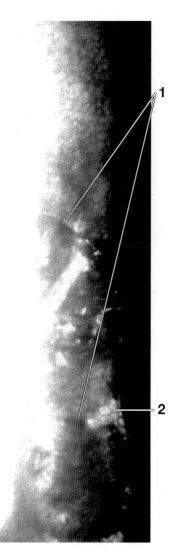

Fig. 7.23 Specular photomicrograph of posterior corneal vesicles. The vesicles (1) are surrounded by normal endothelial cells (2).

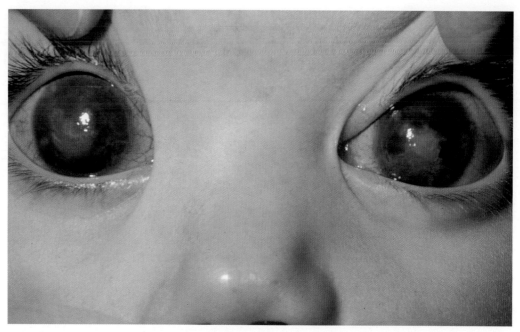

Fig. 7.24 Congenital glaucoma. This child was initially misdiagnosed and developed severe buphthalmos. Central corneal scarring is present.

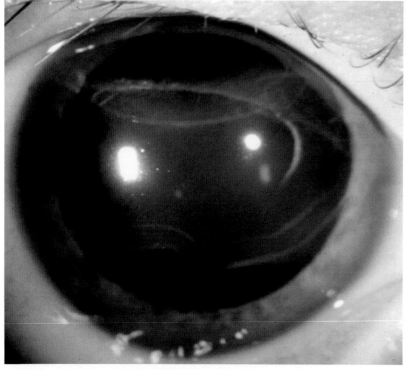

Fig. 7.25 Congenital glaucoma. Breaks in Descemet's membrane (Haab's striae) may occur. The breaks are usually horizontal in the central cornea and become concentric near the limbus. These should be contrasted with breaks in Descemet's membrane occurring from birth trauma, which are usually more vertical (see Fig. 15.33).

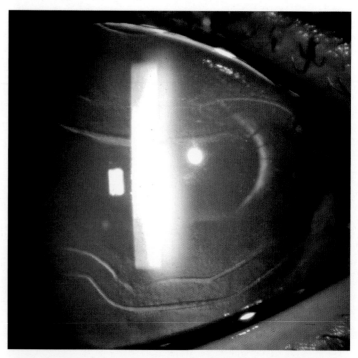

Fig. 7.26 Red reflex view of Haab's striae. The breaks in Descemet's membrane have a railroad track appearance, which is the result of scrolling of Descemet's membrane on both sides of the break.

Anterior Chamber Cleavage Syndromes

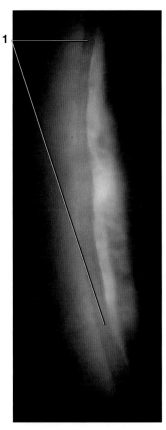

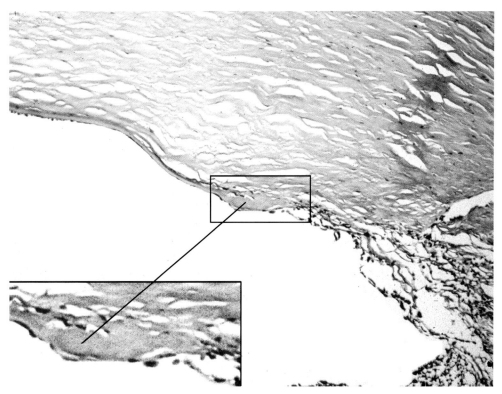

Fig. 7.27 Posterior embryotoxon. This is an enlargement and anterior displacement of Schwalbe's line (1). It is a common finding, present in as many as 30% of normal eyes.

Fig. 7.28 Histopathology of posterior embryotoxon. Schwalbe's line is enlarged at the junction of Descemet's membrane and the nonpigmented trabecular meshwork.

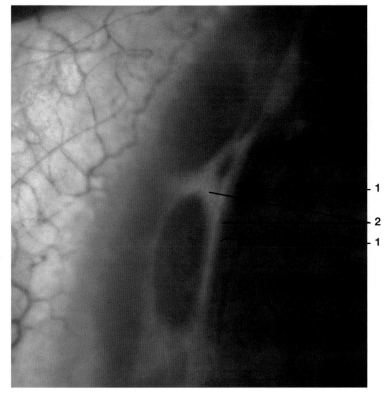

Fig. 7.29 Axenfeld's anomaly. Iris strands (1) adhere to an enlarged Schwalbe's line (2). If the disorder is associated with glaucoma, it is termed Axenfeld's syndrome.

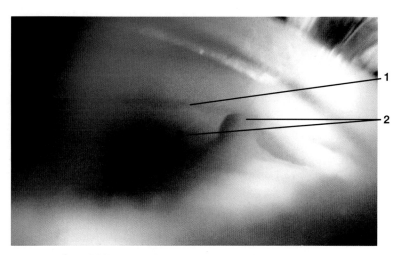

Fig. 7.30 Axenfeld's anomaly. Gonioscopy reveals an enlarged Schwalbe's line (1) with adherent iris strands (2).

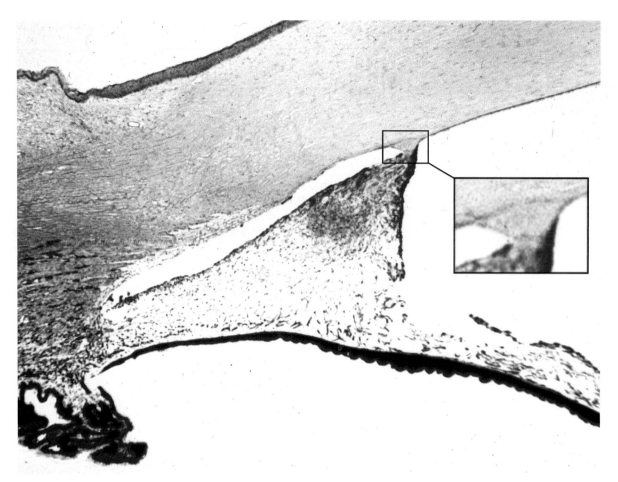

Fig. 7.31 Histopathology of Axenfeld's anomaly. There is an area of adherence between the iris and Schwalbe's line (inset).

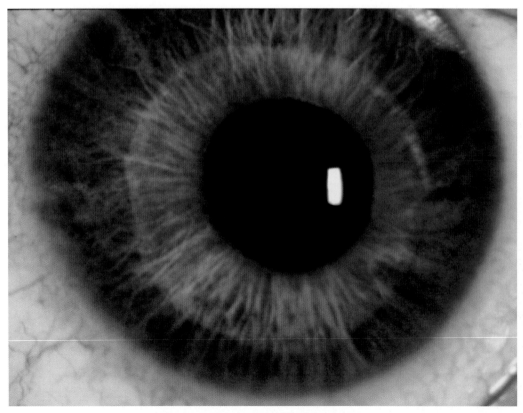

Fig. 7.32 Rieger's anomaly. There is hypoplasia of the iris stroma and mild corectopia. Iris abnormalities are more extensive in Rieger's anomaly compared with those in Axenfeld's anomaly, although both anomalies probably represent a spectrum of disease.

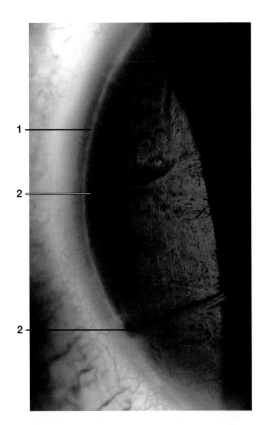

Fig. 7.33 Rieger's anomaly; slit-lamp photo. Similar to Axenfeld's anomaly, there is a prominent Schwalbe's line (1). Thick iris bands (2) are seen approaching Schwalbe's line.

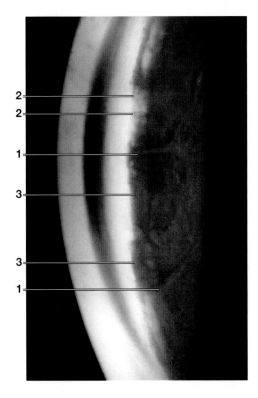

Fig. 7.34 Rieger's anomaly; gonioscopy. The thick iris bands (1) seen in Fig. 7.33, as well as fine (2) and wide (3) iris adhesions, are seen here.

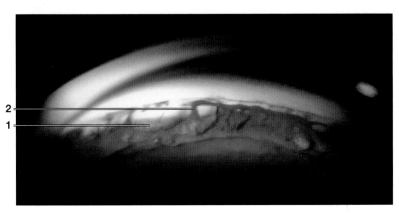

Fig. 7.35 Rieger's anomaly; gonioscopy. Another case illustrates fine iris adhesions covering the trabecular meshwork (1) and large iris adhesions to Schwalbe's line (2).

Normal Anatomy and Developmental Abnormalities of the Cornea **99**

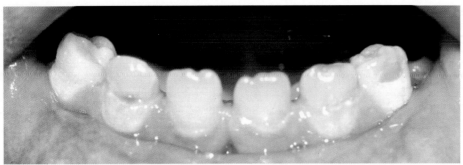

Fig. 7.36

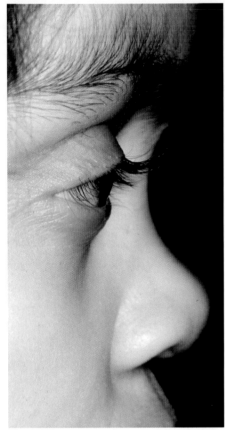

Fig. 7.37

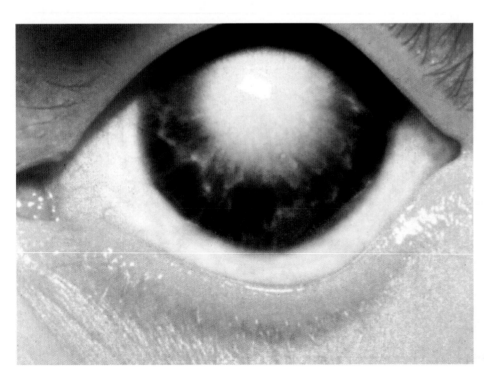

Fig. 7.38

Figs 7.36–7.38 Axenfeld–Rieger syndrome. This is a combination of Rieger's anomaly and systemic abnormalities, which include microdontia (Fig. 7.36), a flat nasal bridge with maxillary hypoplasia (Fig. 7.37), and hypospadias (Fig. 7.38). Inheritance is usually autosomal dominant.

Fig. 7.39 Peter's anomaly. There is central opacification of the corneal stroma with relative clearing in the corneal periphery. In mild cases, adherent strands of iris tissue extend from the pupillary margin to the posterior cornea. In severe cases, the iris is markedly abnormal and the lens may adhere to the posterior cornea. Glaucoma is often present.

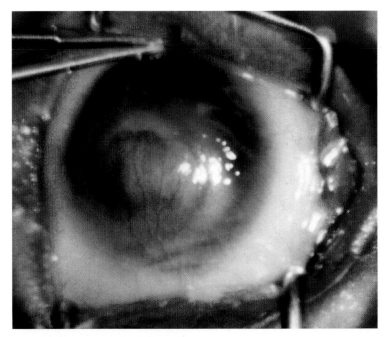

Fig. 7.40 Severe Peter's anomaly. There is marked opacification of the cornea and a superficial vascular pannus.

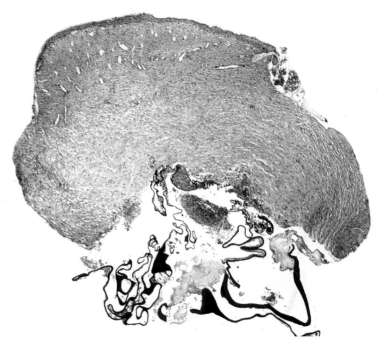

Fig. 7.41 Histopathology of Peter's anomaly. Shown are the increased cellularity and abnormal collagen in the corneal stroma, a loss of normal endothelium and Descemet's membrane, and the adherence of the lens capsule to the posterior cornea.

Chapter 8

Corneal Manifestations of Systemic Disease and Therapy

The corneal manifestations of systemic disease are usually noted in patients with an established systemic diagnosis. Occasionally, however, the clinician has a unique opportunity to diagnose a systemic condition based on the results of the ocular examination. Many of these conditions result in abnormal deposition of material in the cornea. These can easily be discerned because the cornea is normally clear and deposits of any type produce clouding.

Metabolic Disorders

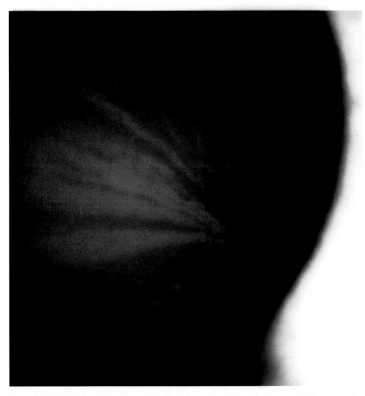

Fig. 8.1 Fabry's disease. This disorder of sphingolipid metabolism results in the deposition of trihexosylceramide in tissues throughout the body. It is transmitted as an X-linked recessive disorder. This male patient has the characteristic deposits in a whorl distribution in the corneal epithelium (cornea verticillata). Nearly all patients with Fabry's disease have this finding.

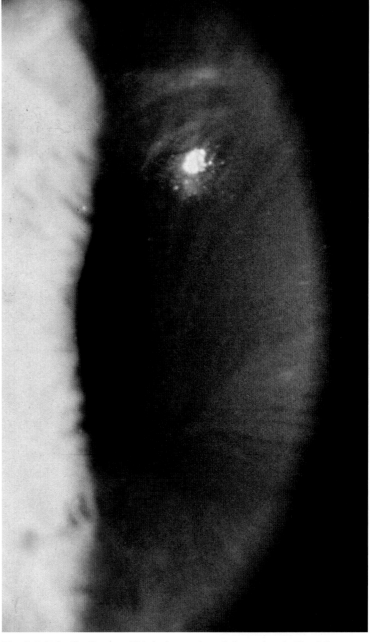

Fig. 8.2 Fabry's disease. This is the mother of the patient in Fig. 8.1. Approximately 90% of female carriers have cornea verticillata.

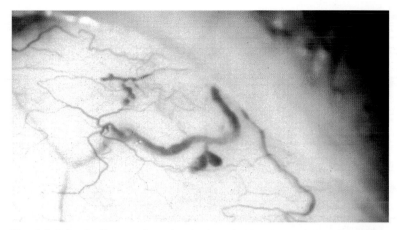

Fig. 8.3 Fabry's disease. Deposits of sphingolipid in the vascular endothelium produce dilated conjunctival vessels with small aneurysms.

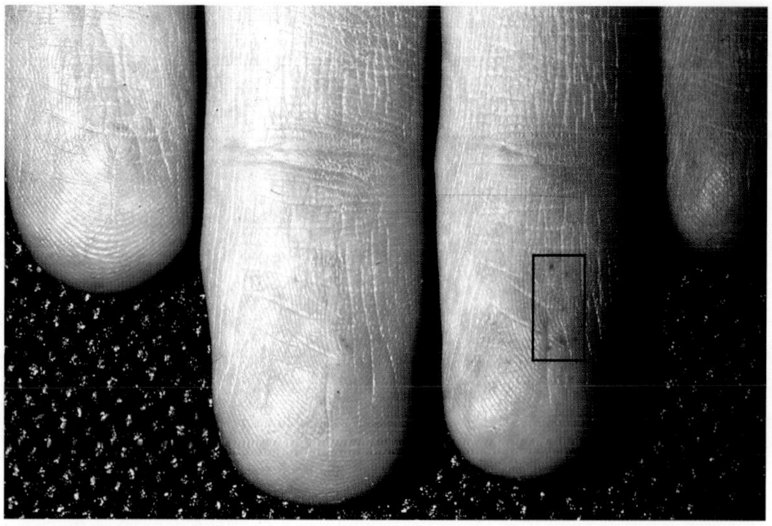

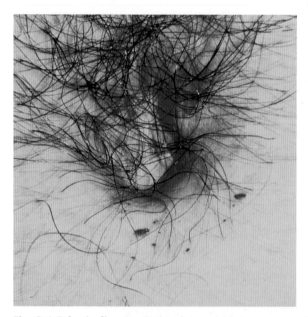

Fig. 8.4 Fabry's disease. Small, punctate, dark red, vascular lesions appear in the skin (box).

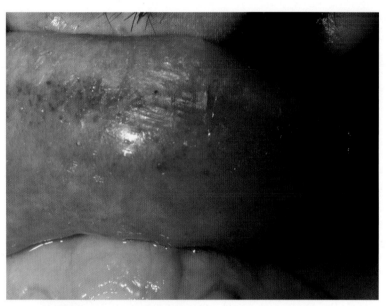

Fig. 8.5 Fabry's disease. There are small, telangiectatic, vascular abnormalities in the buccal mucosa.

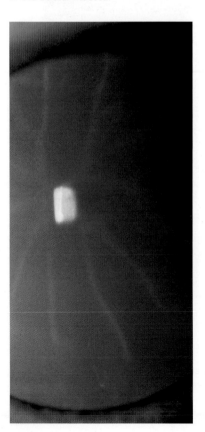

Fig. 8.6 Fabry's disease. Dark red, vascular lesions are seen in the periumbilical skin of this patient.

Fig. 8.7 Fabry's disease. Approximately 50% of patients with this disorder have posterior spoke-like cataracts, possibly representing deposits of sphingolipid along the lens suture lines.

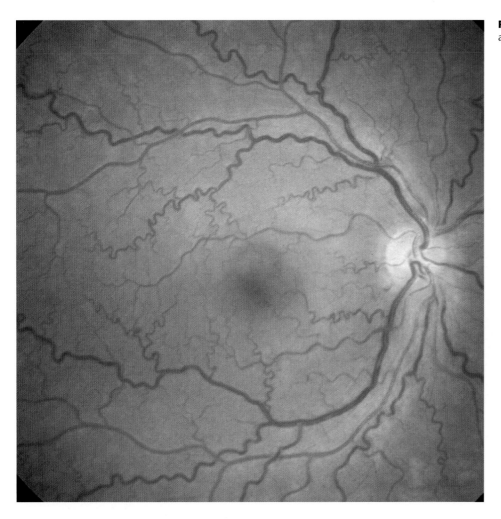

Fig. 8.8 Fabry's disease. The retinal vessels may be dilated and tortuous.

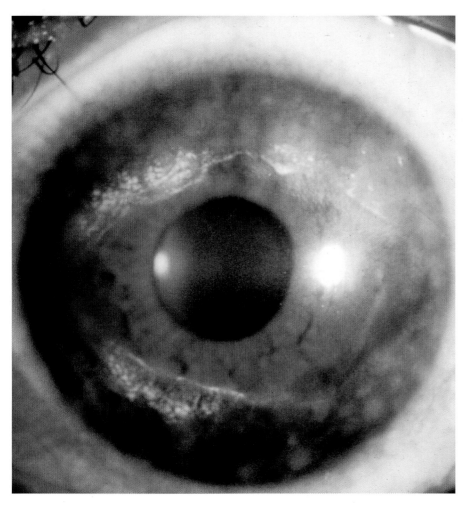

Fig. 8.9 Fish eye disease. This familial condition results in lipid deposition in the cornea. The lipid deposition tends to be denser in the periphery; in advanced forms, diffuse corneal clouding resembling the eyes of boiled fish occurs. Systemically, there is a deficiency in esterification of free cholesterol in high-density a-lipoprotein (HDL). HDL levels are markedly reduced, and triglyceride levels are increased.

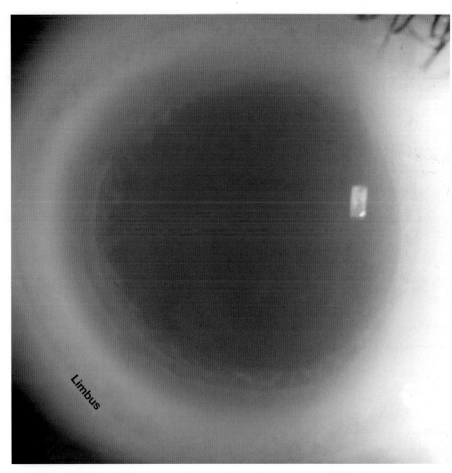

Fig. 8.10 Lecithin–cholesterol acyltransferase (LCAT) deficiency. This autosomal recessive disorder results in lipid deposition in the cornea. The plasma demonstrates raised levels of unesterified cholesterol and lecithin. Systemically, these patients may have renal failure and anemia; however, the corneal findings may precede these manifestations.

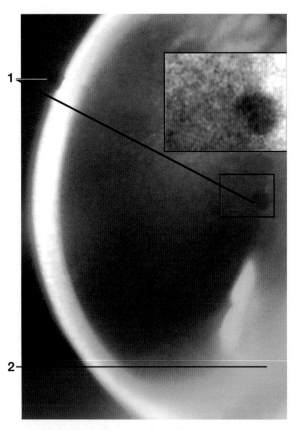

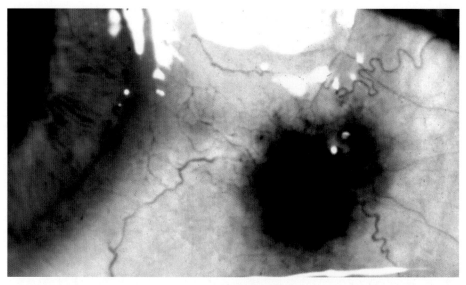

Fig. 8.12 Alkaptonuria. This is an autosomal recessive disorder of phenylalanine and tyrosine metabolism. A metabolic intermediate, homogentisic acid, accumulates throughout the body, causing pigmentary changes. Pigment may accumulate in the eye near the insertion of the recti muscles, particularly the lateral rectus.

Fig. 8.11 LCAT deficiency. Centrally, the deposits are small white dots that may surround clear lacunae (1). In the peripheral cornea the deposits are denser (2) and resemble arcus senilis.

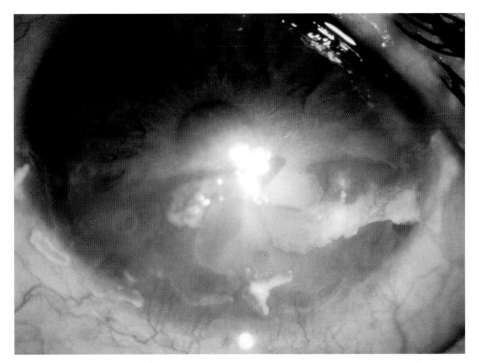

Fig. 8.13 Congenital porphyria. In this disorder of heme biosynthesis, vesicular and ulcerative lesions occur on sun-exposed portions of the skin and eye. In this example the inferior cornea is scarred and vascularized from chronic ulcerations. Other forms of porphyria result in similar blistering and scarring on the conjunctiva and cornea.

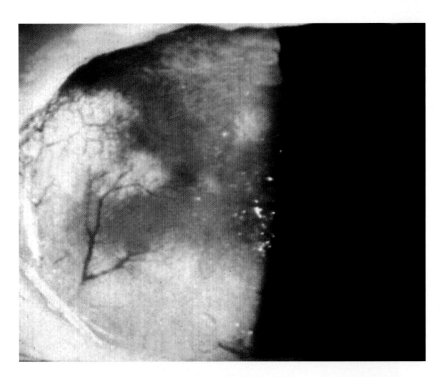

Fig. 8.14 Tangier disease. This systemic abnormality of lipid metabolism is inherited as an autosomal recessive disorder. Systemic abnormalities include an absence of normal HDL in plasma, yellow–orange tonsillar hyperplasia, hepatosplenomegaly, and lymphadenopathy. In this patient, localized lipid deposition in the cornea is associated with vascularization. A white dot-like haze, similar to that seen in LCAT deficiency (see Figs 8.10 and 8.11), has also been described. This patient also had multiple lid abnormalities and corrective surgical procedures owing to lipid infiltration of the lids. The first patients described with this disorder were from Tangier Island, Virginia.

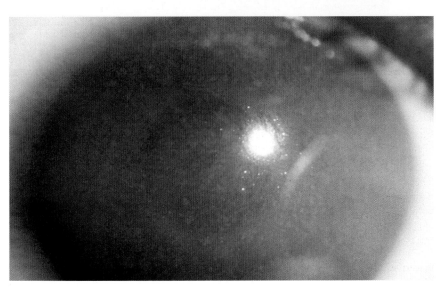

Fig. 8.15 Hurler's syndrome (MPS I-H). An autosomal recessive disorder of mucopolysaccharide (MPS) metabolism, Hurler's syndrome results in the accumulation of dermatan sulfate and heparan sulfate in tissues throughout the body. Corneal clouding begins early in life and is diffuse. The clouding is composed of fine, gray, punctate opacities. Newer treatments with enzyme replacement therapy look promising. Without treatment, death usually occurs by the age of 10 years.

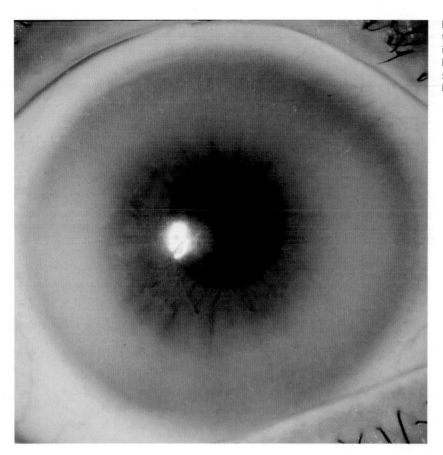

Fig. 8.16 Scheie's syndrome (MPS I-S). Similar to Hurler's syndrome, this autosomal recessive disorder of mucopolysaccharide metabolism results in the accumulation of dermatan sulfate and heparan sulfate throughout the body. The systemic findings are much less severe than those of Hurler's syndrome, and patients have a normal life expectancy. The corneal clouding is densest in the peripheral cornea, and progresses centrally with age.

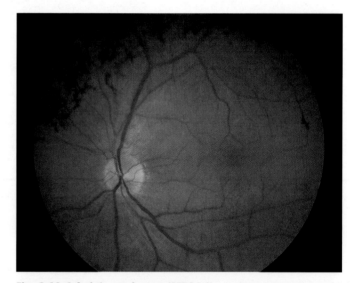

Fig. 8.18 Scheie's syndrome (MPS I-S). A pigmentary retinopathy is commonly seen in Scheie's syndrome.

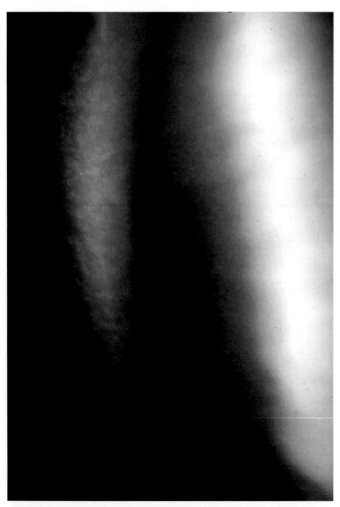

Fig. 8.17 Scheie's syndrome (MPS I-S). The deposits are fine, gray, punctate opacities located throughout the corneal stroma.

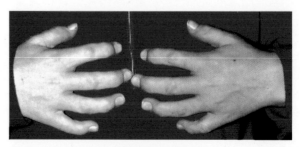

Fig. 8.19 Scheie's syndrome (MPS I-S). The hands are claw-like and the joints are enlarged.

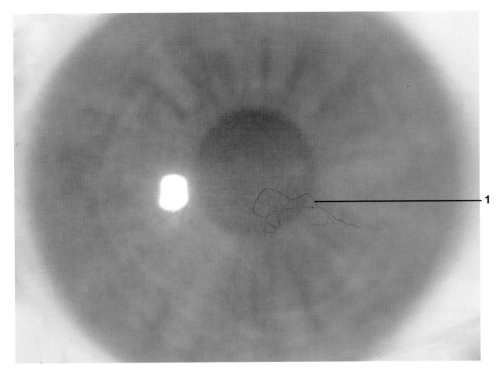

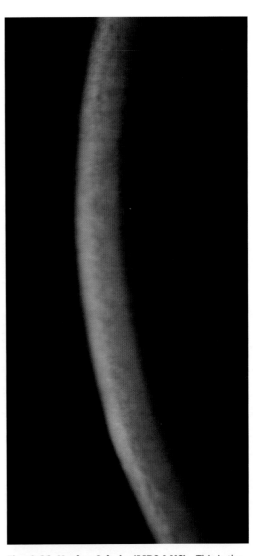

Fig. 8.20 Hurler–Scheie (MPS I-HS). Hurler–Scheie syndrome has the same enzyme defect as that seen in Hurler's syndrome and Scheie's syndrome. There is an accumulation of dermatan sulfate and heparan sulfate in tissues throughout the body. The systemic findings are intermediate between those of Hurler's syndrome and Scheie's syndrome. Diffuse corneal clouding usually develops in the first two decades of life. This is a preoperative photograph of a 12-year-old affected patient prior to corneal transplantation. A superficial corneal blood vessel (1) is seen.

Fig. 8.21 Hurler–Scheie (MPS I-HS). This is the same patient as in Fig. 8.20. The corneal clouding extends throughout the corneal stroma.

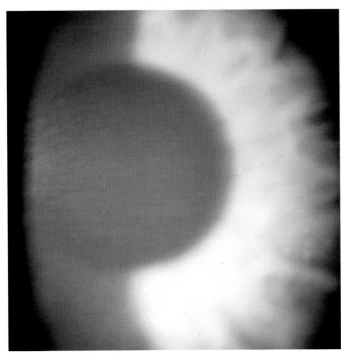

Fig. 8.22 Morquio's syndrome. There is diffuse corneal clouding from keratan sulfate deposition in the corneal stroma. Morquio's syndrome is an autosomal recessive disorder of mucopolysaccharide metabolism.

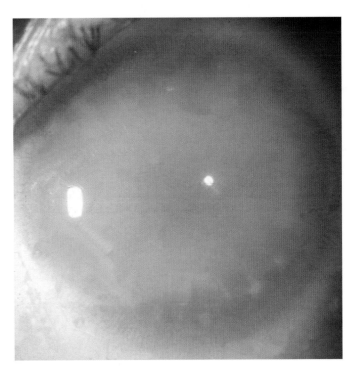

Fig. 8.23 Maroteaux–Lamy syndrome. Corneal clouding is common. Dermatan sulfate accumulates in the corneal stroma. This is an autosomal recessive disorder of mucopolysaccharide metabolism.

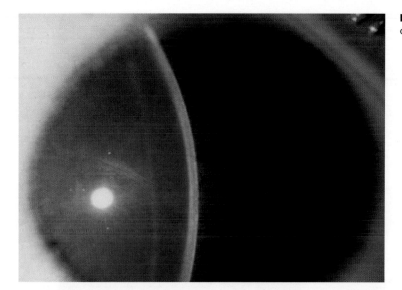

Fig. 8.24 Maroteaux–Lamy syndrome. Slit-beam examination demonstrates corneal haze anterior to posterior, and limbus to limbus.

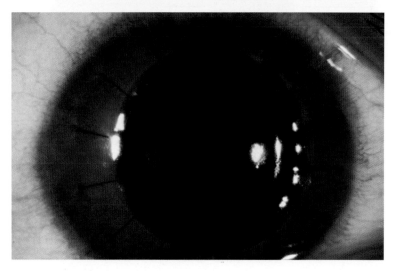

Fig. 8.25 Maroteaux–Lamy syndrome. The donor cornea is dramatically clearer than the host cornea after penetrating keratoplasty.

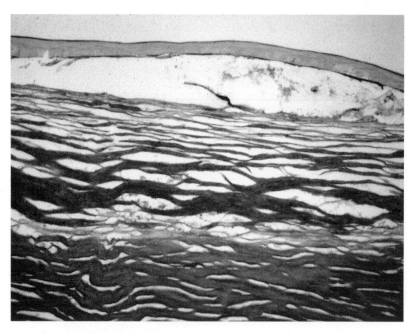

Fig. 8.26 Histopathology of Scheie's syndrome. There are deposits of mucopolysaccharide throughout the corneal stroma. Mucopolysaccharide stains blue with Alcian blue stain.

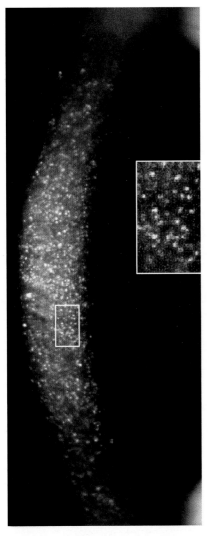

Fig. 8.27 Cystinosis. The corneal crystals are polygonal, refractile, and polychromatic (inset).

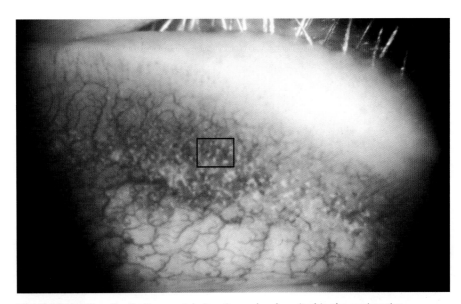

Fig. 8.28 Cystinosis. Cystine crystals (inset) are also deposited in the conjunctiva.

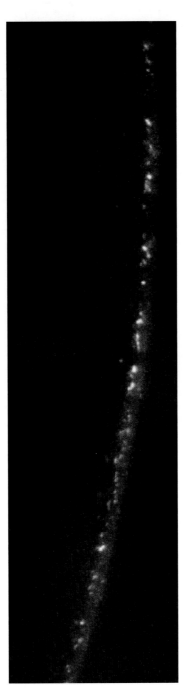

Cystinosis is an autosomal recessive disorder of impaired cystine transport across lysosomal membranes. Cystine is deposited in tissues throughout the body, including the conjunctiva, cornea, and retina. Deposits of crystals in the cornea can cause severe photophobia and episodes of recurrent erosions. The infantile form is the most severe, and death usually occurs in the first decade of life from renal failure. The adolescent form manifests in the second decade of life, and renal involvement is less severe. The adult form is the mildest, and has no renal involvement or retinal changes.

Fig. 8.29 Cystinosis. In addition to corneal crystals, this patient had Fanconi's syndrome caused by cystine deposits in the kidneys.

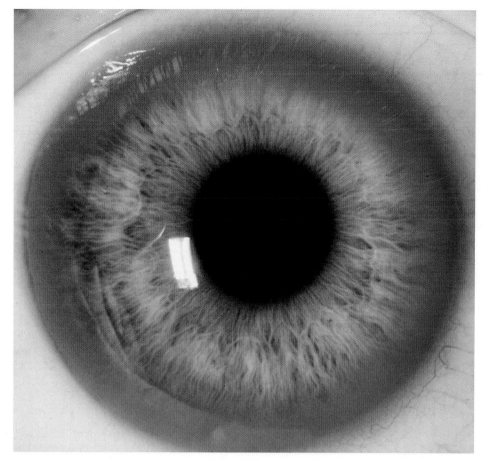

Fig. 8.30 Wilson's disease. There is a defect in copper metabolism, and 95% of patients with Wilson's disease have a Kayser–Fleischer ring. Copper is deposited at the level of Descemet's membrane in the peripheral cornea. The inferior cornea is affected first. The ring is usually dark brown but may appear gold–yellow or green. There is no clear interval separating the ring from the limbus.

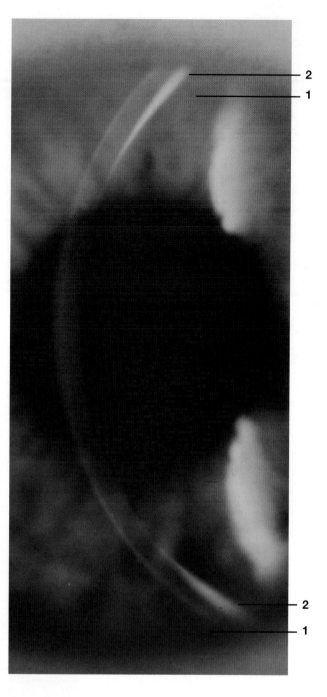

Fig. 8.31 Wilson's disease. The peripheral copper Kayser–Fleischer ring (1) is found by slit-beam illumination to be located in Descemet's membrane (2).

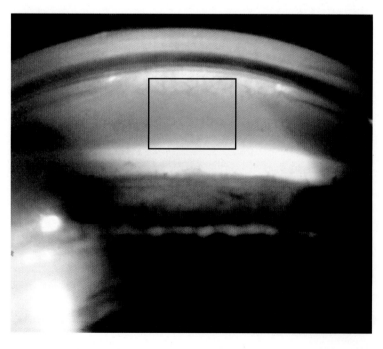

Fig. 8.32 Early Wilson's disease. The copper deposition may be appreciated only with gonioscopy. In this patient there is dark brown pigmentation extending from Schwalbe's line anteriorly (box).

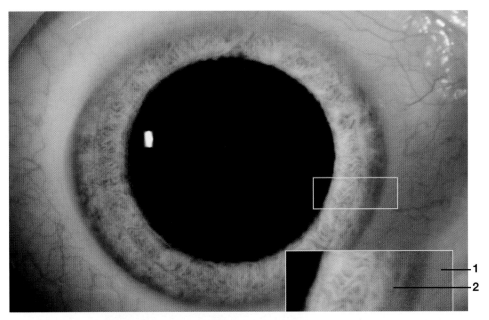

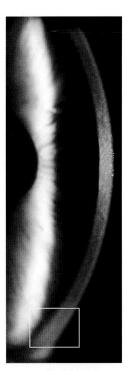

Fig. 8.33 Bilirubin deposits. A Kayser–Fleischer ring should be distinguished from bilirubin deposits in the peripheral cornea. This patient with primary biliary cirrhosis has conjunctival jaundice (1) and peripheral yellow bilirubin deposits in the cornea (2).

Fig. 8.34 Thin slit-lamp view of the patient in Fig. 8.33. The box shows that the bilirubin deposits are more extensive in the posterior stroma but are located throughout the stroma.

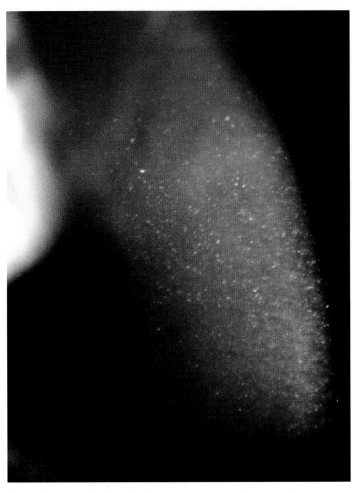

Fig. 8.35 Gout. This patient has urate crystals in the corneal stroma.

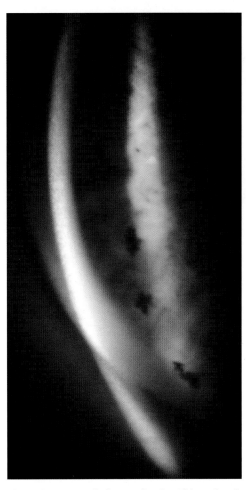

Fig. 8.36 Hypercholesterolemia. This patient has arcus senilis. There is a clear area between the lipid deposits and the limbus.

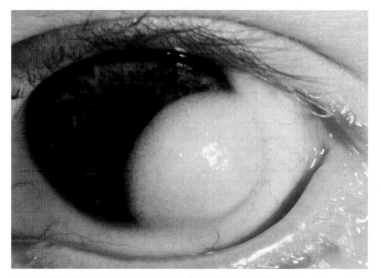

Fig. 8.37 Goldenhar's syndrome. One-third of patients with this syndrome (oculoauriculovertebral dysplasia) have corneal dermoids. The dermoids are usually unilateral and occur most commonly at the inferior temporal limbus.

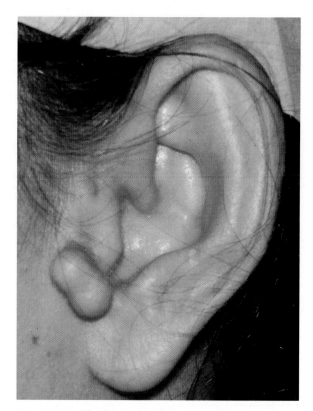

Fig. 8.38 Goldenhar's syndrome. A pretragal appendage is noted.

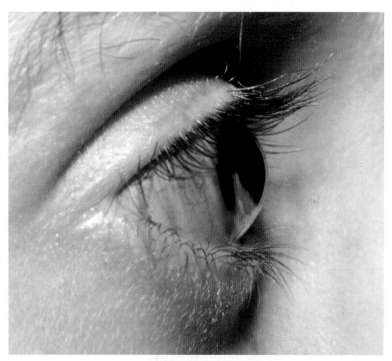

Fig. 8.39 Ehlers–Danlos syndrome. This systemic disorder is characterized by poor cross-linking of collagen molecules. Systemic findings include joint hypermobility, skin hyperextensibility, easy bruising, and propensity toward organ rupture. This patient with Ehlers–Danlos syndrome type VI has keratoglobus and blue sclera. Blue sclera results from scleral thinning and increased visibility of the choroid.

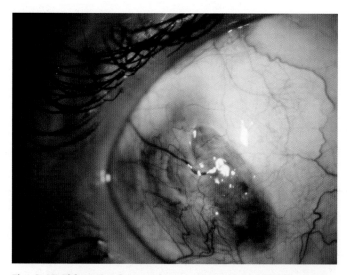

Fig. 8.40 Ehlers–Danlos syndrome. This patient with Ehlers–Danlos syndrome had extreme thinning of the sclera after strabismus surgery.

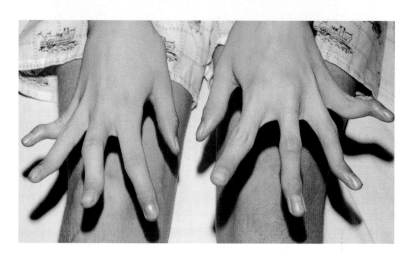

Fig. 8.41 Ehlers–Danlos syndrome. Joint hypermobility is shown.

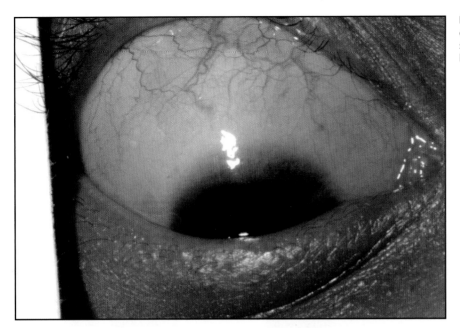

Fig. 8.42 Osteogenesis imperfecta. This inherited disorder is characterized by bone fractures, deafness, and blue scleras. The blue sclera is easily appreciated when compared with the white card on the left of this figure.

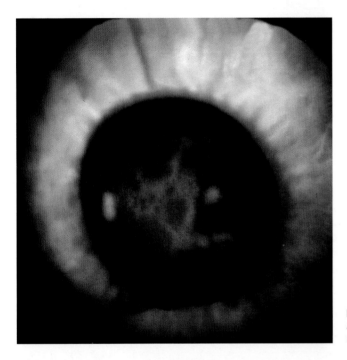

Fig. 8.43 Osteogenesis imperfecta. Central corneal scarring is seen here. Other corneal abnormalities in this disease include decreased central corneal thickness, keratoconus, and megalocornea.

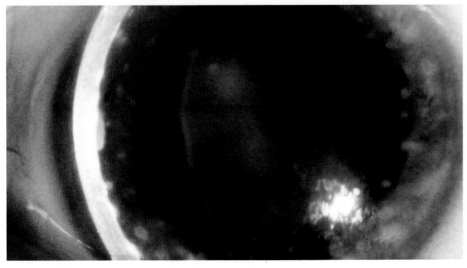

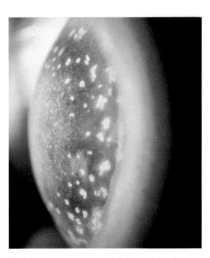

Fig. 8.44 Spondyloepiphyseal dysplasia tarda. In this inherited skeletal dysplasia, multiple deep, grayish white, nodular opacities may be seen in the deep peripheral corneal stroma (some project toward the anterior chamber).

Fig. 8.45 Spondyloepiphyseal dysplasia tarda. Deep peripheral opacities and fine central opacities are noted in the mid and anterior stroma.

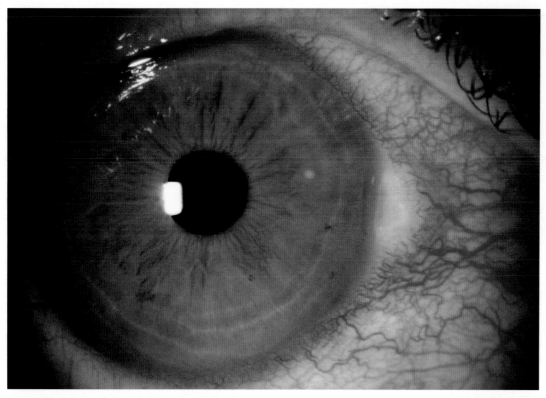

Fig. 8.46 Crohn's disease. This is a chronic inflammatory disease of the gastrointestinal tract. This patient has sclerokeratitis. There is avascularity in the area of infiltration.

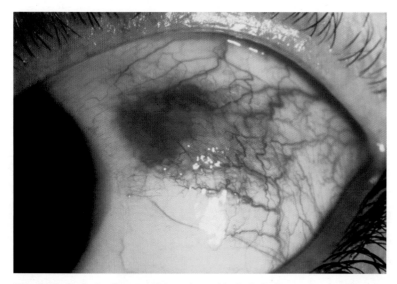

Fig. 8.47 Crohn's disease. This patient with Crohn's disease developed episcleritis.

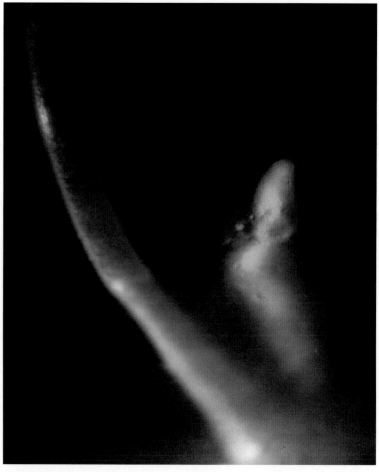

Fig. 8.48 Crohn's disease. There is a marginal noninfected corneal ulcer. Systemic immunosuppression may be needed to control progressive ulceration.

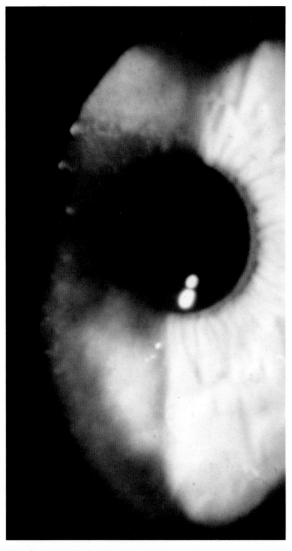

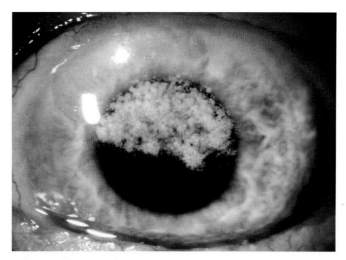

Fig. 8.50 Whipple's disease. Whipple's disease is a multisystem disorder caused by a Gram-positive bacillus, *Tropheryma whippelii*. Intestinal symptoms predominate and include abdominal pain, diarrhea, steatorrhea, anorexia, and weight loss. Ocular signs include stromal keratitis, uveitis, inflammatory vitreous opacities, vitreous or retinal hemorrhage, and diffuse retinal and choroidal vasculitis. In this unusual case there are white "greasy" flocculent precipitates on the back of the cornea.

Fig. 8.49 Crohn's disease. This case demonstrates subepithelial, nebulous keratopathy occurring primarily in the mid-peripheral cornea. The pattern of scarring is distinctive and in some cases has led to the diagnosis of Crohn's disease in patients prior to the development of gastrointestinal symptoms.

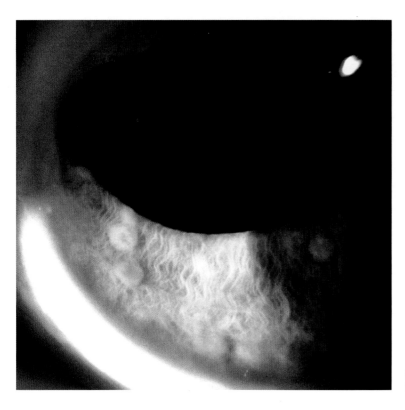

Fig. 8.51 Whipple's disease. The same patient as in Fig. 8.50, demonstrating multiple tan nodules on the iris.

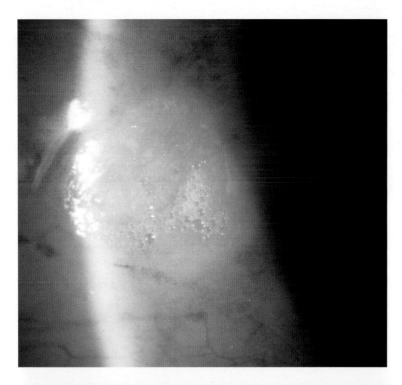

Fig. 8.52 Vitamin A deficiency. Although vitamin A deficiency is rare in the United States, when it occurs, it is usually with cystic fibrosis, severe liver disease, or severe malnutrition (especially in alcoholics) or after intestinal bypass surgery. This is an example of a Bitot spot, a white–gray irregular plaque that usually occurs near the limbus in the interpalpebral region. A gas-producing bacterium, *Corynebacterium xerosis*, is responsible for the foamy appearance of this lesion.

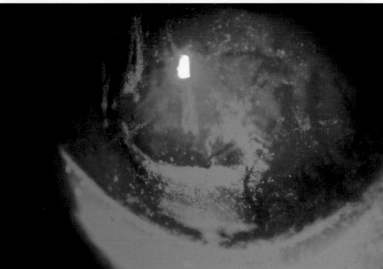

Fig. 8.53 Vitamin A deficiency. Goblet cell function is impaired in this disorder, and there is a lack of mucin. The mucin deficiency leads to an unstable tear film and a rapid tear break-up time, as seen here.

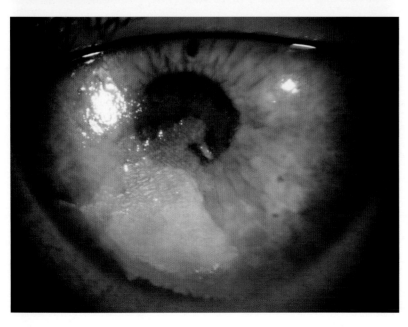

Fig. 8.54 Vitamin A deficiency. This patient has marked keratinization of the inferior cornea. The corneal surface is dry and the light reflex is irregular.

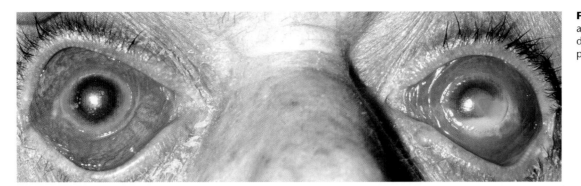

Fig. 8.55 Vitamin A deficiency. In this alcoholic patient, an infected corneal ulcer has developed in the left eye. A hypopyon is present.

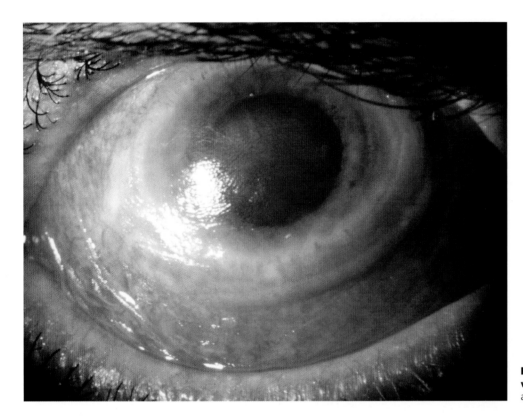

Fig. 8.56 Right eye of the patient in Fig. 8.55 before vitamin A treatment. The corneal light reflex is dulled, and the cornea and conjunctiva lack their normal luster.

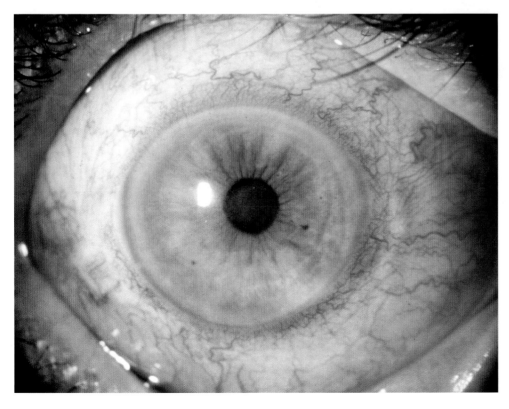

Fig. 8.57 Same patient as in Figs 8.55 and 8.56, 10 days after initiation of vitamin A treatment. The corneal light reflex is sharp, and the surface abnormalities of the conjunctiva and cornea are nearly gone.

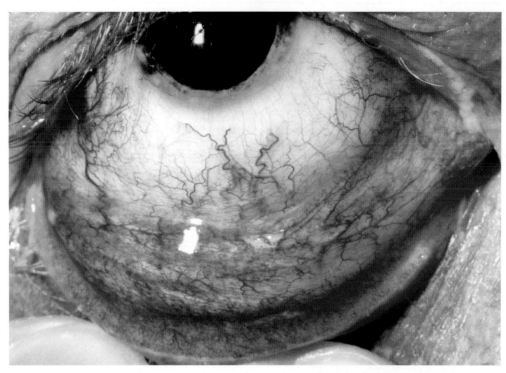

Fig. 8.58 Polycythemia vera. There is an increased red cell mass and hematocrit. Engorged blood vessels can be readily appreciated in the inferior fornix of this patient. These patients may complain of redness of the eyes, allowing the clinician the unique position of establishing the diagnosis.

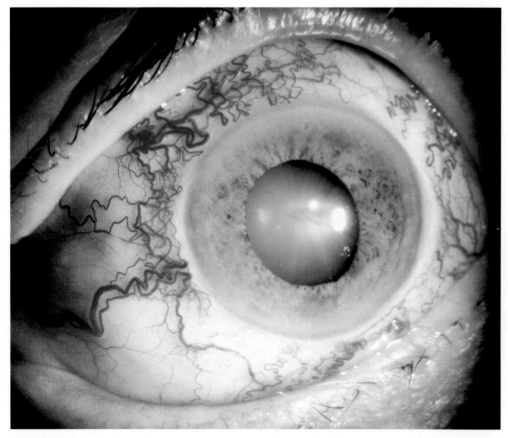

Fig. 8.59 Dural–cavernous fistula. There is a communication between the dural arteries and the cavernous sinus. The conjunctival veins in one eye become markedly enlarged and tortuous, whereas the conjunctival arteries remain normal. Other signs of dural–cavernous fistula include unilateral visual field loss, proptosis, motility disturbances, and raised intraocular pressure.

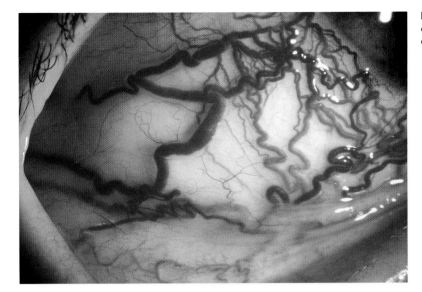

Fig. 8.60 Dural–cavernous fistula. This is a higher magnification of the conjunctiva in a different patient. There is marked enlargement and tortuosity of the conjunctival veins.

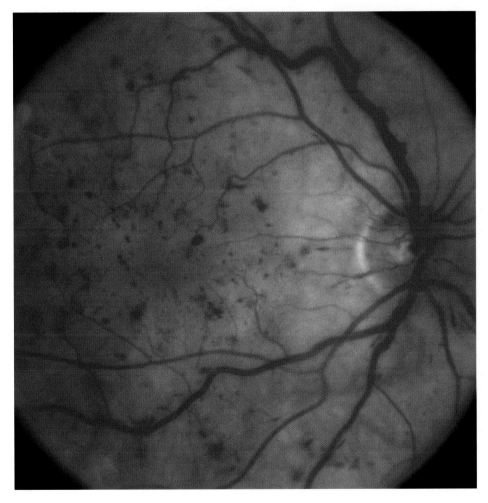

Fig. 8.61 Dural–cavernous fistula. This is the retina of the patient seen in Fig. 8.60. The retinal veins are enlarged, and there are scattered retinal hemorrhages from venous stasis retinopathy.

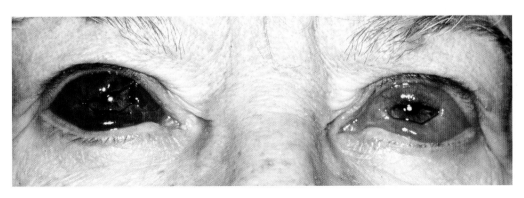

Fig. 8.62 Primary amyloidosis. In primary amyloidosis there is deposition of abnormal proteins throughout the body. The protein material is usually composed of immunoglobulin light chains. This patient with end-stage systemic amyloidosis has diffuse amyloid infiltration of the conjunctiva.

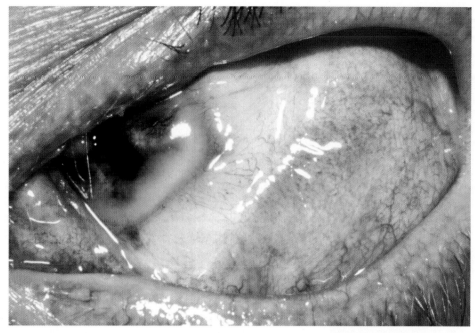

Fig. 8.63 Primary amyloidosis. Amyloid deposits are seen infiltrating the conjunctiva and cornea.

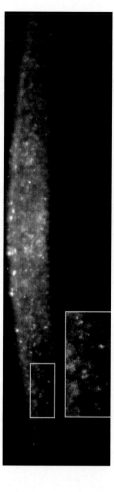

Fig. 8.64 Multiple myeloma. There is systemic deposition of entire immunoglobulin molecules and an excess of light chains. Systemic findings include anemia, hypercalcemia, and osteolytic bone lesions. This patient with multiple myeloma has immunoglobulin crystals in the cornea (inset).

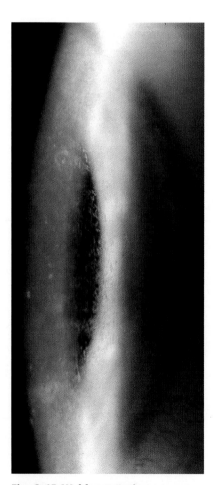

Fig. 8.65 Waldenström's macroglobulinemia. There is systemic deposition of IgM. This patient demonstrates immunoglobulin deposition in the cornea. In direct illumination these deposits are white; in indirect illumination, they appear crystalline.

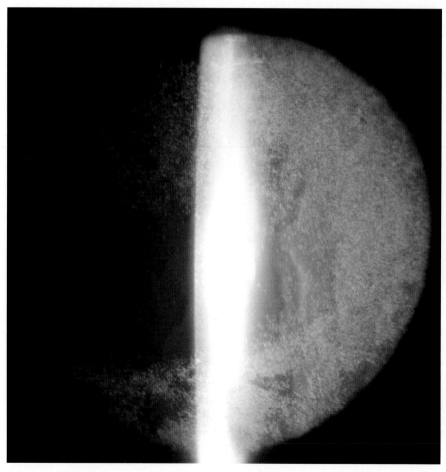

Fig. 8.66 Waldenström's macroglobulinemia. In the patient in Fig. 8.65, the red reflex demonstrates the refractile and crystalline nature of deposits.

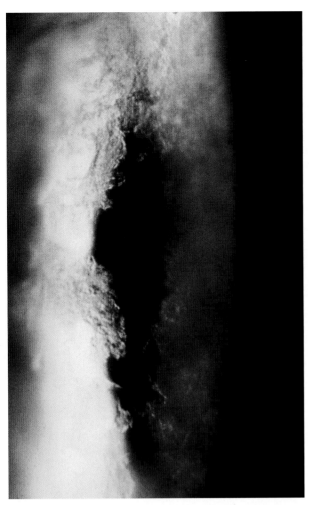

Fig. 8.67 Benign monoclonal gammopathy. Immunoglobulin crystals are seen in the cornea.

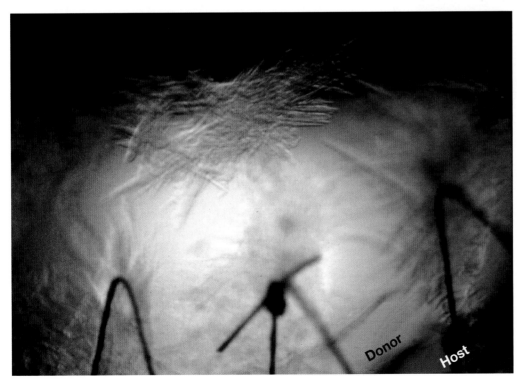

Fig. 8.68 Benign monoclonal gammopathy. This patient had a recurrence of immunoglobulin crystals in a graft. Although usually a benign process, some patients develop multiple myeloma.

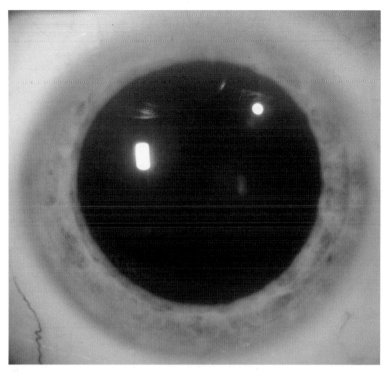

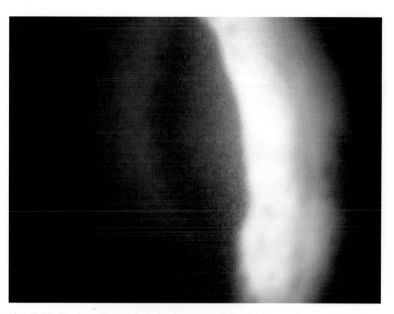

Fig. 8.70 Benign monoclonal gammopathy. This is another pattern of corneal clouding observed with benign monoclonal gammopathy. There are fine particulate opacities, which are best seen with indirect illumination.

Fig. 8.69 Benign monoclonal gammopathy. Patients with benign monoclonal gammopathy may have a diffuse stromal haze, as seen here. This was an incidental finding and the visual acuity was 20/20.

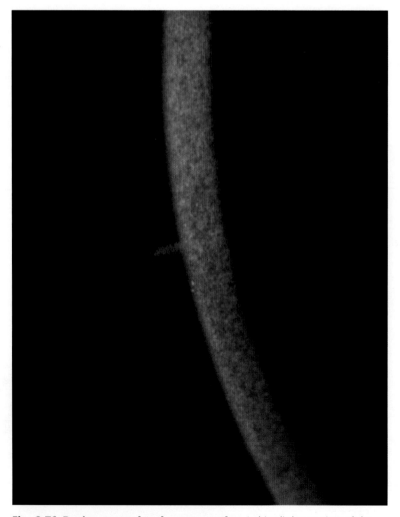

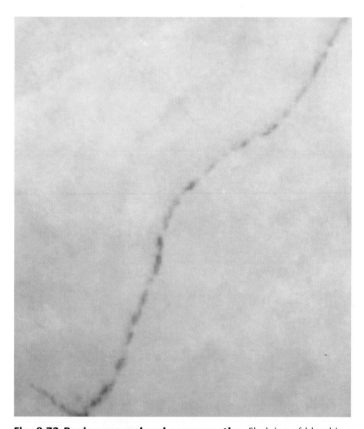

Fig. 8.72 Benign monoclonal gammopathy. Sludging of blood in a conjunctival vessel is seen in a patient with benign monoclonal gammopathy.

Fig. 8.71 Benign monoclonal gammopathy. A thin slit-beam view of the patient in Fig. 8.70 shows opacities through the entire depth of the cornea.

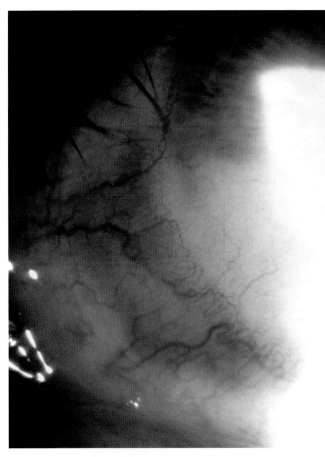

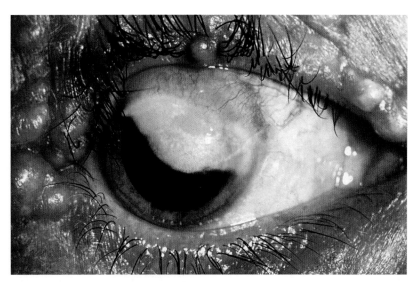

Fig. 8.74 Hand–Schüller–Christian disease. A disseminated form of eosinophilic granuloma, this disease can be fatal and comprises a triad of lytic lesions in the skull, exophthalmos from orbital involvement, and diabetes insipidus. The histology is identical to that of eosinophilic granuloma. Here the tumor has extended into the subcutaneous tissue of the skin and into the conjunctiva and cornea.

Fig. 8.73 Eosinophilic granuloma. This benign tumor composed of eosinophils and histiocytes usually begins in one of the bones of the orbital rim (most commonly the frontal bone). Here the tumor has infiltrated anteriorly into the conjunctiva and cornea.

Endocrine Disorders

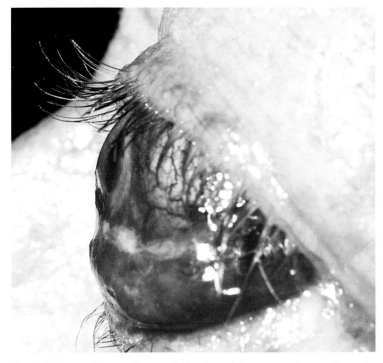

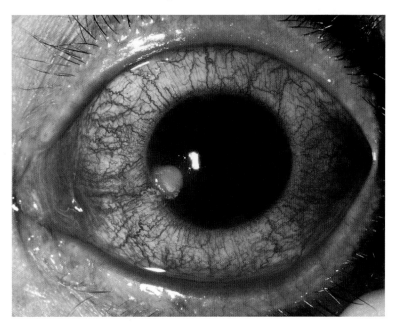

Fig. 8.76 Thyroid eye disease. This patient had chronic exposure keratitis and developed an indolent ulcer. Exophthalmos and lid retraction predispose to corneal exposure.

Fig. 8.75 Thyroid eye disease. Infiltration of the extraocular muscles and connective tissue can result in severe proptosis and orbital inflammation.

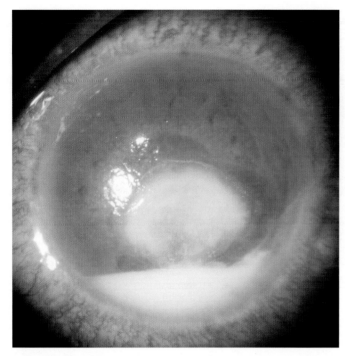

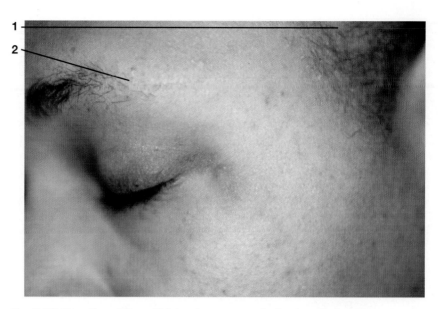

Fig. 8.78 Hypothyroidism. Hair loss is a common finding in patients with hypothyroidism. In this patient there is loss of scalp hair (1) and loss of lateral brow hair (2).

Fig. 8.77 Thyroid eye disease. There is an infected corneal ulcer with hypopyon in this patient with exposure keratitis caused by thyroid eye disease.

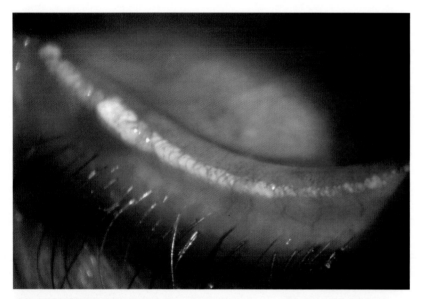

Fig. 8.79 Primary hyperparathyroidism. Calcium is deposited throughout the body in hyperparathyroidism. Here, calcium deposits are seen on the lid margin.

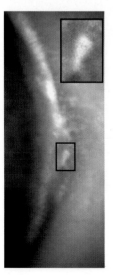

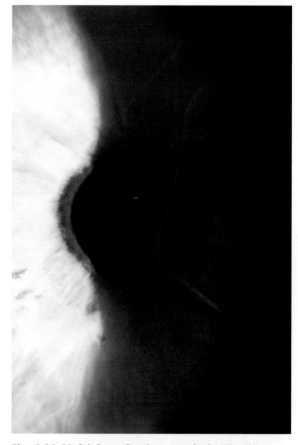

Fig. 8.81 Multiple endocrine neoplasia IIB. This syndrome consists of multiple tumors of organs of neural crest cell origin including medullary carcinoma of the thyroid, pheochromocytoma, mucosal neruomas, and intestinal neurogangliomas. Prominent, thickened, corneal nerves are present in all cases and can be a useful sign to assist the clinician in establishing the diagnosis.

Fig. 8.80 Chronic renal failure. The inset shows limbal calcium deposits in this patient.

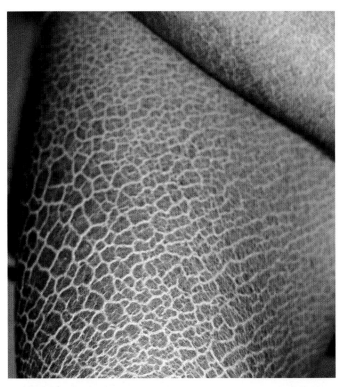

Fig. 8.82 X-linked ichthyosis. There are large brown hyperkeratotic scales on the skin.

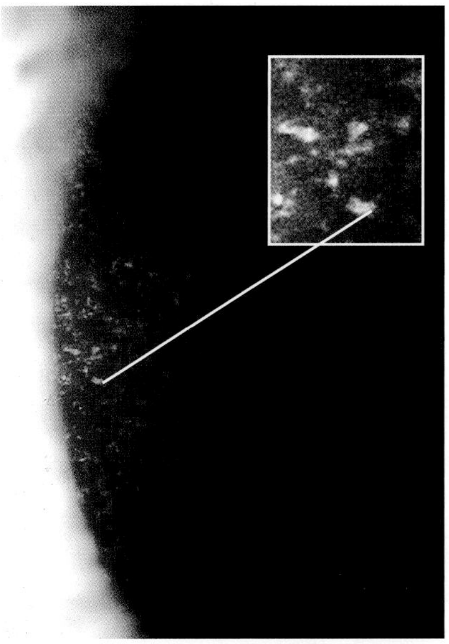

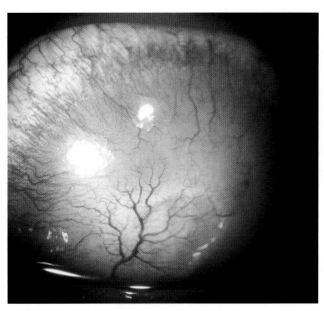

Fig. 8.83 X-linked ichthyosis. There are fine white deposits just anterior to Descemet's membrane (inset). Other forms of ichthyosis do not have these deposits.

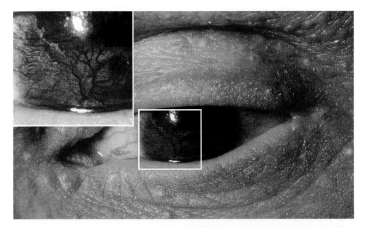

Fig. 8.84 Keratitis, ichthyosis, and deafness (KID) syndrome. This rare inherited disorder may be autosomal dominant or sporadic. Hair is scant or absent, and in this patient there is an absence of eyelashes. Corneal findings include superficial pannus (inset), diffuse punctate keratopathy, stromal scarring, and vascularization.

Fig. 8.85 KID syndrome. In the same patient as in Fig. 8.84, the cornea is scarred and vascularized.

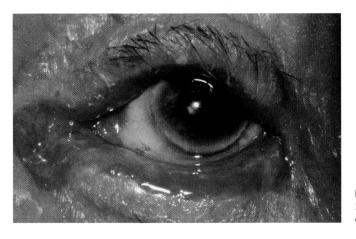

Fig. 8.86 Lamellar ichthyosis. Lamellar ichthyosis is a rare autosomal recessive disorder. Scales cover the entire skin surface. Lid involvement with cicatricial ectropion can lead to exposure keratitis.

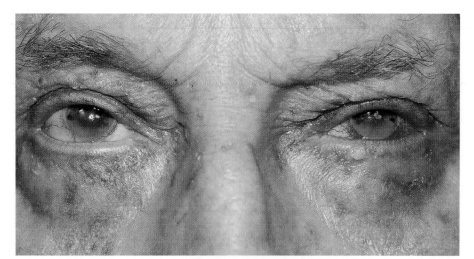

Fig. 8.87 Psoriasis. This chronic skin disease is characterized by scaling papules or plaques. This patient with involvement of the skin of the eyelids has lash loss and a nonspecific conjunctivitis.

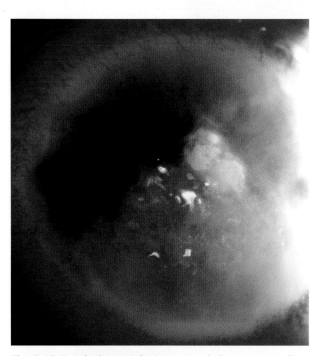

Fig. 8.88 Psoriasis. An infectious corneal ulcer is seen in this patient with psoriasis of the lids. Other corneal findings include sterile ulceration, superficial vascularization, and corneal scarring.

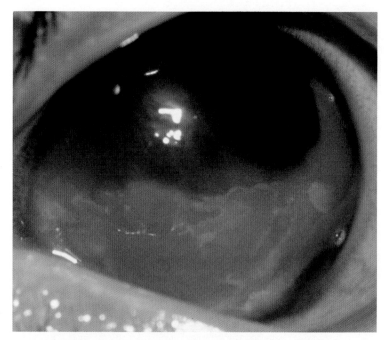

Fig. 8.89 Epidermolysis bullosa. There is poor epithelial adhesion to the basement membrane. Recurrent erosion with ulceration is common.

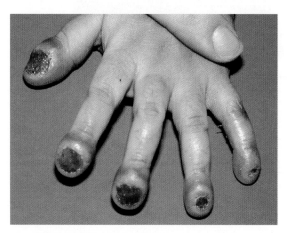

Fig. 8.90 Epidermolysis bullosa. Poor epithelial adhesion causes bullous lesions of the skin after minor trauma. The fingernails can be dystrophic, and the distal digits may be encased in a keratinized shell.

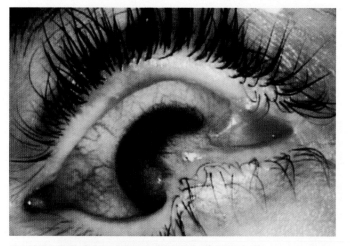

Fig. 8.91 Ectodermal dysplasia. Ectodemal dysplasia is a congenital, inherited abnormality of the skin and appendages (hair, nails, teeth, and sweat glands). Various inheritance patterns with different clinical presentations have been described. Multiple lid and anterior segment abnormalities have been described, including lash loss, absence of meibomian glands, ankyloblepharon (seen here), hypoplastic lacrimal ducts, severe dry eye, pterygia, corneal scarring (also seen here), cataract, uveitis and glaucoma.

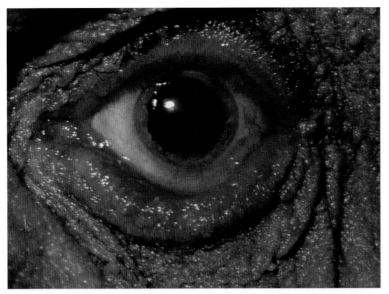

Fig. 8.92 Acanthosis nigricans. Acanthosis nigricans is characterized by papillary hypertrophy and hyperpigmentation of the face, neck, axillae, groin, antecubital and popliteal fossae, umbilicus, and anus. There are several causes including an autosomal dominant form, a form associated with obesity and insulin-resistant states, and a form seen with adenocarcinomas of various organs. These conditions produce a factor that over-stimulates keratinocytes and dermal fibroblasts. Ocular findings include lid thickening and hyperpigmentation, ectropion, conjunctival hypertrophy, canalicular obstruction, and corneal scarring and vascularization due to chronic exposure keratitis.

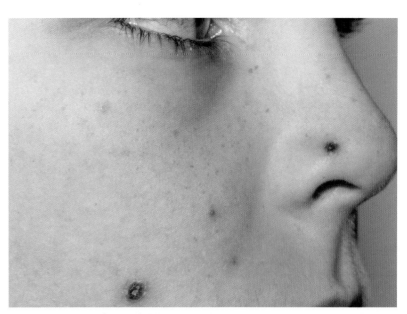

Fig. 8.93 Hydroa vacciniforme. Hydroa vacciniforme is a skin disease of childhood associated with sun exposure. Papules or nodules develop within hours of sun exposure, and over several days develop into vesicles that necrose and scar. Here, two lesions are seen on the skin of the cheek and nose.

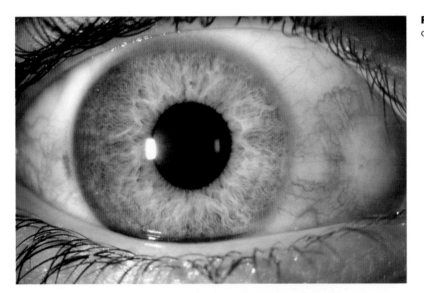

Fig. 8.94 Hydroa vacciniforme. The same patient as in Fig. 8.93 has a conjunctival lesion near the plica semilunaris of the right eye.

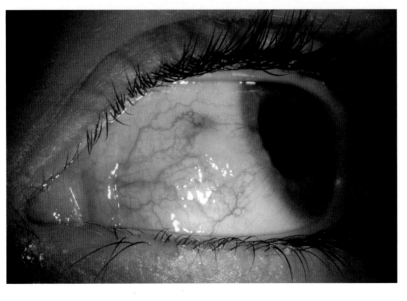

Fig. 8.95 Hydroa vacciniforme. The same patient as in Figs 8.93 and 8.94 has a second conjunctival lesion near the limbus of the left eye.

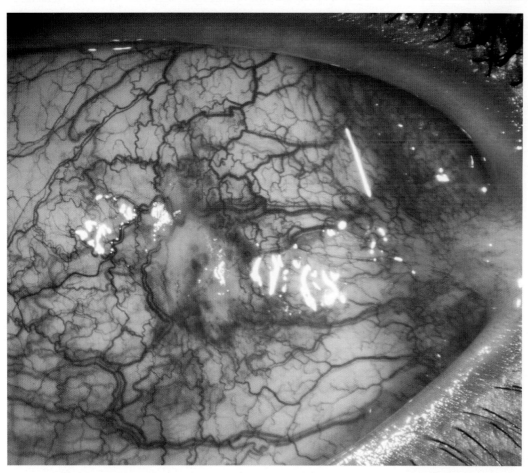

Fig. 8.96 Varicella (chickenpox). This is a common viral infection of young children. The rash spreads in waves and begins as flat macules that progress to papules and vesicles. A pock in the conjunctiva can be seen here.

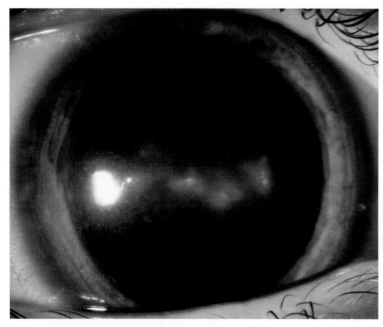

Fig. 8.97 Varicella (chickenpox). This 8-year-old boy developed disciform keratitis at the time of systemic varicella infection. The keratitis improved with topical corticosteroids, but the child was left with stromal scarring after a protracted course.

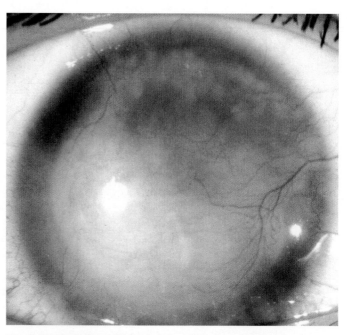

Fig. 8.98 Varicella (chickenpox). Rarely, this disease is associated with interstitial keratitis. This patient has extensive corneal scarring and vascularization.

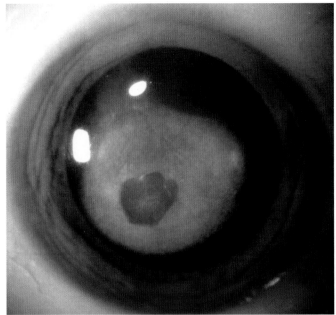

Fig. 8.99 Variola (smallpox). This patient demonstrates a central corneal scar from a smallpox or variola infection. Fortunately, the variola virus has been eradicated, and complications of this type are rarely seen today. The threat of biological warfare has renewed the possibility of this virus emerging again.

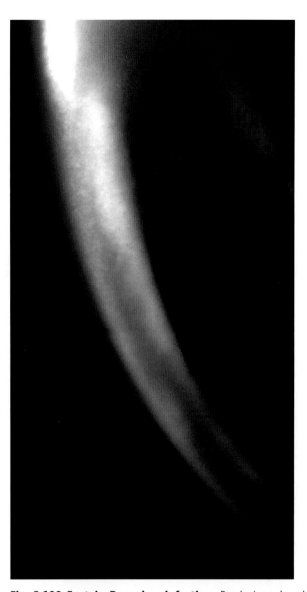

Fig. 8.100 Epstein–Barr virus infection. Rarely, irregular white opacities can be found throughout the corneal stroma. These opacities can occur in patients with active mononucleosis or in the absence of systemic disease with only serologic evidence of infection. They usually respond to topical corticosteroids.

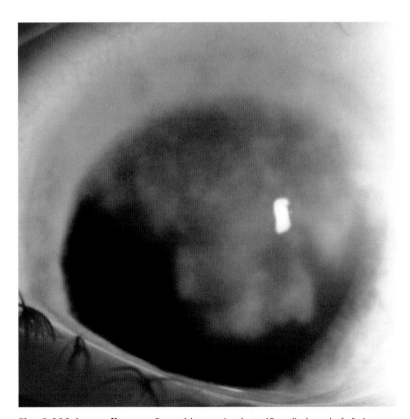

Fig. 8.101 Lyme disease. Caused by a spirochete (*Borrelia burgdorferi*), Lyme disease is transmitted by ticks. In the acute infection, patients develop fever, chills, malaise, and an enlarging red rash on the thighs, buttocks, or trunk (chronicum migrans). Months later, patients may experience a relapsing migratory polyarthritis. Patients may develop an interstitial keratitis characterized by multiple corneal infiltrates with indistinct borders in all levels of the stroma. Corneal vascularization is limited, and the conjunctiva is usually uninflamed.

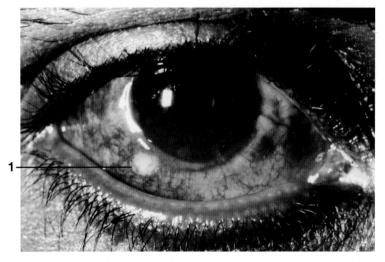

Fig. 8.102 Tuberculosis. Tuberculosis is caused by *Mycobacterium tuberculosis*. Many ocular manifestations of tuberculosis have been described, but the characteristic lesion is the conjunctival (1) or, in some cases, corneal phlyctenule. This is presumed to be an allergic hypersensitivity of the conjunctival or corneal epithelium to an endogenous toxin.

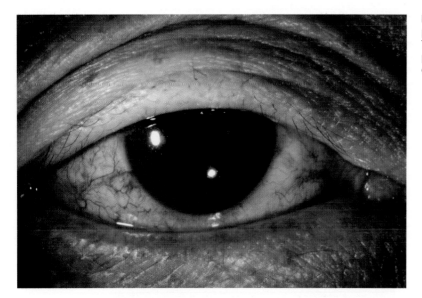

Fig. 8.103 Leprosy. Worldwide it is estimated that there are six to eight million people with leprosy, with most cases occurring in Asia, Africa, and Latin America. The causative agent, *Mycobacterium leprae*, is an acid-fast bacillus that has a predilection for skin and peripheral nerves. Madarosis, loss of the eyelashes or eyebrows, is one of the earliest and most universal signs of leprosy.

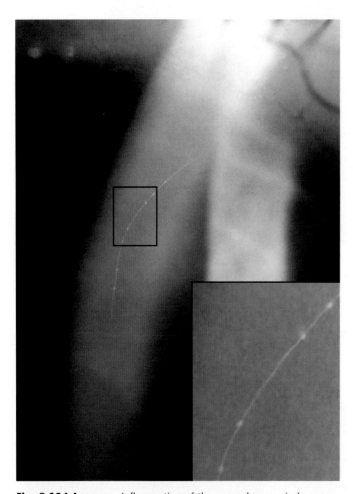

Fig. 8.104 Leprosy. Inflammation of the corneal nerves in leprosy causes the nerves to enlarge. There are focal areas of nerve beading (inset) from inflammatory cell aggregation near active bacillus.

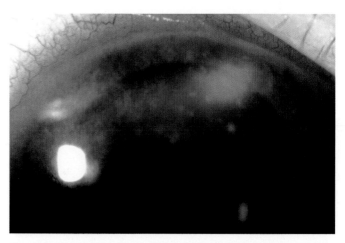

Fig. 8.105 Leprosy. The keratitis in leprosy usually begins in the superior temporal cornea. This is the coolest area of the cornea and the bacillus replicates better in a cooler environment. The inflammation is mostly subepithelial and the lesions have a chalky white coloration. The initial inflammation is avascular.

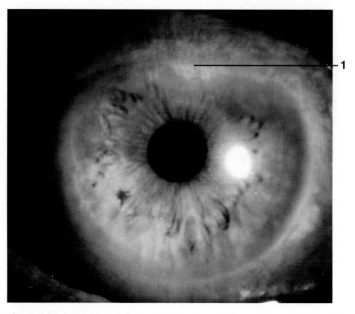

Fig. 8.106 Leprosy. With repeated bouts of inflammation there is destruction of Bowman's layer, and a superficial panus develops. The pannus (1) begins in the superficial temporal cornea. Calcium deposition may also occur.

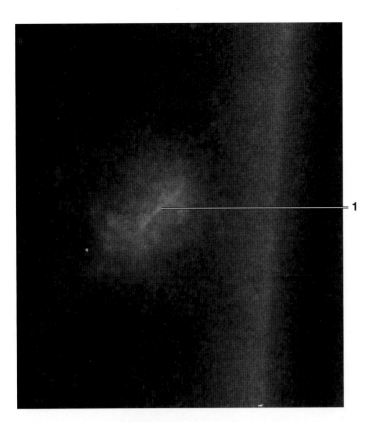

Fig. 8.107 Onchocerciasis. Onchocerciasis or "river blindness" is a parasitic infection caused by the nematode, *Ochocerca volvulus*, which is spread between human hosts by the *Simulium* blackfly. Once established in the host, the worm produces 10 000 microfilariae a day. These microfilariae spread throughout the body causing an intense host inflammatory reaction. Seen here is an inflammatory reaction surrounding dead microfilariae (1) in the cornea.

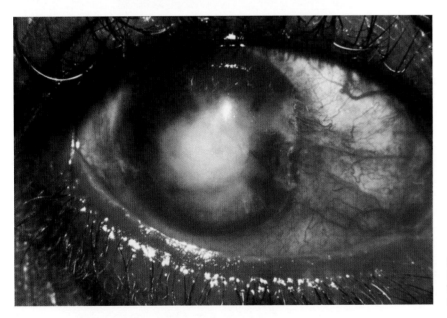

Fig. 8.108 Onchocerciasis. In patients with high skin counts of disease, blindness results from corneal scarring. Shown here is sclerosing keratitis of the cornea. This inflammation begins peripherally and spreads centrally as a reaction to dead microfilariae.

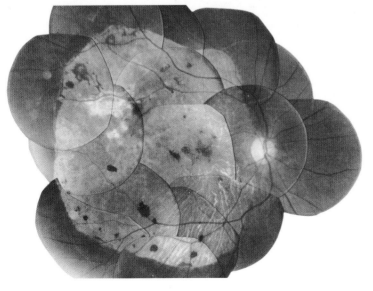

Fig. 8.109 Onchocerciasis. In patients with lower skin counts of disease, blindness results from chorioretinal atrophy. The microfilariae produce a chorioretinitis that leads to diffuse atrophy of the retinal pigment epithelium. The end-stage appearance, as seen here, resembles retinitis pigmentosa.

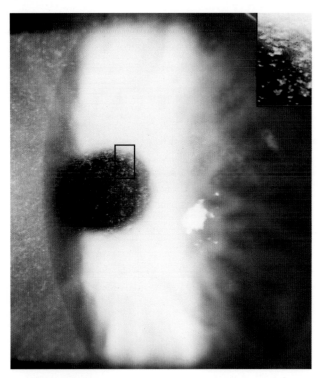

Fig. 8.110 Microsporidia. In immunocompromised patients, microsporidia can cause a diffuse epithelial keratitis. There are multiple, white, intraepithelial infiltrates (inset), which represent active organisms.

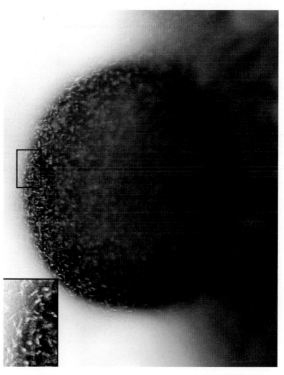

Fig. 8.111 Iritis associated with cytomegalovirus (CMV) retinitis. Stellate keratic precipitates (inset) are a common finding in patients with advanced CMV retinitis.

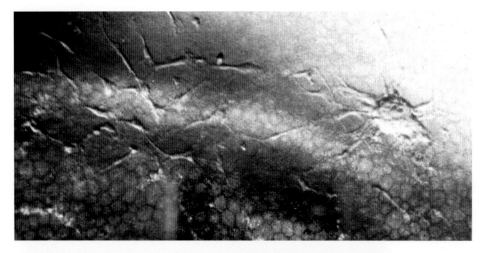

Fig. 8.112 Iritis associated with CMV retinitis. The relief mode of a specular photomicrograph shows the fine branching pattern of these stellate deposits. Histologically, they are composed of macrophages and fibrin.

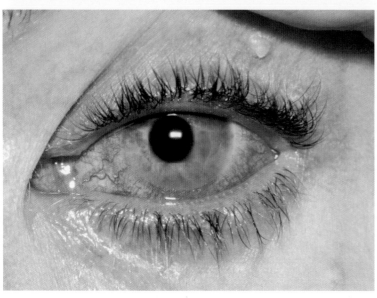

Fig. 8.113 Molluscum contagiosum. Molluscum lesions are more common in individuals with HIV infection. Their altered immune status makes them more susceptible to viral infections. This patient with AIDS had multiple molluscum lesions on the periocular skin and a chronic toxic conjunctivitis.

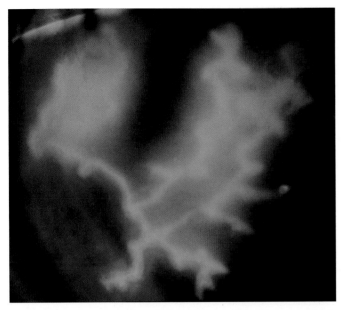

Fig. 8.114 Herpes simplex virus (HSV) geographic corneal ulcer. HSV infection in HIV-infected patients differs from infection in immunocompetent patients in that there is an increased frequency of disease recurrence and the disease is more refractory to standard antiviral treatments.

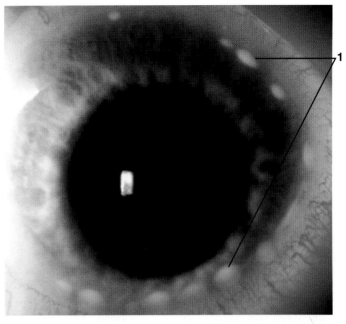

Fig. 8.115 Reiter's syndrome in AIDS. There is an increased incidence of Reiter's syndrome in individuals with AIDS. In this patient with both disorders, multiple peripheral sterile corneal infiltrates (1) can be seen.

Corneal Manifestations of Local and Systemic Therapies

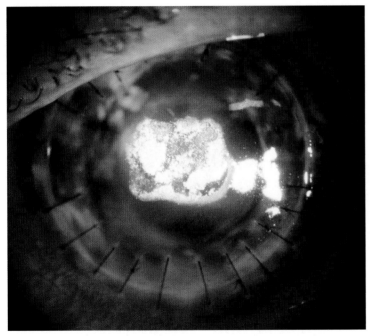

Fig. 8.116 Ciprofloxacin deposits. Topical ciprofloxacin precipitates at physiologic pH. Chalky white deposits accumulate in areas of absent epithelium.

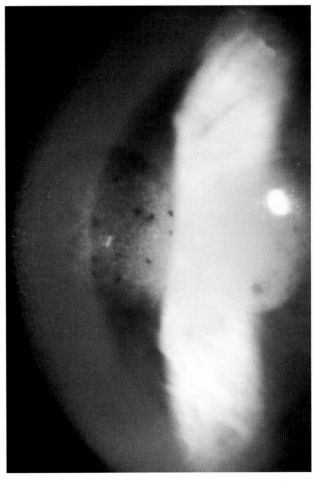

Fig. 8.117 Mercury deposits. Noncalcific band keratopathy can result from mercury deposits in Bowman's layer. These are orange–brown and most commonly the result of mercury preservatives in ophthalmic drops (in this case, pilocarpine).

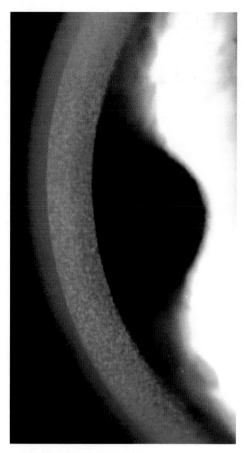

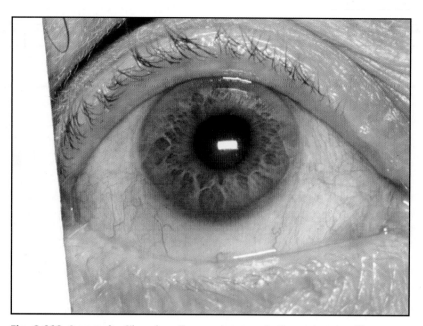

Fig. 8.119 Argyrosis. Silver deposits may also occur in the conjunctiva. The conjunctiva is gray when compared with the white card on the left. Here and in Fig. 8.118, the silver deposits are secondary to the topical medication Argyrol, a silver nitrate compound. Argyrol is no longer in clinical use.

Fig. 8.118 Argyrosis. This is the accumulation of silver in tissues in the body. Silver deposits in the cornea occur in the deepest portion near Descemet's membrane; they have a slate-gray appearance.

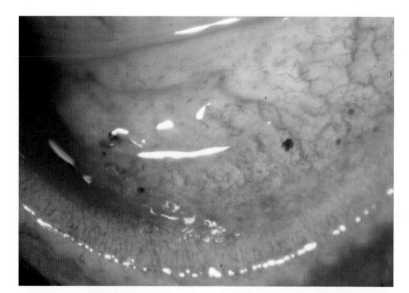

Fig. 8.120 Adrenochrome deposits. These dark black deposits are commonly found in the conjunctiva of patients treated with epinephrine eye-drops for glaucoma.

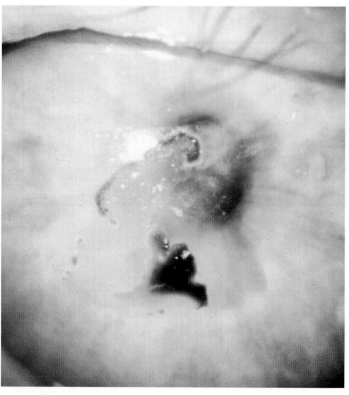

Fig. 8.121 Adrenochrome deposits. These may develop on the cornea.

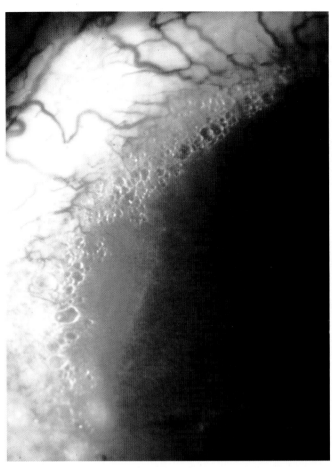

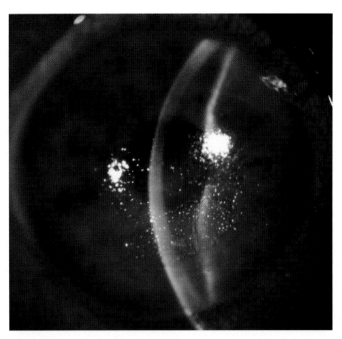

Fig. 8.123 Preservative toxicity. Frequent use of topical medications with preservatives can cause a breakdown of the surface epithelium. This is more likely to occur in patients with preexisting corneal surface abnormalities, such as dry eye.

Fig. 8.122 Intraepithelial ointment. Rarely, ophthalmic ointment preparations can become entrapped in the epithelium after corneal abrasion healing. Here, they appear as refractile deposits near the limbus.

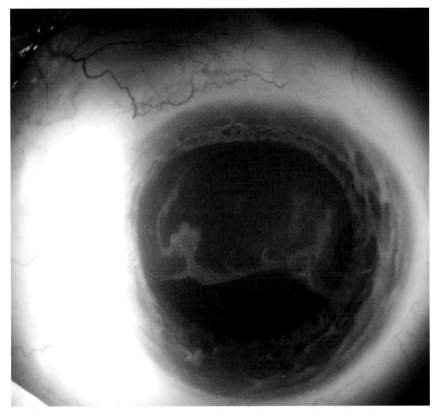

Fig. 8.124 Limbal stem cell deficiency from mitomycin. This patient developed a localized limbal stem cell deficiency after a trabeculectomy with mitomycin. This is the appearance of the eye 9 weeks after the procedure. The superior epitheilium is irregular and hazy.

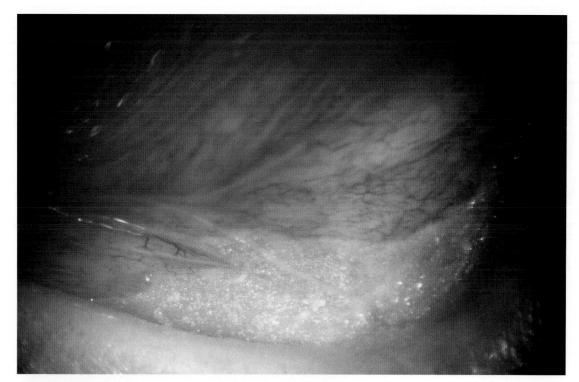

Fig. 8.125 Radiation therapy. Extensive keratinization of the palpebral conjunctiva is noted after local radiation treatment for an angiosarcoma. Another example of radiation effects is seen in Fig. 13.25.

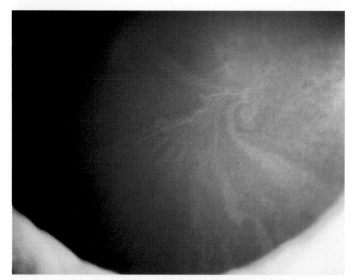

Fig. 8.126 Chloroquine deposits. Whorl opacities in the corneal epithelium are termed cornea verticillata.

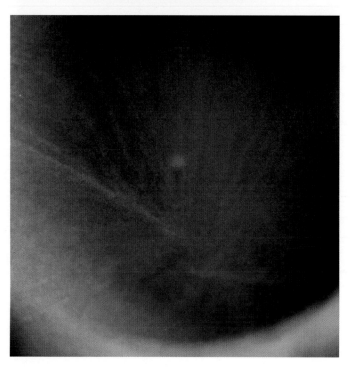

Fig. 8.127 Amiodarone deposits. A cornea verticillata pattern occurred after a total cumulative dose of 56 g amiodarone.

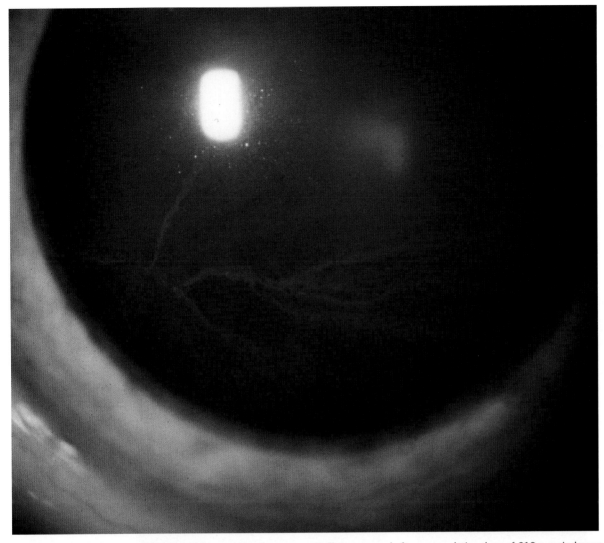

Fig. 8.128 Amiodarone deposits. This example of cornea verticillata occurred after a cumulative dose of 219 g amiodarone.

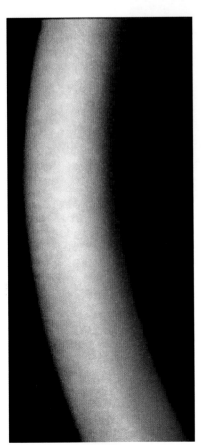

Fig. 8.129 Gold accumulation in the cornea. Termed corneal chrysiasis, this occurs in patients treated with both oral and intramuscular gold therapy for arthritis. The deposits are yellow–brown granules in the deep corneal stroma.

Figs 8.130–8.134 highlight the anterior segment findings associated with systemic phenothiazine use. The location in the anterior lens and deep cornea suggests that these compounds (or breakdown products) enter tissue via the aqueous. Light exposure probably plays a role in the pathogenesis, as the deposits are more intense in the interpalpebral region.

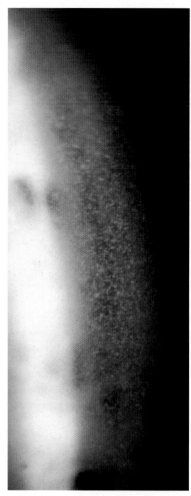

Fig. 8.130 Thorazine deposits. Extensive deposits are noted throughout the entire corneal stroma, although they are more numerous in the posterior stroma.

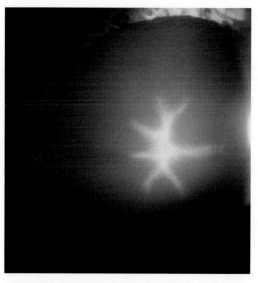

Fig. 8.131 Stellate thorazine deposits beneath the anterior lens capsule.

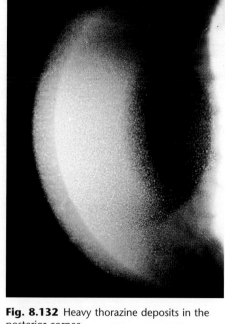

Fig. 8.132 Heavy thorazine deposits in the posterior cornea.

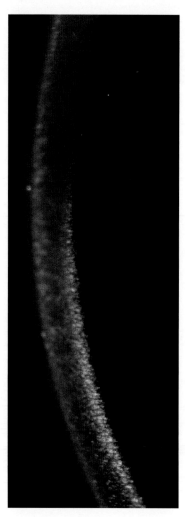

Fig. 8.133 Stellazine deposits. Brown deposits in the posterior corneal stroma are primarily in the interpalpebral region.

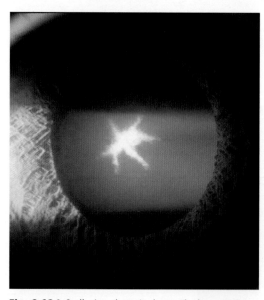

Fig. 8.134 Stellazine deposits beneath the anterior lens capsule.

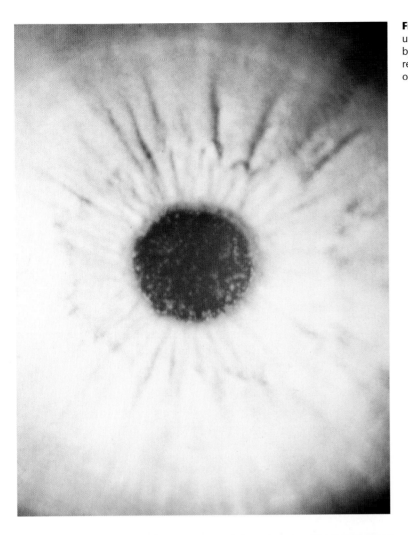

Fig. 8.135 Cytarabine-associated cysts. Cytarabine (Ara-C) is an antimetabolite used to treat systemic malignancies. Its use is associated with a keratitis characterized by multiple intraepithelial cysts and a diffuse conjunctivitis. The cysts may develop in response to altered epithelial cell metabolism. With direct illumination, the cysts are opaque. Symptoms include irritation, decreased vision, and photophobia.

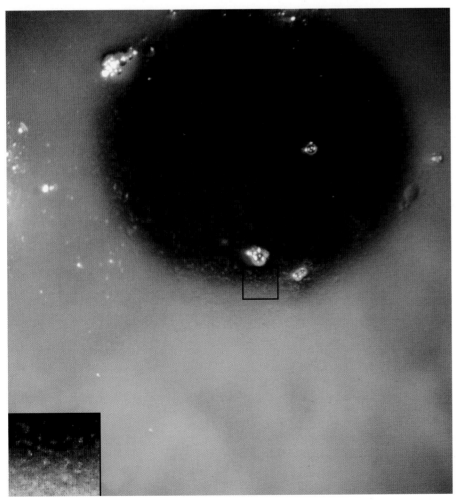

Fig. 8.136 Cytarabine-associated cysts. These are seen with indirect illumination. (inset). In addition, there are white globs of mucus on the cornea from dry eye syndrome.

Chapter 9

Lid, Conjunctival, and Corneal Manifestations of Chemical and Biological Warfare

Unfortunately we live in a world where the specter of biological warfare remains a real threat. Healthcare providers must be able to recognize the signs and symptoms of these potentially devastating diseases to help ensure the best chance of victim survival.

Anthrax

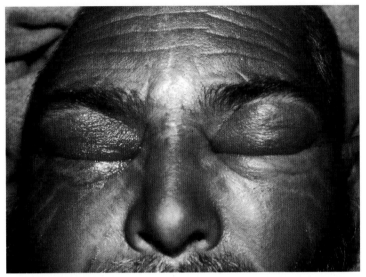

Fig. 9.1 Anthrax. Anthrax is caused by *Bacillus anthracis*, a spore-forming, Gram-positive rod. This Afghani patient has acute lid edema from cutaneous exposure.

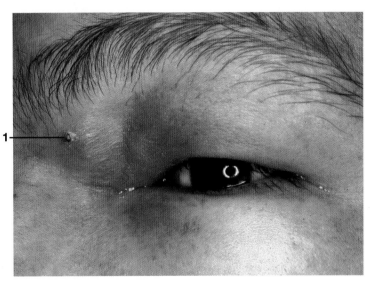

Fig. 9.2 Anthrax. As the cutaneous lesion progresses, a papule forms which then ruptures to form a vesicle (1).

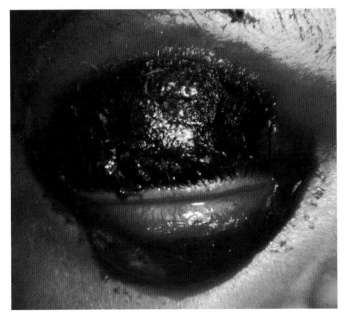

Fig. 9.3 Anthrax. As the cutaneous lesion progresses, a coal-black eschar forms. Anthrax is derived from the Greek word, anthrakos, meaning "coal."

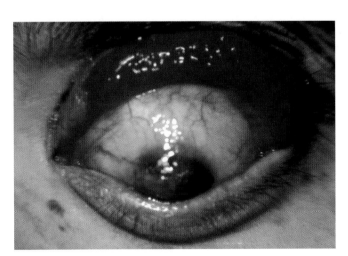

Fig. 9.4 Healed anthrax pustule. After 2–4 weeks, the eschar sloughs and the area heals with scar tissue. This results in a cicatricial ectropion of the upper lid and exposure keratitis.

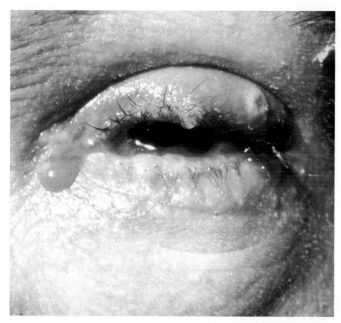

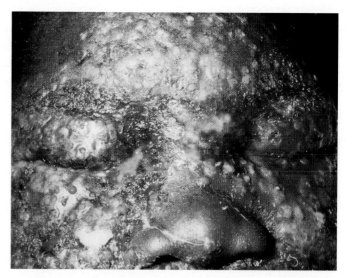

Fig. 9.6 Eczema vaccinatum. Patients with a history of eczema or atopic dermatitis are at risk of developing eczema vaccinatum following smallpox vaccination. Extensive vaccinial lesions form on areas previously affected with eczema or atopic disease.

Fig. 9.5 Vaccinia blepharoconjunctivitis. Smallpox was successfully eradicated in 1977. The vaccinia virus is a live virus used to help the body gain immunity to smallpox. It is injected into the deltoid muscle. Vaccination complications occur when the vaccination site is touched and the eye and lid are then rubbed. In this patient, the vaccinia virus was autoinnoculated into the eye. There is a diffuse blepharoconjuctivitis and an umbilicated pustule on the upper lid. Corneal involvement is rare, but in severe cases can result in necrotizing keratitis and perforation.

Chapter 10

Corneal Dystrophies, Ectatic Disorders, and Degenerations

Corneal dystrophies are bilateral inherited disorders not usually associated with any other systemic conditions. Most are autosomal dominant disorders. Patients exhibit a spectrum of pathologic conditions, so the examination of multiple family members may help to establish the diagnosis. Degenerations, in contrast, are bilateral aging changes of the cornea and are not inherited or associated with systemic disease. Ectatic disorders are often characterized by a great reduction in vision because they alter the shape of the primary refractive element of the eye.

Anterior Membrane Dystrophies

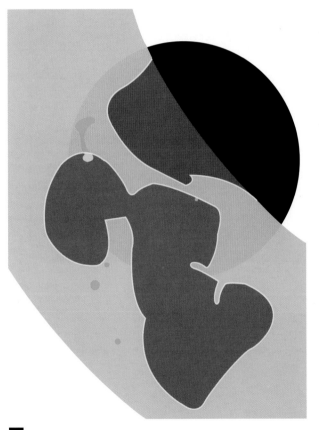
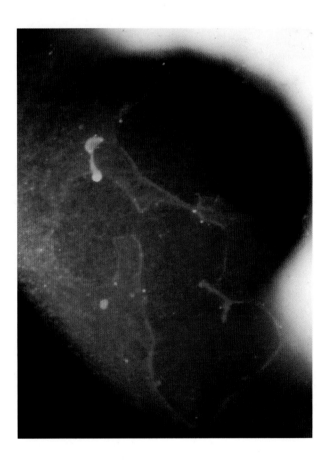

■ **Pupil**

Area containing intraepithelial extra basement membrane material

Area where there is a lack of intraepithelial extra basement membrane material

Intraepithelial cysts containing pyknotic nuclei and cytoplasmic debris = "dots"

Portion of a dot extruding out from under intraepithelial extra basement membrane material

Border between intraepithelial extra basement membrane material and lack thereof = "maps"

Fig. 10.1 Epithelial basement membrane dystrophy (map–dot–fingerprint dystrophy). This is the most common corneal dystrophy seen in clinical practice. The geographic figures in this disorder are caused by reduplications of basement membrane. Similar geographic reduplications of basement membrane may be seen in the area of a healed epithelial defect; therefore, these changes may represent a response of the cornea to various insults. This disorder is usually bilateral and occasionally seen with an autosomal dominant pattern of inheritance. Patients are frequently asymptomatic; however, if the lesions extend into the visual axis, blurred vision and monocular diplopia may develop. Patients may also have symptoms and signs of recurrent erosion. This figure demonstrates a large, gray area with scattered, putty-like dots. The large dot is slightly darker superiorly, where it lies under additional basement membrane material.

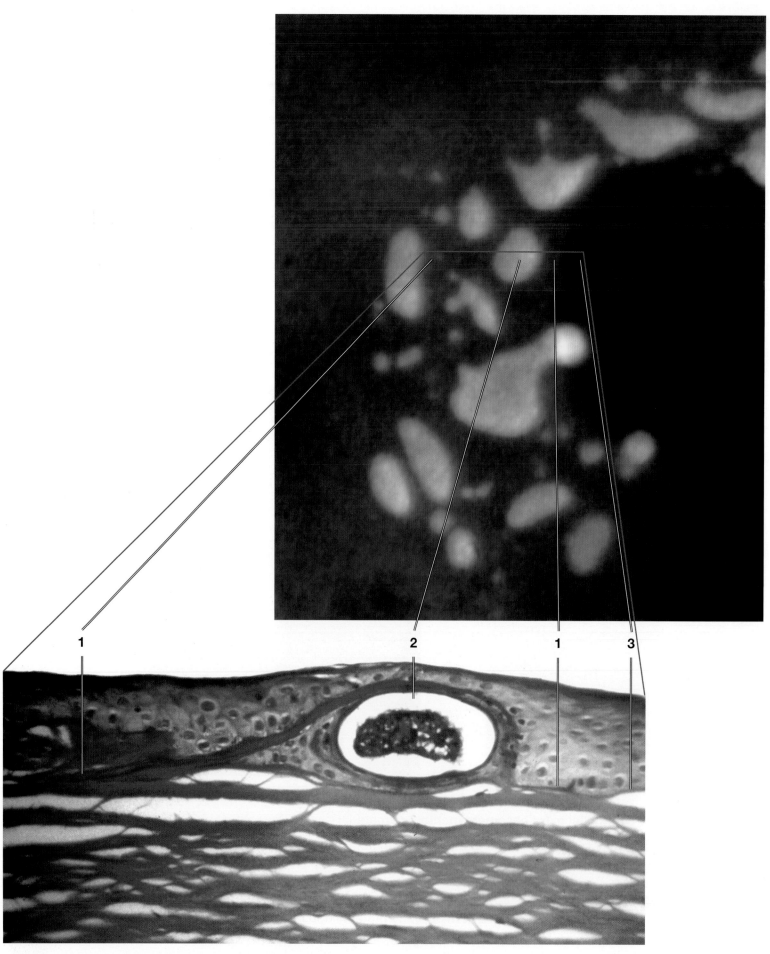

Figs 10.2 and 10.3 Epithelial basement membrane dystrophy. The high-magnification slit-lamp photo (Fig. 10.2) shows an area of dystrophy with pathologic features that could correspond to the cross-sectioned pathologic specimen shown in Fig. 10.3. The specimen is not from the same patient. (1) Area containing intraepithelial extra basement membrane. (2) Intraepithelial microcyst containing pyknotic nuclei and cytoplasmic debris ("dot"). Note how the cyst is trapped by surrounding basement membrane material. (3) Area where there is a lack of extra basement membrane material.

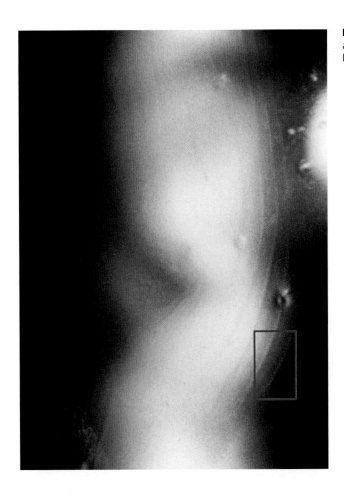

Fig. 10.4 Epithelial basement membrane dystrophy, fingerprint lines. These lines (box) are formed when extra basement membrane material forms folds that extend into the epithelial layer.

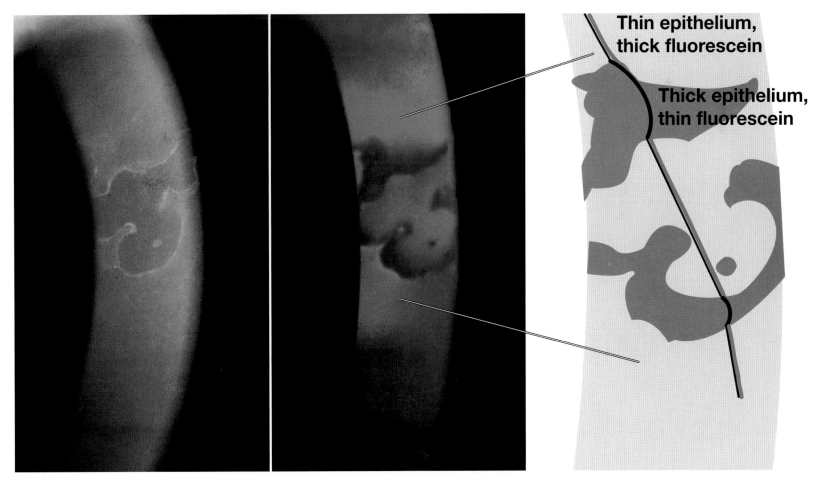

Thin epithelium, thick fluorescein

Thick epithelium, thin fluorescein

Fig. 10.5 Epithelial basement membrane dystrophy, negative staining. The left slit-lamp photograph shows a scalloped or map-like lesion representing the edge of a thickened epithelial layer. Thickening is due to extra basement membrane material. Fluorescein in the tear film rolls off these locations, resulting in relatively dark areas (negative staining). The tear film, containing fluorescein, is thin and dark over these thickened epithelial areas, but thick and bright over the thinner (more normal) epithelial areas.

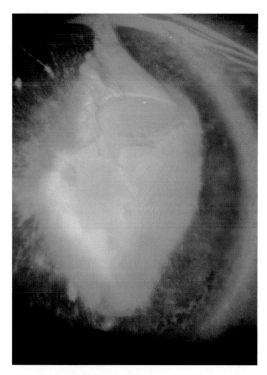

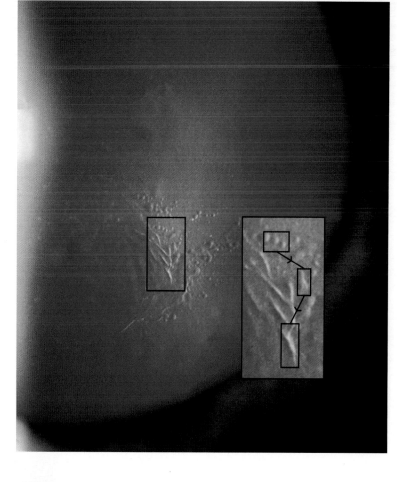

Fig. 10.6 Epithelial basement membrane dystrophy. Patients occasionally develop recurrent corneal erosions.

Fig. 10.7 Epithelial basement membrane dystrophy. Blebs are fine, bubble-like structures that appear clear with retro-illumination. These blebs can coalesce to form groups with a linear branching pattern (inset).

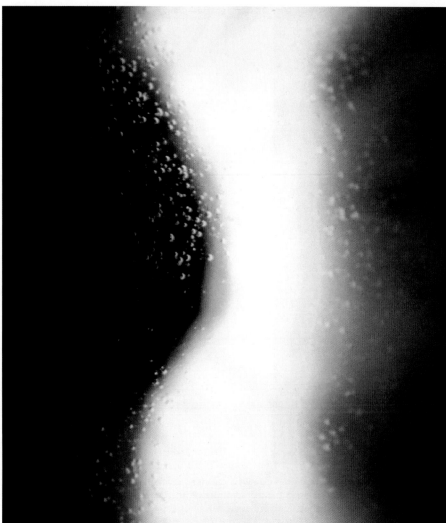

Fig. 10.8 Meesmann's dystrophy. This autosomal dominant disorder is characterized by the appearance of multiple vesicular or bleb-like structures within the corneal epithelium. They tend to be more numerous in the interpalpebral zone. The cysts occasionally rupture onto the ocular surface and can cause pain and decreased vision. The cysts appear as gray dots with direct illumination and as small vesicles with indirect illumination. The genetic abnormality for Meesmann's dystrophy is due to mutations in the *Keratin 3* and *Keratin 12* genes, located on chromosomes 12 and 17 respectively.

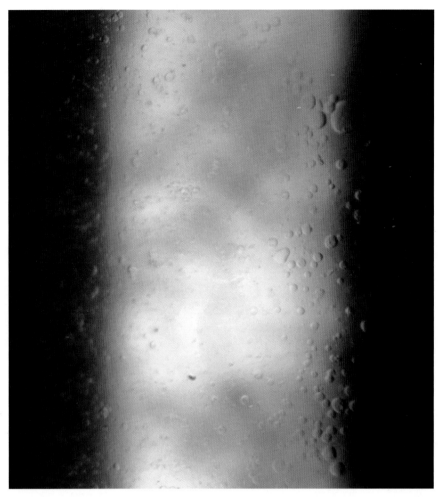

Fig. 10.9 Meesmann's dystrophy. This high-power view shows the cysts of Meesmann's dystrophy. The cysts vary in size.

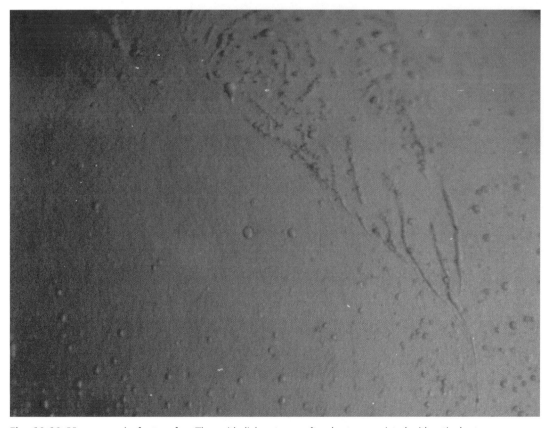

Fig. 10.10 Meesmann's dystrophy. The epithelial cysts are often best appreciated with retinal retro-illumination. Here single cysts are seen; centrally, there are linear areas where the cysts have coalesced.

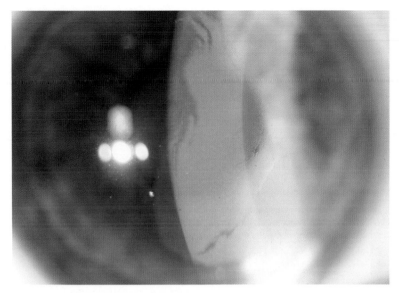

Fig. 10.11 Band-shaped and whorled microcystic dystrophy of the corneal epithelium. This rare corneal dystrophy is characterized by an abnormal microcystic corneal epithelium in whorled patterns with feathery edges. If the lesions are central, vision is usually diminished. The inheritance pattern in one family was autosomal dominant; other patients with this dystrophy have not had pedigree analysis. Histopathology shows vacuolization of the epithelial cells cytoplasm.

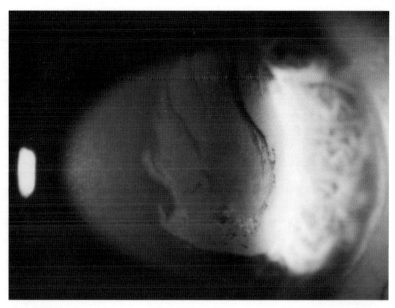

Fig. 10.12 Band-shaped and whorled microcystic dystrophy of the corneal epithelium. A broad oblique beam shows the texture of this epithelial dystrophy.

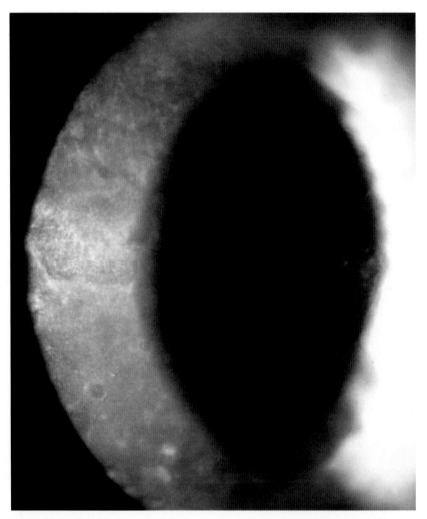

Fig. 10.13 Reis–Bücklers' dystrophy (corneal dystrophy of Bowman's layer type I or CDBI). This autosomal dominant dystrophy is characterized by irregular gray–white opacities beneath the epithelium. It begins in childhood and visual loss is progressive. Recurrent erosions occur periodically. The genetic abnormality is due to mutations in the *beta-transfoming growth factor*-induced gene human clone 3 (*BigH3*) located on chromosome 5.

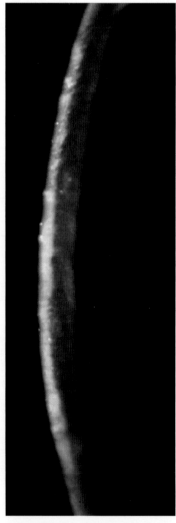

Fig. 10.14 Reis–Bücklers' dystrophy. A thin slit-beam view demonstrates the opacification beneath the epithelium and the irregularity of the corneal surface.

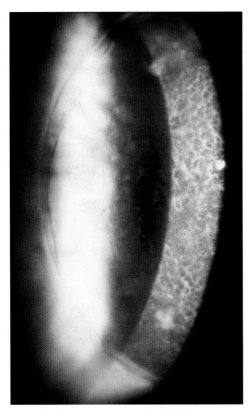

Fig. 10.15 Reis–Bücklers' dystrophy. This disorder often recurs in a graft. Peripherally, there is a fine granular pattern, and centrally the opacification is denser and the surface more irregular.

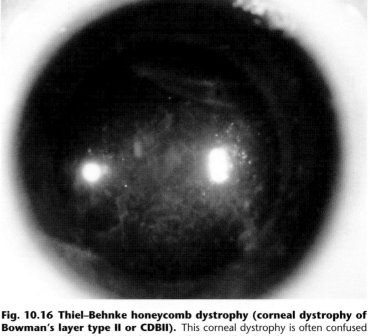

Fig. 10.16 Thiel–Behnke honeycomb dystrophy (corneal dystrophy of Bowman's layer type II or CDBII). This corneal dystrophy is often confused with Reis–Bücklers' dystrophy because it has a similar clinical appearance. Both dystrophies are autosomal dominant with recurrent erosions starting early in childhood. The visual impairment in Thiel–Behnke dystrophy begins much later in life than the visual impairment in Reis–Bücklers' dystrophy. Transmission electron microscopy differentiates these two dystrophies. In Reis–Bücklers' dystrophy rod-like bodies are seen in the region of Bowman's layer, and in Thiel–Behnke dystrophy "curly" fibers are seen in the region of Bowman's layer. Similar to Reis–Bücklers' dystrophy, Thiel–Behnke dystrophy is due to mutations in the *beta-transfoming growth factor*-induced gene human clone 3 (*BigH3*) located on chromosome 5, but the mutations occur with different amino acids at different sites within the gene.

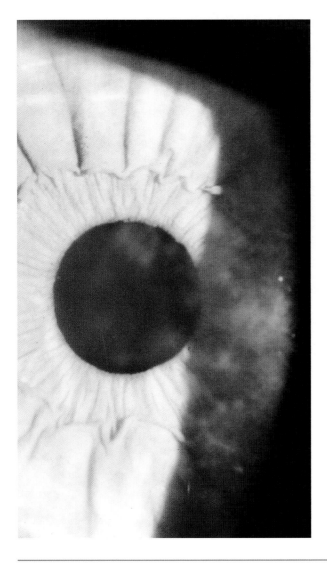

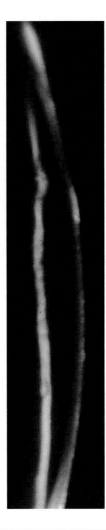

Figs 10.17 and 10.18 Subepithelial mucinous dystrophy. This autosomal dominant disorder is characterized by subepithelial deposits of gray–white material between which there is a generalized subepithelial haze. The cornea is involved limbus to limbus. Patients experience multiple recurrent erosions, which begin in childhood. Visual loss can become significant later in life.

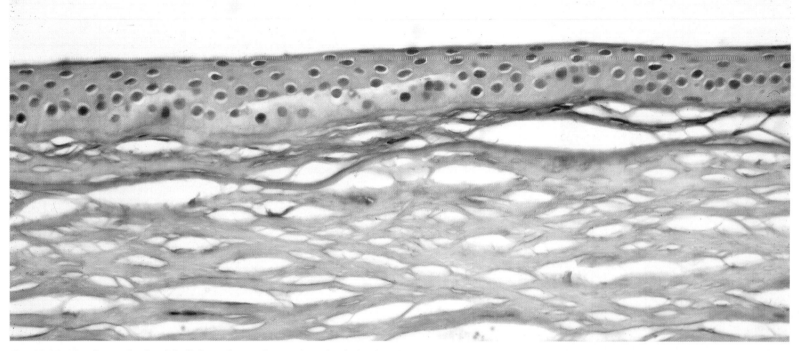

Fig. 10.19 Histology of subepithelial mucinous dystrophy. The thick subepithelial layer stains with Alcian blue. The deposits are composed of chondroitin 4-sulfate and dermatan sulfate.

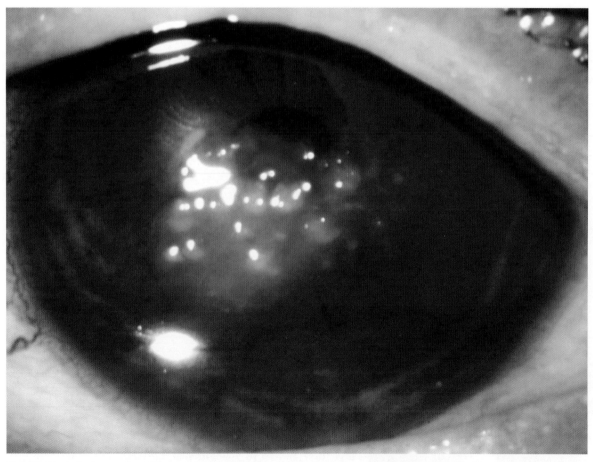

Fig. 10.20 Gelatinous drop-like corneal dystrophy. In this dystrophy, subepithelial gelatinous deposits composed of amyloid form on the surface of the cornea. The corneal surface develops a "mulberry" appearance. Symptoms of photophobia and decreased vision begin in the first two decades of life. The disorder recurs in corneal grafts. The inheritance pattern is autosomal recessive and the genetic abnormality is due to mutations in the *M1S1* (tumor-associated calcium signal transducer 2) gene located on chromosome 1.

Stromal Dystrophies

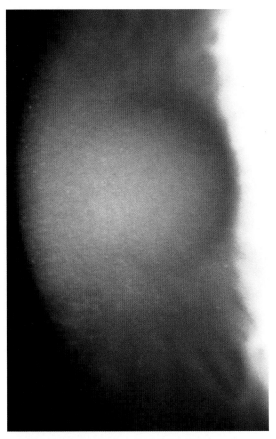

Fig. 10.21 Early lattice dystrophy type I. The corneal findings are subtle. Three findings have been described: central stromal haze (as seen here), subepithelial white spots, and filamentary lines. This is a 13-year-old girl with central stromal haze.

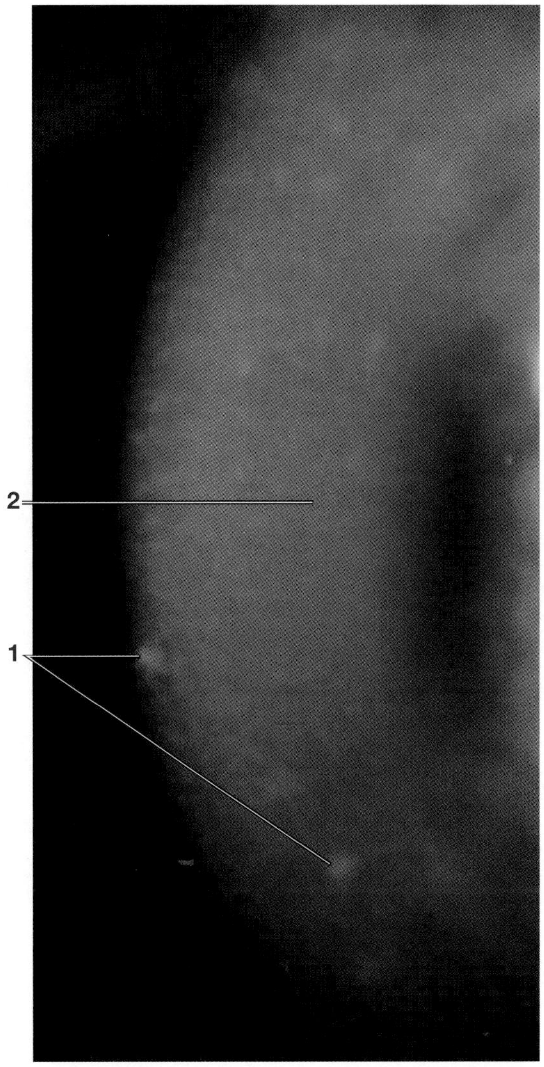

Fig. 10.22 Early lattice dystrophy type I. This 4-year-old boy has several subepithelial white spots (1) and central stromal haze (2).

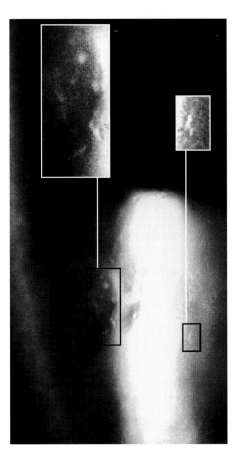

Fig. 10.23 Early lattice dystrophy type I. Refractile filamentary lines (inset) are seen in a 13-year-old girl.

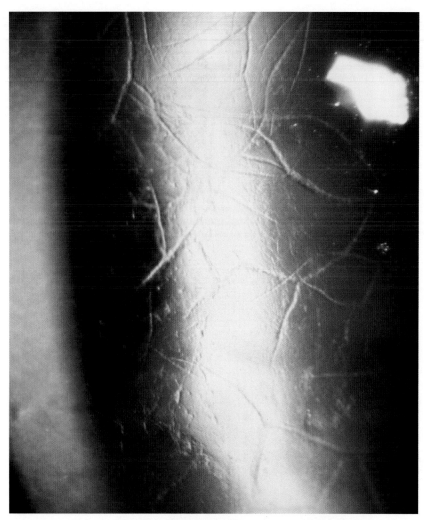

Fig. 10.24 Lattice dystrophy type I in an adult. There are refractile filamentary lines with nodular dilations. The deposits are more common in the anterior stroma. Usually, there is a limbal clear zone. A fine central anterior stromal haze may be present. The inheritance pattern is autosomal dominant. The genetic abnormality is due to mutations in the *beta-transfoming growth factor*-induced gene human clone 3 (*BigH3*) located on chromosome 5.

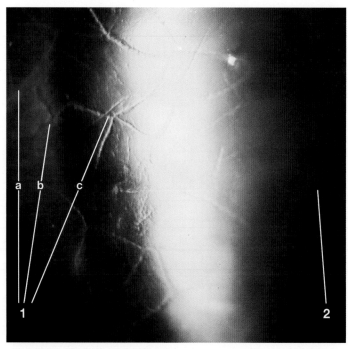

Fig. 10.25 Lattice dystrophy type I. (1) Lattice lines are white (a) or dark (b) in direct light, and translucent, almost crystalline, in indirect light (c). (2) Lattice lines do not reach the limbus except in advanced cases.

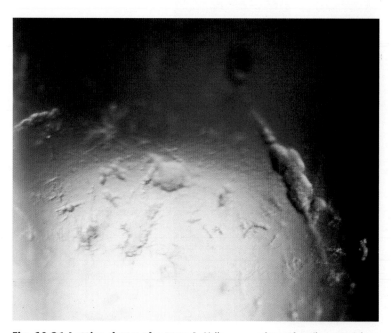

Fig. 10.26 Lattice dystrophy type I. Yellow or amber refractile material can be seen in subepithelial areas in some cases. The histopathology of these areas shows elastoid degeneration.

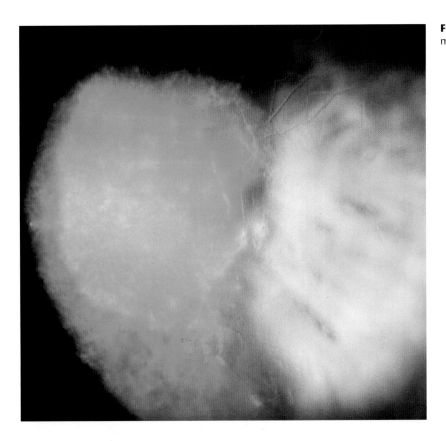

Fig. 10.27 Epithelial erosion in lattice dystrophy type I. Visual acuity may be markedly decreased in patients with epithelial involvement.

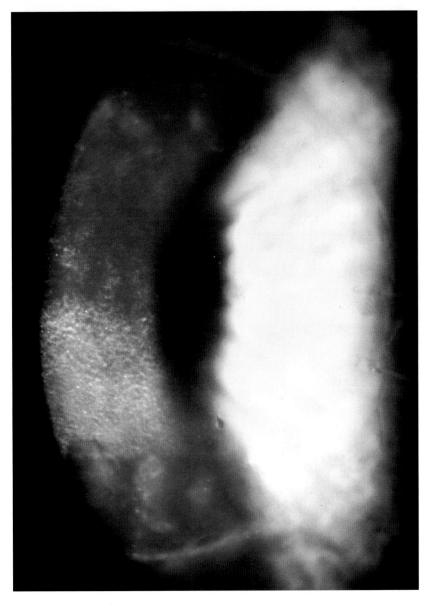

Fig. 10.28 Lattice dystrophy type I. This commonly recurs in the graft, beginning in the periphery and spreading centrally. Typically there are elevated subepithelial opacities, fine lattice lines, and diffuse haze in the anterior stroma. Occasionally, adequate vision can be maintained by scraping the superficial subepithelial deposits.

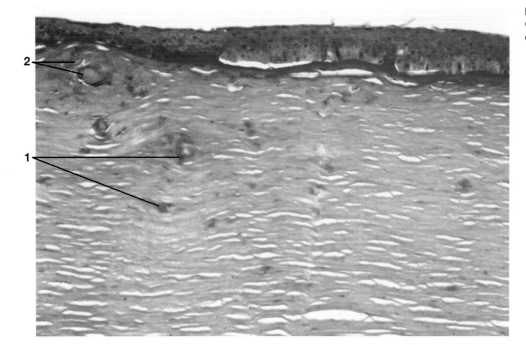

Fig. 10.29 Advanced lattice dystrophy type I.
Congo red stain reveals extracellular fusiform deposits of congophilic material (1) and elastoid degeneration (2).

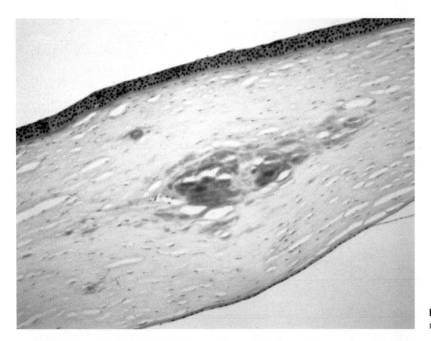

Fig. 10.30 Histopathology of lattice corneal dystrophy type I. Congo red stain reveals large fusiform stromal lesion.

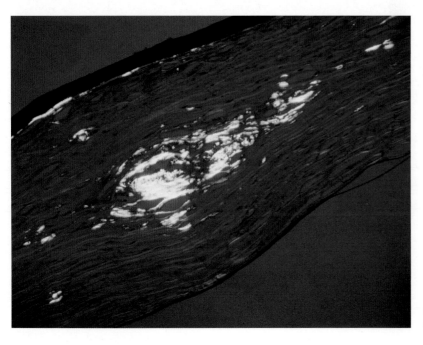

Fig. 10.31 Same patient as in Fig. 10.30. Birefringence of the Congo red stain is seen with polarized light.

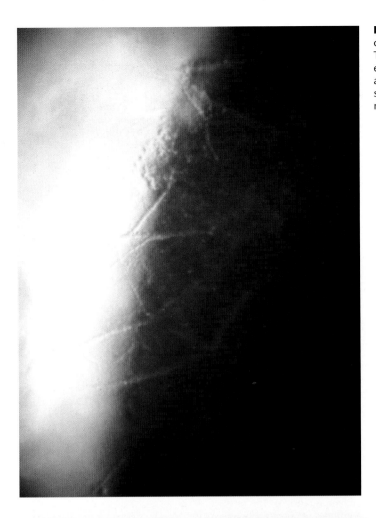

Fig. 10.32 Lattice dystrophy type II (Meretoja's syndrome). There are refractile corneal deposits that differ in several respects from those seen in lattice dystrophy type I. The deposits are fewer, coarser, and most dense in the corneal mid-periphery, and generally extend to the limbus with a more radial orientation. The central cornea is usually spared, and the cornea is relatively clear between the lines. In contrast to lattice type I, there are systemic findings, including blepharochalasis, bilateral facial nerve palsies, peripheral neuropathy, and systemic amyloidosis.

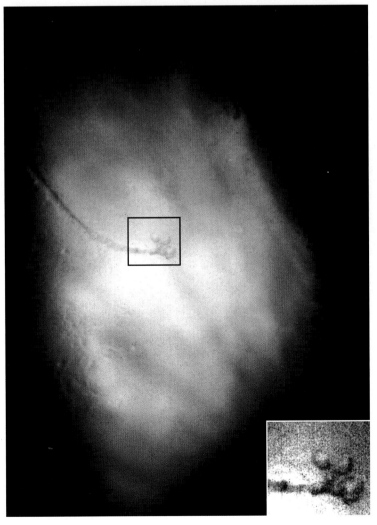

Fig. 10.33 Lattice dystrophy type II. In this patient the lattice lines are coarse and there are prominent terminal bulbs (inset). Despite the phenotypic similarities between lattice dystrophy type I and type II, the genetic bases for the diseases is very different. Lattice dystrophy type I is caused by mutations in the *beta-transfoming growth factor-*induced gene human clone 3 (*BigH3*) located on chromosome 5. Lattice dystrophy type II is caused by an abnormality in an actin-binding protein coded for by the *gelsolin* gene on chromosome 9.

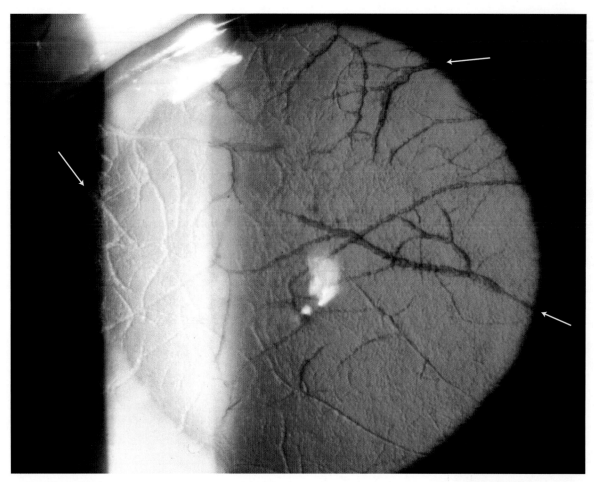

Fig. 10.34 Lattice dystrophy type IIIA. Coarse lattice lines traverse the cornea from limbus to limbus (arrows). This rare form of lattice dystrophy is inherited as an autosomal dominant disorder, has an adult onset, and includes frequent episodes of recurrent corneal erosions. The genetic abnormality is due to mutations in the *beta-transfoming growth factor*-induced gene human clone 3 (*BigH3*) located on chromosome 5.

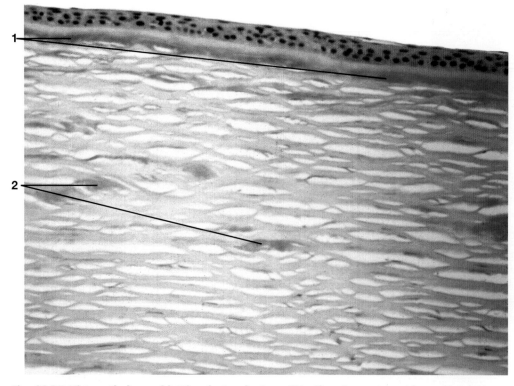

Fig. 10.35 Histopathology of lattice dystrophy type IIIA. There is a prominent layer of amyloid deposition just posterior to Bowman's layer (1) and irregular deposits in the stroma (2). The amyloid deposits stain with Congo red.

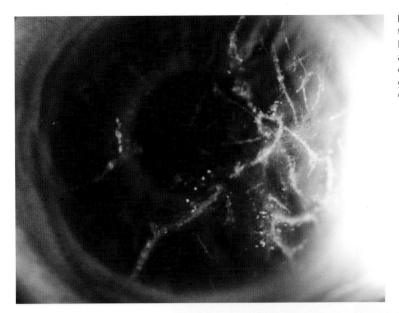

Fig. 10.36 Lattice dystrophy type IV. This 69-year-old man has lattice dystrophy type IV. Thick lattice lines are seen coming in from limbus in the mid and deep stroma. In this form of lattice dystrophy there is a lack of epithelial involvement and erosions are not seen. The onset is late in life. Similar to lattice dystrophy types I and IIIA, lattice dystrophy type IV is due to mutations in the *beta-transfoming growth factor*-induced gene human clone 3 (*BigH3*) located on chromosome 5, but the mutations occur with different amino acids at different sites within the gene.

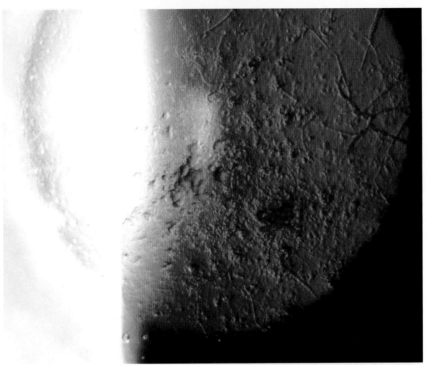

Fig. 10.37 Lattice dystrophy type IV. This 74-year-old man has deep linear and drop-like deposits in the cornea of his right eye. The left eye was not involved. The best corrected vision was 20/60.

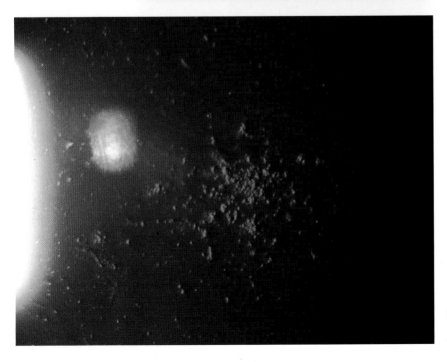

Fig. 10.38 Lattice dystrophy type IV. In this 62-year-old man there are multiple droplike opacities in the deep cornea but no linear opacities. The visual acuity is 20/30.

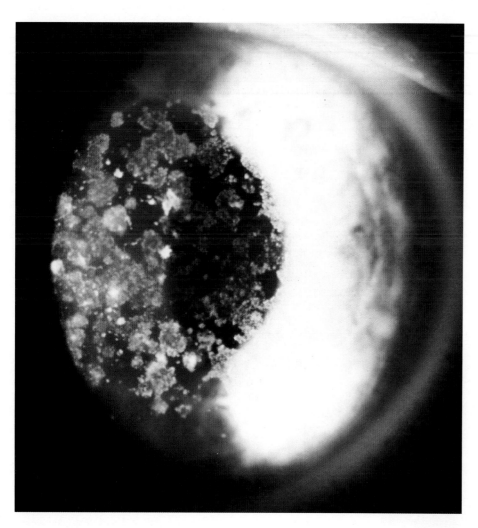

Fig. 10.39 Granular dystrophy. In this autosomal dominant condition, there are numerous "breadcrumb" white deposits in the corneal stroma. The deposits are concentrated centrally and in the anterior stroma. There is a peripheral clear zone of 2–3 mm that remains free of deposits. Visual impairment usually begins after the fifth decade of life. The genetic abnormality is due to mutations in the *beta-transfoming growth factor*-induced gene human clone 3 (*BigH3*) located on chromosome 5.

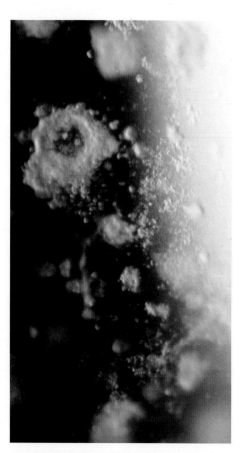

Fig. 10.40 Granular dystrophy. In this high-magnification view, some of the lesions are opaque with clear centers. There are small refractile deposits as well.

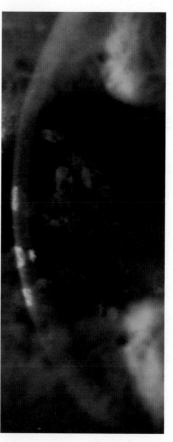

Fig. 10.41 Thin slit-beam view of granular dystrophy. The deposits are primarily in the anterior stroma, and the overlying epithelium is disrupted occasionally. Recurrent erosions can occur but are uncommon.

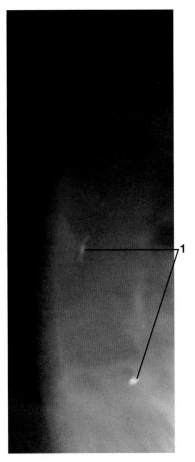

Fig. 10.42 Granular dystrophy in a 15-month-old child. The earliest sign of granular dystrophy is fine dots in the superficial stroma (1).

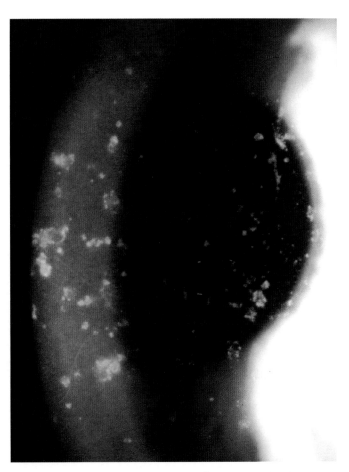

Fig. 10.43 Granular dystrophy in a 7¹/₂-year-old child. As the disease progresses, there are focal white opacities with variable shapes in the anterior stroma.

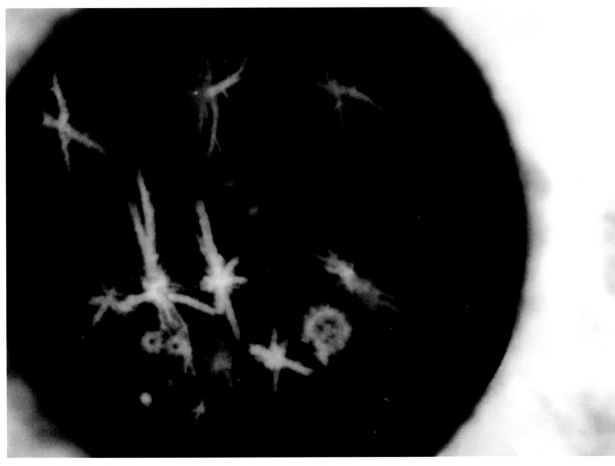

Fig. 10.44 Granular dystrophy. In this unusual case of granular dystrophy, the deposits resemble snowflakes.

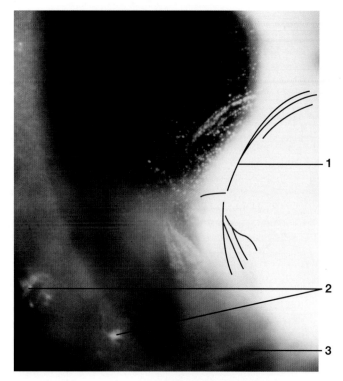

Fig. 10.45 Recurrence of granular dystrophy in a graft. The most common pattern is a superficial cornea verticillata pattern (1). Suture track scar (2) and corneal wound (3) are shown.

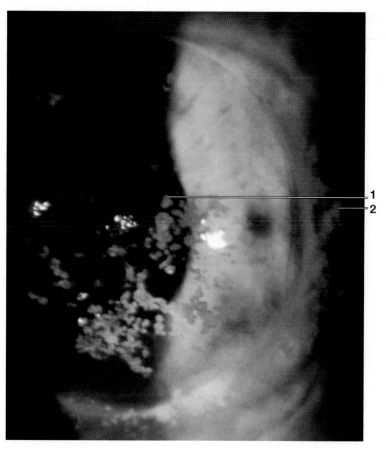

Fig. 10.46 Advanced recurrence of granular dystrophy in a graft. Multiple white granular opacities are seen in the graft (1). Granular deposits are also seen in the host tissue (2).

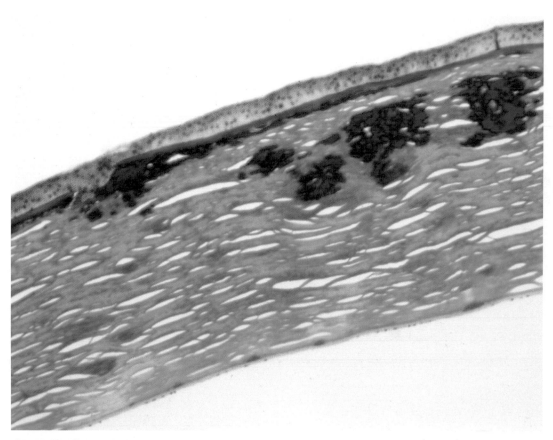

Fig. 10.47 Histopathology of granular dystrophy. There are deposits of extracellular hyaline material in the corneal stroma. These deposits are primarily in the anterior stroma and have a breadcrumb appearance. The hyaline material stains red with Masson's trichrome stain.

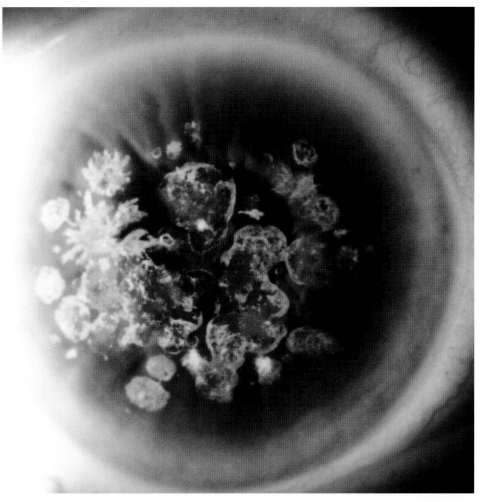

Fig. 10.48 Avellino dystrophy. This autosomal dominant disorder has features of both granular and lattice dystrophy clinically and on histopathologic examination. The lattice lesions develop after the granular deposits. Granular dystrophy, lattice dystrophies types I, IIIA, and IV, and Avellino dystrophy are all due to mutations in the *beta-transforming growth factor*-induced gene human clone 3 (*BigH3*) located on chromosome 5 (see Fig. 10.53).

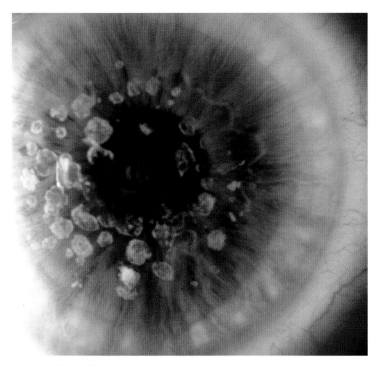

Fig. 10.49 Avellino dystrophy. Another patient with Avellino dystrophy demonstrates the variable appearance characteristic of dominantly inherited disorders. These patients, like those with lattice and granular dystrophy, can have recurrent erosions.

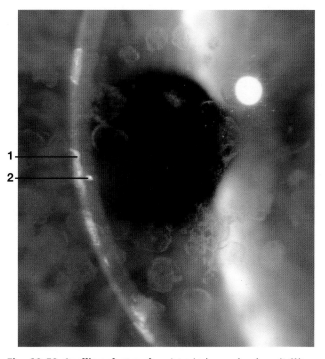

Fig. 10.50 Avellino dystrophy. A typical granular deposit (1) appears as hyaline material on histopathologic examination. This deposit (2) corresponds to amyloid material on histopathologic examination.

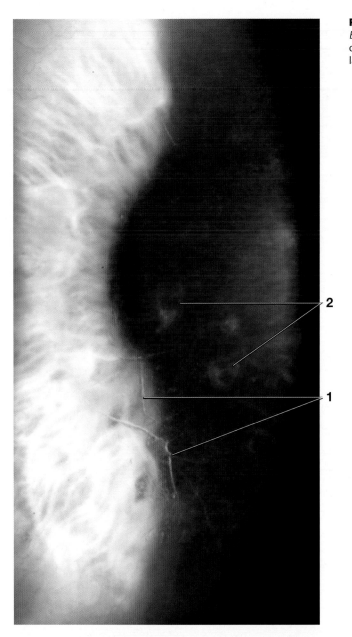

Fig. 10.51 Avellino dystrophy. This 29-year-old woman has an Arg124His mutation of the *BigH3* gene. Note the typical lattice lines (1) representing the lattice dystrophy component and donut-shaped opacities (2), which probably represented the granular portion of this combined lattice/granular dystrophy.

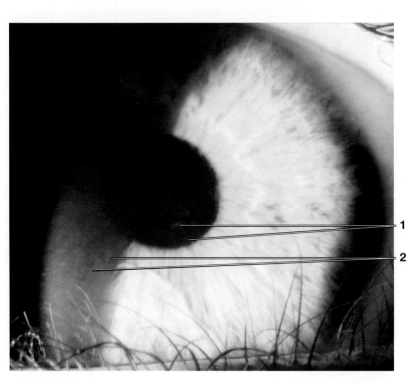

Fig. 10.52 Avellino dystrophy. This is the 34-month-old son of the patient in Fig. 10.51, also with an Arg124His mutation of the *BigH3* gene. The child began having erosions at 18 months of age. Anterior, variously shaped, spots (1) and haze (2) were noted. The spots could be seen to reach the limbus.

The BIGH3 - Associated Corneal Dystrophies

The transforming growth factor beta-inducing gene (TGFBI), also known as keratoepithelin or BIGH3, a gene on chromosome 5q31, when mutant, produces abnormal proteins which accumulate in the cornea with varying presentations (phenotypes). Below are 7 resultant corneal dystrophies. Also illustrated (lower right) are some examples of opacities found in lattice type I and granular type I.

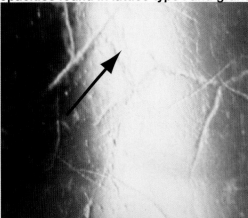

Lattice type I

Most common mutation
Arg124Cys
A. dominant
Onset 1st decade
(Seen by authors as early as age 3 years)
Chords of amyloid begin centrally and branch toward limbus
Most deposition in the anterior and mid stroma
To limbus if severe

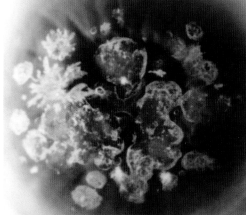

Granular type II
(Avellino)

Most common mutation
Arg124His
A. dominant
Onset 1st decade

Clinically and histologically a combination of lattice (amyloid) and granular (hyaline) dystrophies
Not to limbus

Lattice type IIIA

Most common mutation
Pro501Thr

A. dominant

Onset 5th decade

Chords of amyloid begin at limbus and branch centrally
Deposition is mainly anterior (with erosions)
To limbus

Reis-Bücklers

Most common mutations
Arg124Leu
Gly623Asp
A. dominant

Onset 1st decade

Subepithelial and Bowman's level rings and haze

Early and frequent erosions
Rods on EM
To limbus

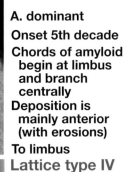

Lattice type IV

Most common mutation
Leu527Arg

A. dominant

Onset 5th decade

Clumping of small, mostly central deposits or large branches in from the limbus

All levels but mainly deep

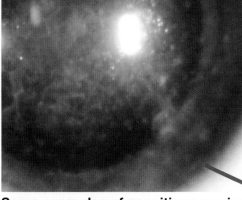

Thiel-Behnke

Most common mutation
Arg555Gln

A. dominant

Onset 1st decade

Subepithelial and Bowman's level honeycomb shapes
Early and frequent erosions
Curls on EM
To limbus

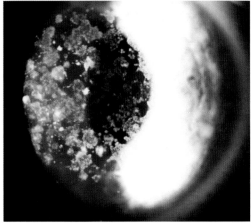

Granular type I

Most common mutation
Arg555Trp
A. dominant
Onset 1st decade
(Seen by authors as early as age 15 months)
Deposition is mainly anterior and mid stroma
Snowflakes, crumbs, dots, etc.
Erosions vary with patients
Not to limbus

Some examples of opacities seen in:
Lattice dystrophy type I   Granular dystrophy type I

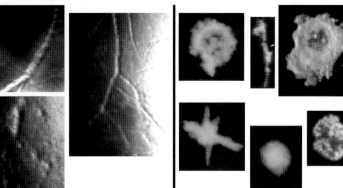

Fig. 10.53 *Big3H* gene mutation dystrophy table.

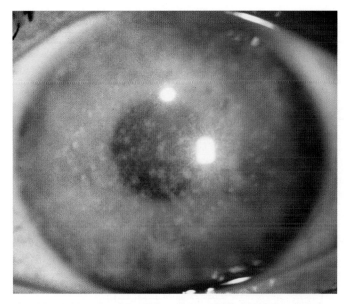

Fig. 10.54 Macular dystrophy. This autosomal recessive disorder is characterized by a diffuse stromal haze extending limbus to limbus and throughout the corneal stroma. Multiple, irregular, gray–white, nodular lesions are found within the diffuse haze. Recurrent erosions can occur, although less frequently than in lattice dystrophy. Photophobia may be out of proportion to the clinical findings. Visual acuity is usually markedly decreased by the third and fourth decades of life. A defect in the *carbohydrate sulfotransferase* gene on chromosome 16 is the cause of this dystrophy.

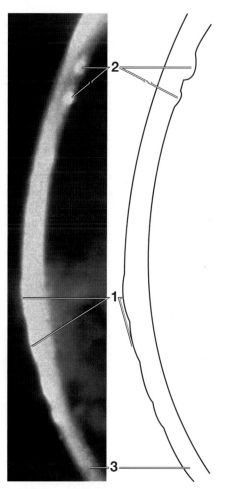

Fig. 10.55 Thin slit-beam view of macular dystrophy. The central lesions are more anterior (1) and the peripheral white lesions are more posterior (2). The cornea is thinner than normal (3).

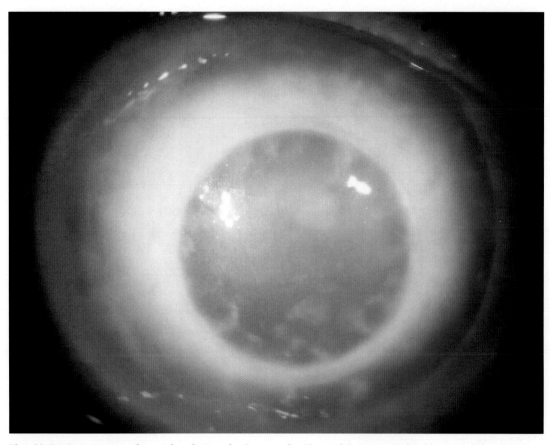

Fig. 10.56 Recurrence of macular dystrophy in a graft. The graft has a generalized haze, and there are focal white nodular deposits.

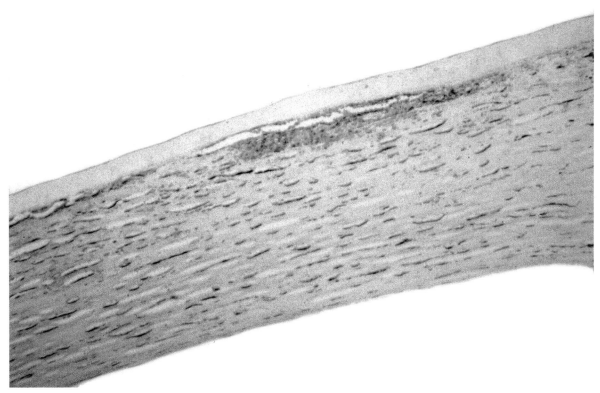

Fig. 10.57 Histopathology of macular dystrophy. Alcian blue staining of extracellular and intracellular mucopolysaccharides occurs in all layers of the cornea, including the epithelium, endothelium, and Descemet's membrane.

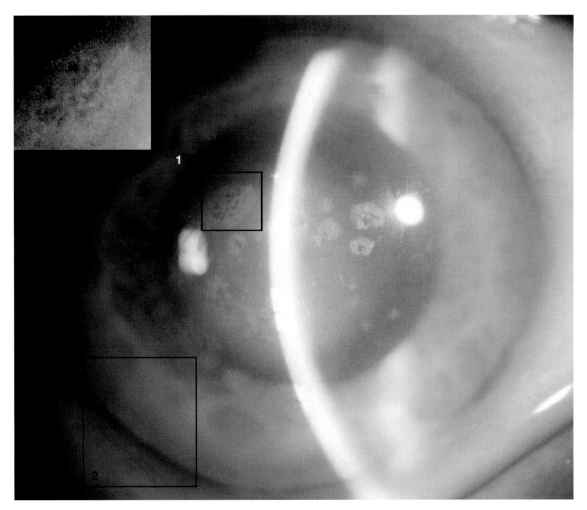

Fig. 10.58 Schnyder's crystalline dystrophy. In this autosomal dominant disorder, there is central anterior stromal corneal opacity. The peripheral edge is irregular and crystalline (1). The crystals are composed of cholesterol, and patients may have systemic hyperlipidemia. Arcus (2) is often present.

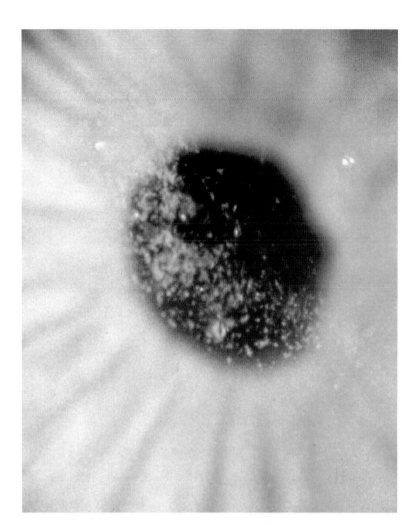

Fig. 10.59 The 16-year-old son of the patient in Fig. 10.58. Small, white, crystalline opacities are seen in the central anterior stroma.

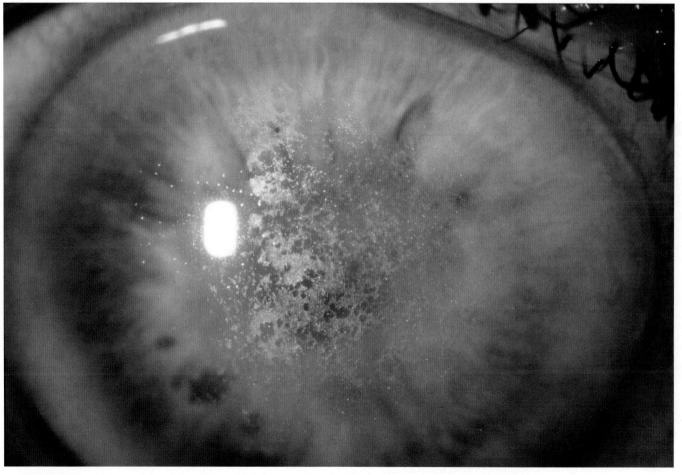

Fig. 10.60 Schnyder's crystalline dystrophy. Multiple central crystalline deposits and peripheral arcus are seen.

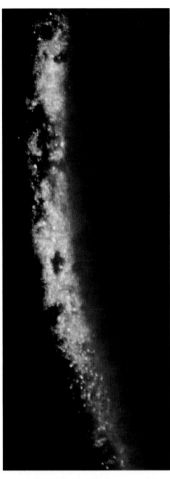

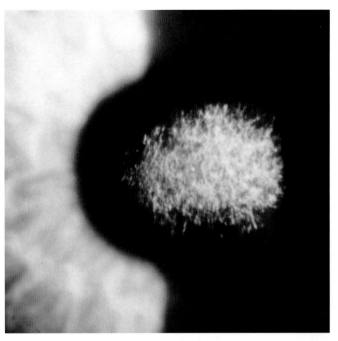

Fig. 10.62 Schnyder's crystalline dystrophy. Crystals are seen in the central cornea.

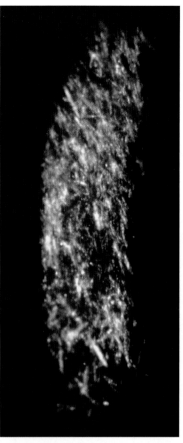

Fig. 10.63 Schnyder's crystalline dystrophy. A slit-beam view shows crystals with a spicular pattern in another patient.

Fig. 10.61 Thin slit-beam view of the patient in Fig. 10.60. There is a crystalline pattern in the anterior corneal stroma.

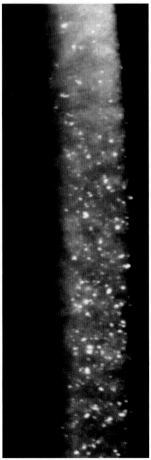

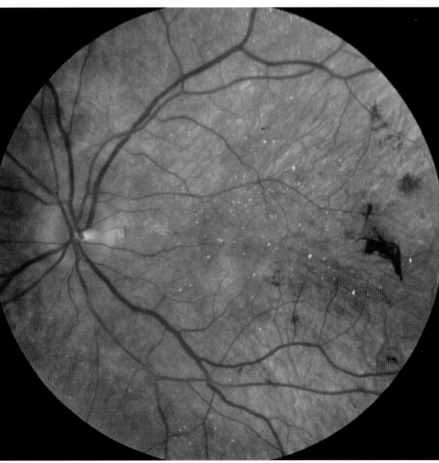

Figs 10.64 and 10.65 Bietti's crystalline corneal–retinal dystrophy. This autosomal recessive disorder is characterized by crystalline deposits in the peripheral cornea (Fig. 10.64) and retina (Fig. 10.65). As the disease progresses, pigment changes occur within the retina and the choriocapillaris atrophies. Patients may have symptoms of nyctalopia, poor dark adaptation, peripheral visual field loss, and central visual acuity loss. The corneal crystals resemble cholesterol or other lipid deposits histologically, and the disorder may represent a systemic defect in lipid metabolism.

Fig. 10.64   **Fig. 10.65**

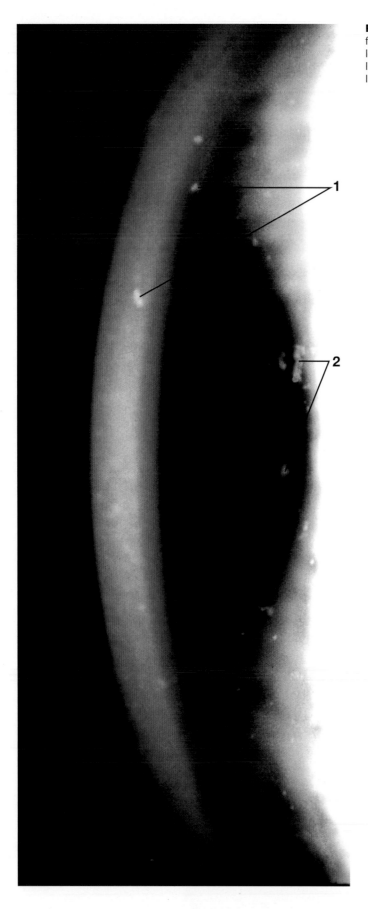

Fig. 10.66 Fleck dystrophy. This autosomal dominant disorder is seen as an incidental finding. There are white, comma-shaped, stellate, circular, and wreath-like opacities at all levels of the corneal stroma. The opacities are white in direct light (1) and gray in indirect light (2). Histologically, the deposits are formed by distended keratocytes filled with complex lipids and glycosaminoglycans. Vision is not affected.

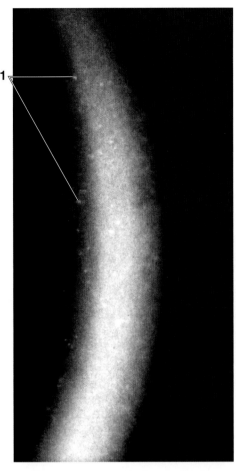

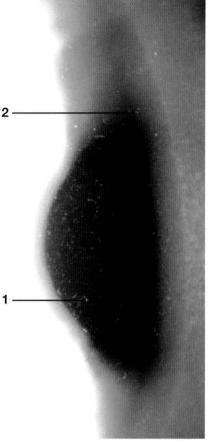

The deep white stromal opacities in pre-Descemet's dystrophy resemble those seen in X-linked ichthyosis (see Fig. 8.83). They may also resemble the deposits in cornea farinata (see Fig. 10.138), although in cornea farinata the deposits are much finer.

Fig. 10.67 Pre-Descemet's dystrophy. There are fine, white opacities in the deep stroma just anterior to Descemet's membrane (1).

Fig. 10.68 Pre-Descemet's dystrophy. This is the 30-year-old daughter of the patient in Fig. 10.67. Deep white stromal opacities are seen in indirect light (1) and direct light (2).

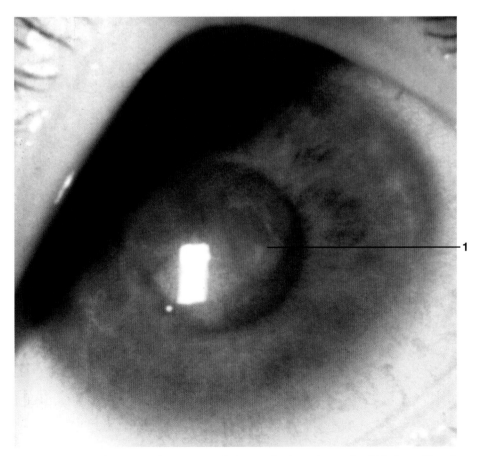

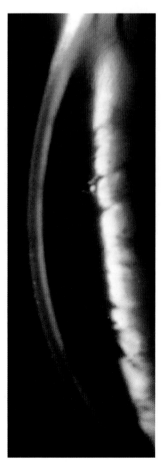

Fig. 10.70 Posterior amorphous stromal dystrophy. This thin slit-beam view demonstrates deep stromal opacification. The corneas in this disorder are thin, and the corneal topography is flat, leading to hyperopia. Iris anomalies may be present. The inheritance pattern is autosomal dominant. The presence of anomalies in infants and occasional iris abnormalities suggest that this may be a congenital disorder of anterior segment differentiation. Vision is not usually greatly affected but rarely can be reduced enough to require corneal transplantation.

Fig. 10.69 Posterior amorphous stromal dystrophy in a 6-month-old infant. There is central corneal opacification (1).

Posterior Membrane Dystrophies

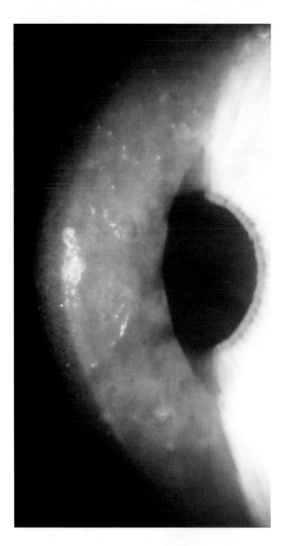

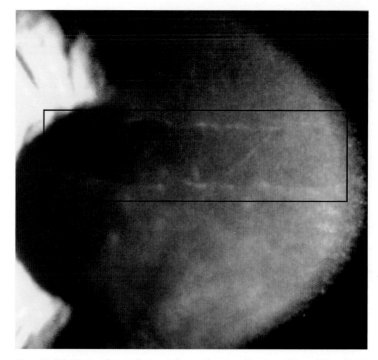

Fig. 10.71 Posterior polymorphous dystrophy. This autosomal dominant disorder of the corneal endothelium is almost always bilateral, although it can be extremely asymmetric or unilateral. This is an example of posterior corneal vesicles, the most common finding in this disorder.

Fig. 10.72 Posterior polymorphous dystrophy. Broad band-like opacities can occur at the level of Descemet's membrane and the endothelium (box).

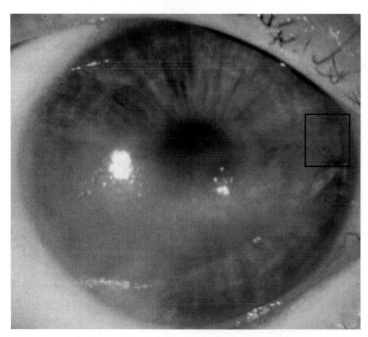

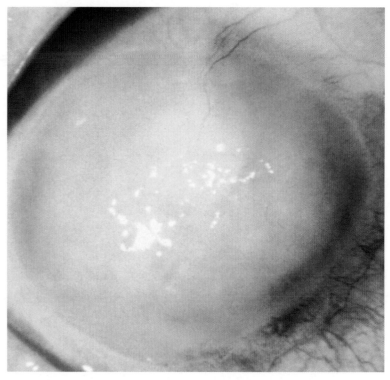

Fig. 10.73 Diffuse corneal edema in a 12-year-old girl with posterior polymorphous dystrophy. Most patients do not develop corneal edema; however, if edema develops, it can occur early or late in the course of the disease or even at birth. This patient also has calcific band keratopathy (box).

Fig. 10.74 Posterior polymorphous dystrophy. This is the 74-year-old grandfather of the patient in Fig. 10.73. There is extensive corneal edema, as well as calcific and lipid degeneration.

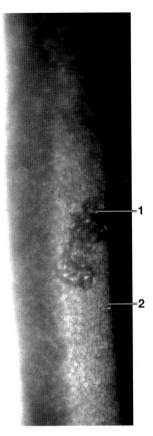

Fig. 10.75 Specular photomicrograph of posterior polymorphous dystrophy. Vesicles with abnormal endothelium (1) are surrounded by relatively normal endothelium (2).

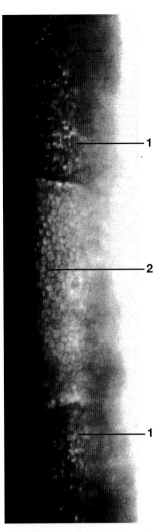

Fig. 10.76 Specular photomicrograph of posterior polymorphous dystrophy. Markedly abnormal endothelium (1) with intervening relatively normal endothelium (2) is seen. There is a sharp demarcation between the normal and abnormal regions.

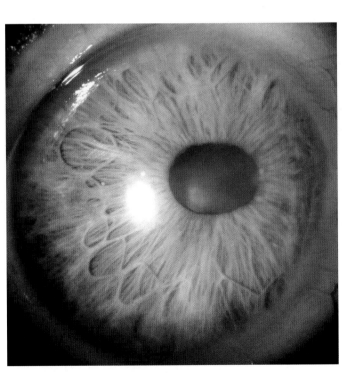

Fig. 10.77 Posterior polymorphous dystrophy. The abnormal endothelium can grow across the trabecular meshwork and onto the iris. Iris traction can result in peripheral anterior synechiae and corectopia. Iris atrophy is not usually present.

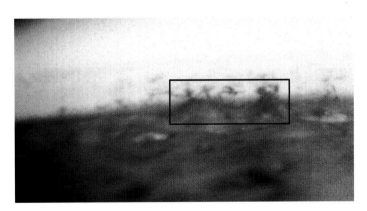

Fig. 10.78 Posterior polymorphous dystrophy. Peripheral anterior synechiae (box) are seen only with gonioscopy. The prognosis for penetrating keratoplasty in these cases is relatively good.

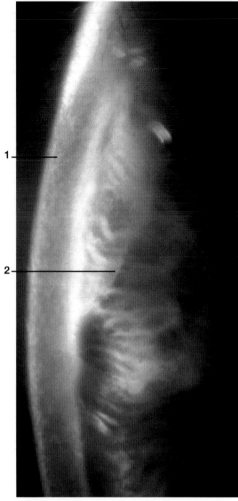

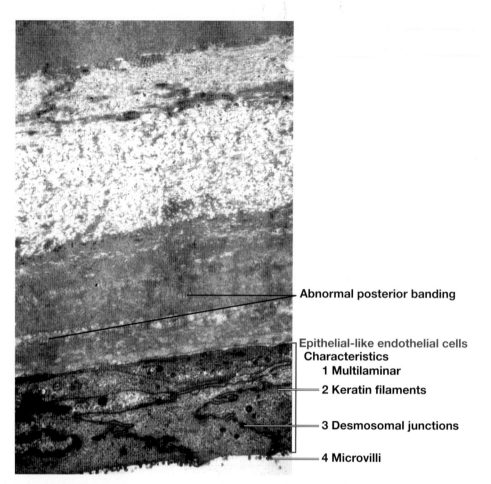

Abnormal posterior banding

Epithelial-like endothelial cells
Characteristics
1 Multilaminar
2 Keratin filaments
3 Desmosomal junctions
4 Microvilli

Fig. 10.80 Electron photomicrograph of the posterior cornea in posterior polymorphous dystrophy. Abnormal banding occurs in the posterior aspect of Descemet's membrane, and endothelial cells with epithelial-like characteristics, including a multilaminar architecture (1), keratin filaments (2), desmosomal junctions (3), and microvilli (4), are seen.

Fig. 10.79 Posterior polymorphous dystrophy. Corneal edema is noted (1). Visible peripheral anterior synechiae are associated with a sheet of epithelial-like endothelial cells (2). The prognosis for keratoplasty in these cases with easily visualized peripheral anterior synechiae is worse because of postoperative glaucoma.

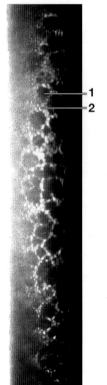

Fig. 10.81 Endothelial dystrophy. Dark holes (1) in the endothelial mosaic (2) represent guttata.

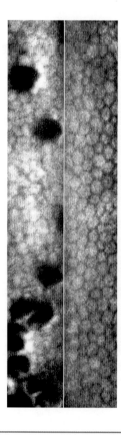

Fig. 10.82 Pseudoguttata. The photomicrograph on the left is of a patient with iritis. Swollen endothelial cells appear as pseudoguttata in the mosaic. Normal endothelial mosaic is found in the same patient when the iritis has resolved (right).

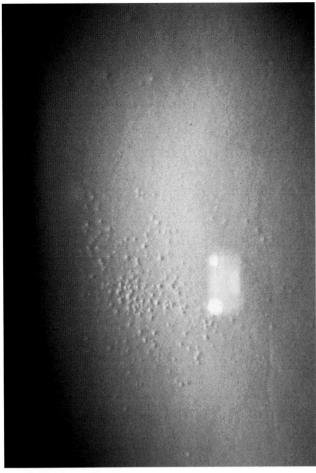

Fig. 10.83 Endothelial dystrophy. Corneal guttata are seen with red reflex.

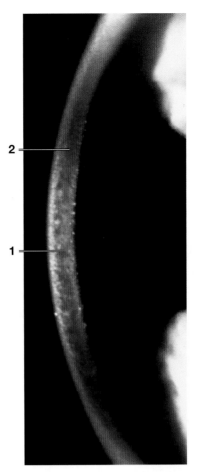

Fig. 10.84 Fuchs' dystrophy. A thicker central cornea (normally thinner) (1) and thinner peripheral cornea without edema (2) are seen.

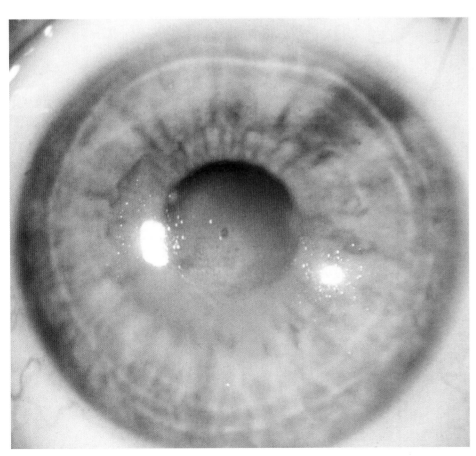

Fig. 10.85 Fuchs' dystrophy with stromal and epithelial edema. The term Fuchs' dystrophy, seen here, implies corneal guttata with corneal edema. The term endothelial dystrophy is reserved for patients with corneal guttata and no evidence of corneal edema (see Fig. 10.83).

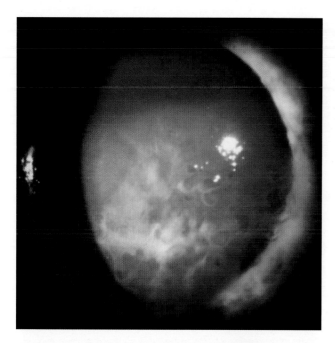

Fig. 10.86 Fuchs' dystrophy. Patients with chronic corneal edema may develop subepithelial fibrosis, as seen here. At this stage, corneal sensation is often decreased.

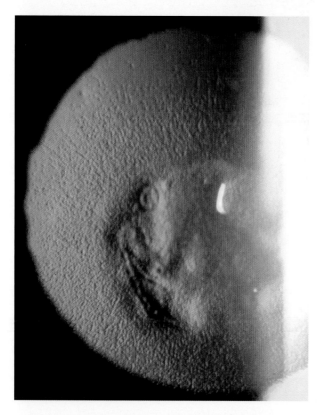

Fig. 10.87 Red reflex of Fuchs' dystrophy. Peripherally there are numerous guttata, and centrally there is localized corneal edema with bullae.

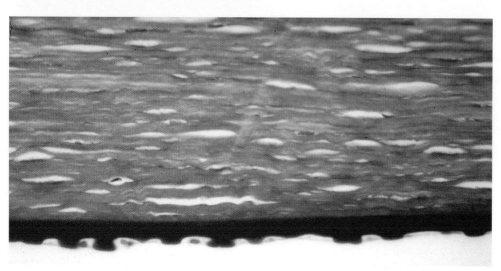

Fig. 10.88 Histopathology of the posterior cornea in Fuchs' dystrophy. The thickened Descemet's membrane with nodular excrescences (cornea guttata) is seen. Endothelial cells are sparse.

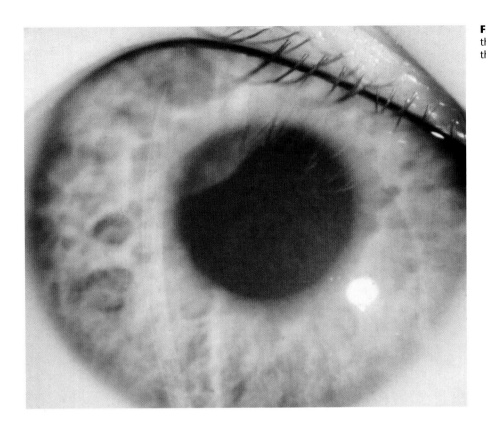

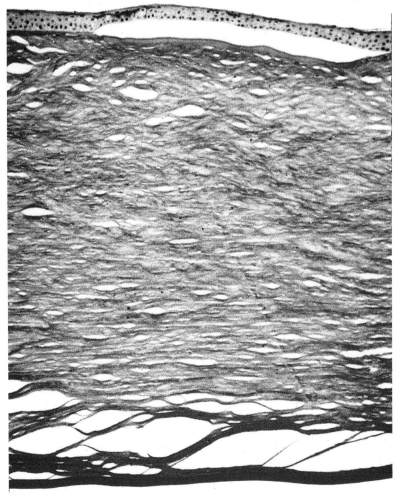

Fig. 10.89 Congenital hereditary endothelial dystrophy. In this condition, diffuse stromal edema is present at birth or develops in the first decade of life, and there is no evidence of cornea guttata.

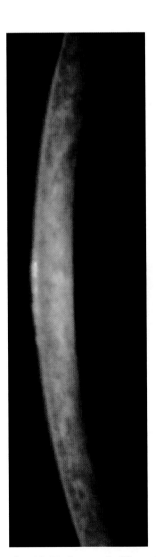

Fig. 10.90 Congenital hereditary endothelial dystrophy. A thin slit-beam view of the patient in Fig. 10.89 shows diffuse stromal edema. The central cornea is thicker than the peripheral cornea.

Fig. 10.91 Histopathology of congenital hereditary endothelial dystrophy. There is an absence of endothelial cells, and Descemet's membrane is thickened. There is corneal edema, with loss of the artifactual stromal clefting and random orientation of collagen lamellae. Epithelial bullae are present.

Noninflammatory Ectatic Disorders

Keratoconus is a noninflammatory progressive thinning of the cornea. The cornea assumes a cone shape. Keratoconus is usually bilateral but often asymmetric. Most cases are sporadic, but approximately 10% of patients have a positive family history.

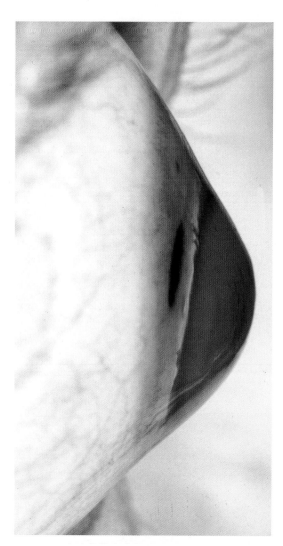

Fig. 10.92 Keratoconus. The thinning is most pronounced at the apex of the cone, which is usually inferior to the visual axis. As the thinning progresses, patients develop increasing degrees of irregular myopic astigmatism. In this case, the angle structures can be directly visualized because of the extreme protrusion of the cornea.

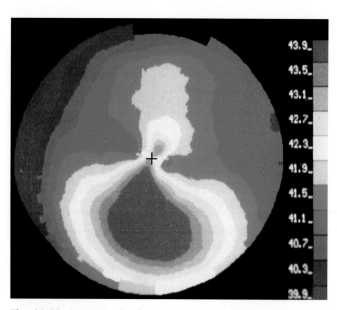

Fig. 10.93 Computerized topography in early keratoconus. The corneal curvature is 43.90 diopters inferior to fixation.

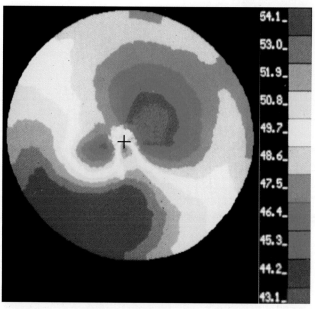

Fig. 10.94 Computerized topography in advanced keratoconus. The corneal curvature is 54.10 diopters inferior to fixation.

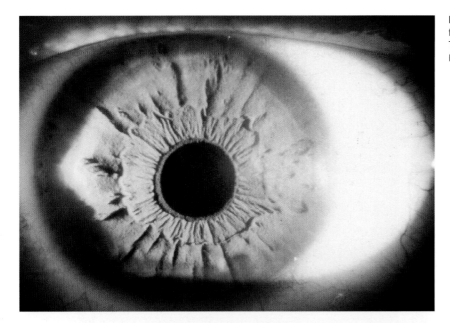

Fig. 10.95 Keratoconus. In this case the observer is shining a penlight from the right, resulting in a triangle of light on the left portion of the iris. The triangle is formed from focused light from the cone. This is known as Rizutti's sign.

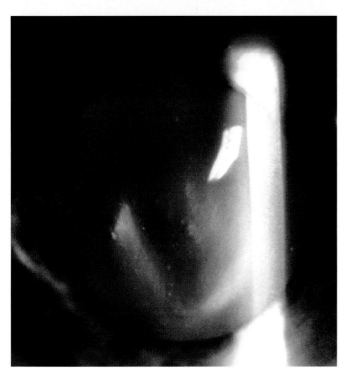

Fig. 10.96 Keratoconus. Munson's sign is a late finding. When the patient looks down, the lower lid protrudes conically.

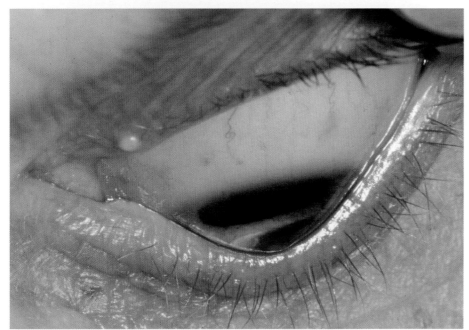

Fig. 10.97 Keratoconus. The central red reflex is irregular because of the steepness of the cone and irregular astigmatism. Dynamic retinoscopy results in a scissoring reflex.

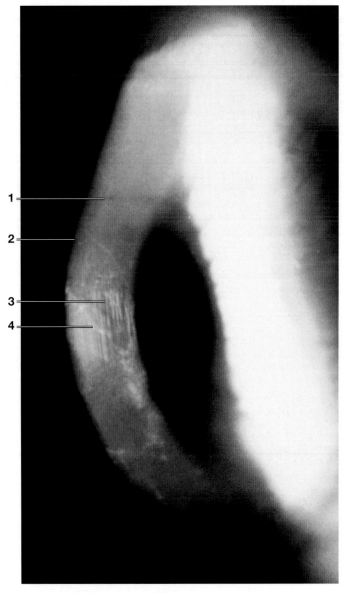

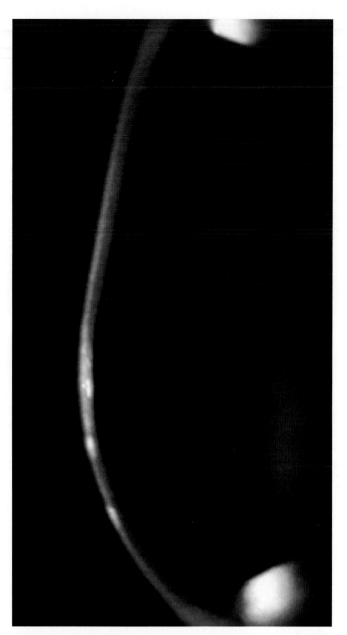

Fig. 10.98 Keratoconus. Fleischer ring (1), protrusion of the cone (2), Vogt's striae (3), and anterior stromal scarring (4) are shown.

Fig. 10.99 Thin slit-beam view of keratoconus. The cornea is thinnest at the region of maximal protrusion.

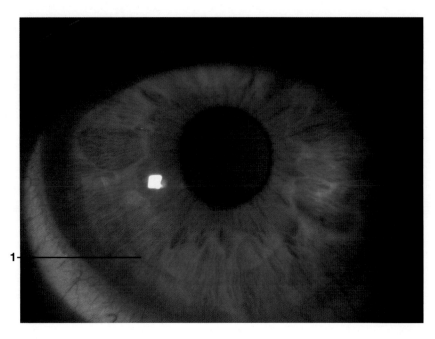

Fig. 10.100 Keratoconus. A Fleischer ring (1) is composed of iron in the corneal epithelium. The ring configuration is produced by an irregular distribution of tears at the base of the cone and resultant iron deposition. It is easier to see the line of iron with the cobalt blue light.

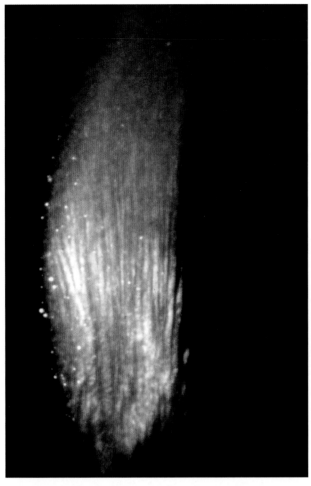

Fig. 10.101 Keratoconus. Vogt's striae are stress lines in the posterior cornea stroma and occur near the apex of the cone.

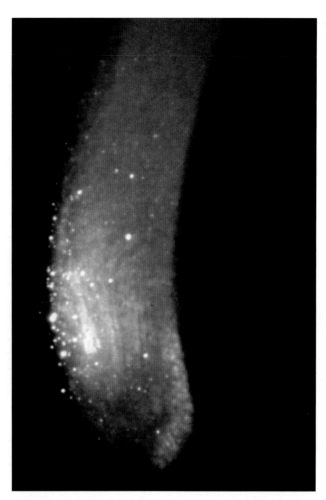

Fig. 10.102 Keratoconus. When digital pressure is applied to the globe, Vogt's striae disappear.

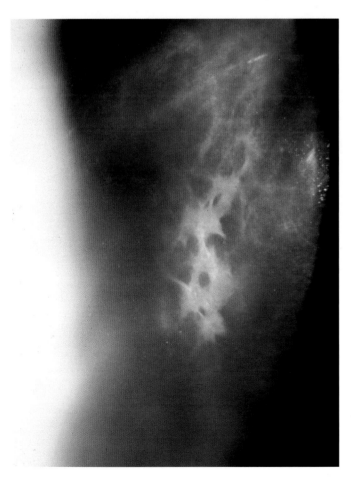

Fig. 10.103 Keratoconus. Breaks in Bowman's membrane result in anterior stromal scarring.

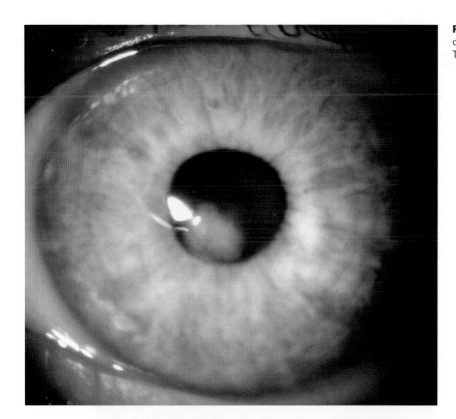

Fig. 10.104 Keratoconus. Occasionally, an elevated subepithelial nodule occurs from chronic rubbing of a contact lens on the apex of the cone. These nodules can usually be scraped from the surface of the cornea.

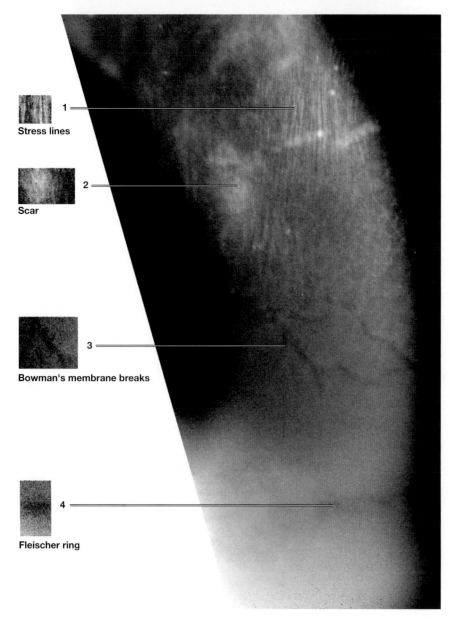

Stress lines

Scar

Bowman's membrane breaks

Fleischer ring

Fig. 10.105 Keratoconus. Vogt's striae in the deep stroma (1), scarring in the anterior stroma from old breaks in Bowman's membrane (2), fresh breaks in Bowman's membrane with clear areas between breaks (3), and iron deposition in the epithelium (Fleischer ring) (4) are shown.

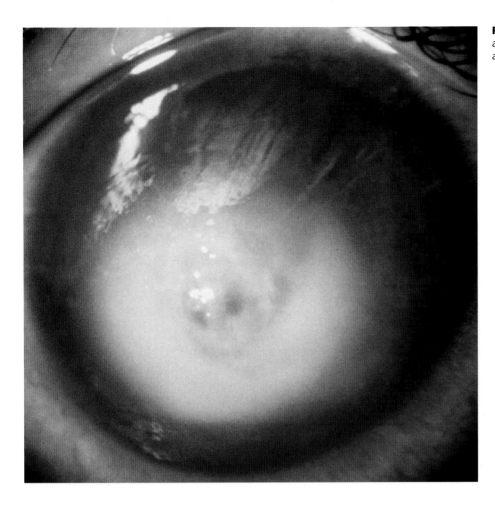

Fig. 10.106 Keratoconus. Corneal hydrops occurs when there is an acute break in Descemet's membrane. The cornea is edematous, and patients complain of pain and sudden decreased vision.

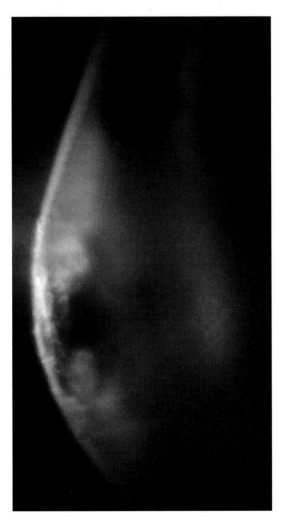

Fig. 10.107 Keratoconus. This is a thin slit-beam view of hydrops. The cornea is markedly edematous. With time, the edema resolves and stromal scarring occurs. Rarely, the visual acuity can improve if the scar flattens the cone.

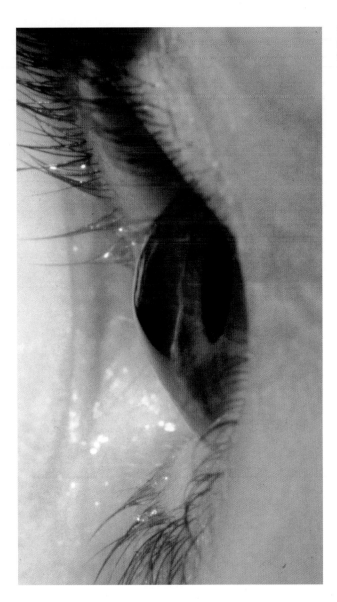

Fig. 10.108 Keratoconus in a patient with Leber's congenital amaurosis. The cone is more central and superior in this case. Patients with Leber's congenital amaurosis frequently rub their eyes (the oculodigital sign), and this may predispose the development of keratoconus.

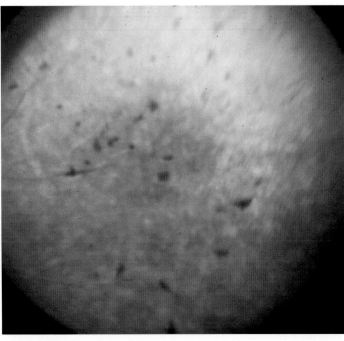 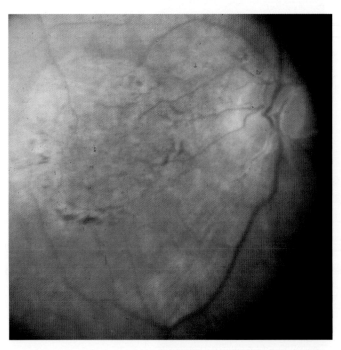

Figs 10.109 and 10.110 Keratoconus in a patient with Leber's congenital kamaurosis. The peripheral retina (Fig. 10.109, left) and central retina (Fig. 10.110, right) in the same patient as in Fig. 10.108 are shown. There is a diffuse pigmentary retinopathy. Both pictures are slightly out of focus because of the difficulty in focusing the image through an irregularly shaped cornea.

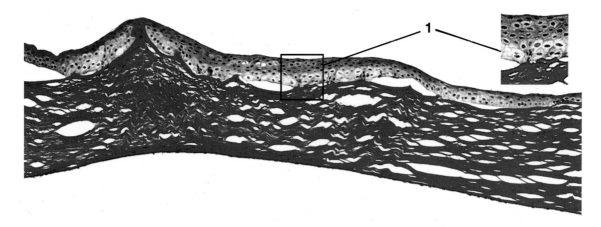

Fig. 10.111 Keratoconus. There is an irregular thickness of the epithelium and a rupture of Bowman's membrane with epithelial stromal apposition (1). The stroma is thinner in the central portion (cone) of the specimen. The endothelium is normal.

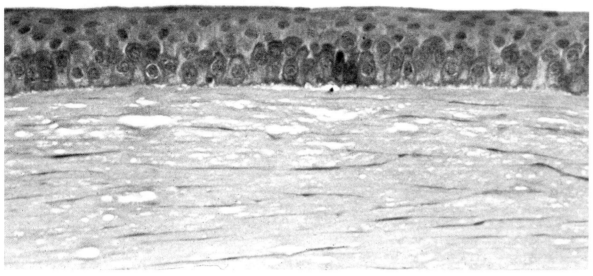

Fig. 10.112 Keratoconus. Prussian blue stains iron deposits in the epithelium, especially the basal cells. The loss of Bowman's membrane is demonstrated.

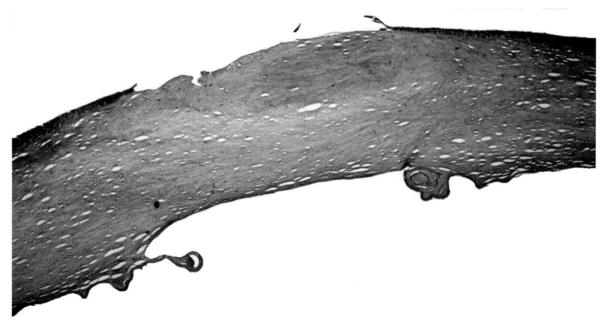

Fig. 10.113 Keratoconus. Corneal hydrops and the break in Descemet's membrane with scrolled edges are shown. There is scarring in the central stroma, and a large epithelial defect is present.

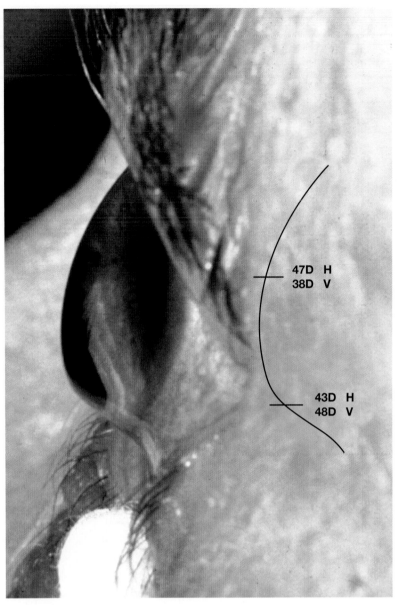

Fig. 10.114 Pellucid marginal degeneration. This is an inferior thinning of the cornea that usually extends from 4 to 8 o'clock. The thinning is 1–2 mm wide and located 1–2 mm from the inferior limbus. It is not associated with vascularization. It typically begins between the ages of 20 and 40 years, and the progression may be slow. Unlike keratoconus, there is no Fleischer ring or Vogt's striae. Centrally, there is against-the-rule astigmatism (in this example, 47 diopters horizontally, 38 diopters vertically), and inferiorly, there is with-the-rule astigmatism (in this example, 43 diopters horizontally, 48 diopters vertically).

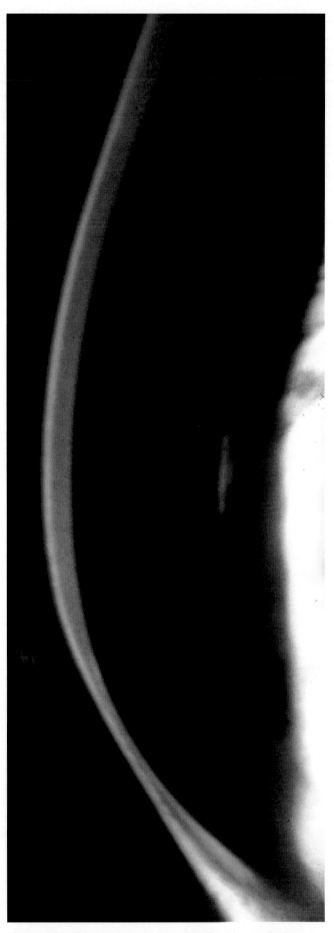

Fig. 10.115 Thin slit-beam view of pellucid marginal degeneration. There is marked thinning of the cornea inferiorly, well below the area of maximal corneal protrusion. In contrast, the thinning in keratoconus is in the area of maximal corneal protrusion (see Fig. 10.99).

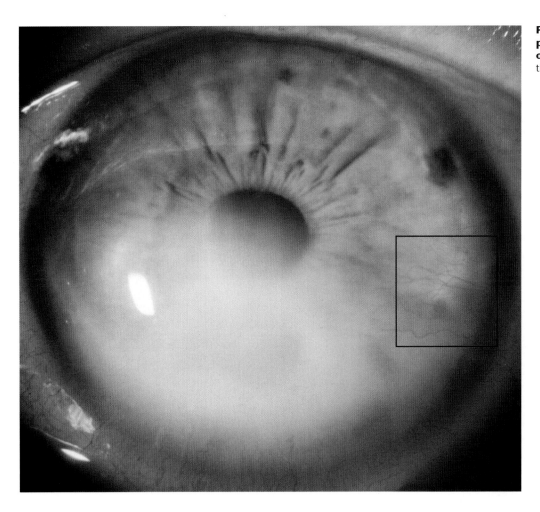

Fig. 10.116 Corneal scarring in a patient with pellucid marginal degeneration after an episode of acute hydrops. There is peripheral vascularization of the cornea in reaction to the hydrops (box).

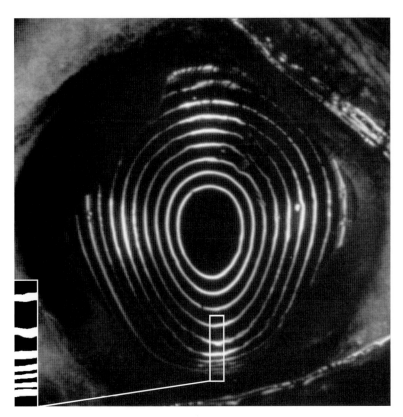

Fig. 10.117 Photokeratoscopy of pellucid marginal degeneration.
Typically, the central mire has an egg shape. Centrally, the horizontal rings are closer together than the vertical rings; this indicates corneal steepening in the horizontal axis (against-the-rule astigmatism). Inferiorly (inset), the vertical rings become close together, indicating a shift in steepening to the vertical axis (with-the-rule astigmatism).

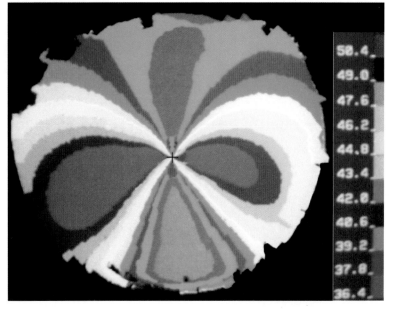

Fig. 10.118 Computerized topography of pellucid marginal degeneration. Centrally, there is corneal steepening in the horizontal meridian (against-the-rule astigmatism). The shift to with-the-rule astigmatism inferiorly cannot be seen in this photograph, as the corneal imaging system does not image the far peripheral cornea.

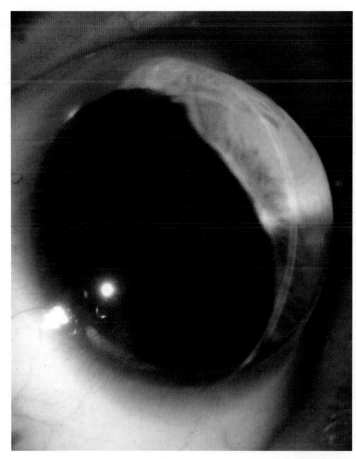

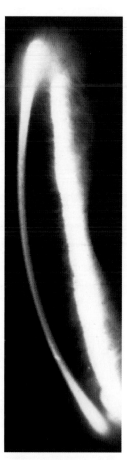

Fig. 10.119 Keratoglobus. This is a diffuse thinning of the cornea to one-third to one-fifth of normal thickness. In this case the thinning is more pronounced in the periphery, as seen in the inferior portion of the slit beam. It is noted in early life, and progression is minimal.

Fig. 10.120 Thin slit-beam view of keratoglobus. The cornea is diffusely thin.

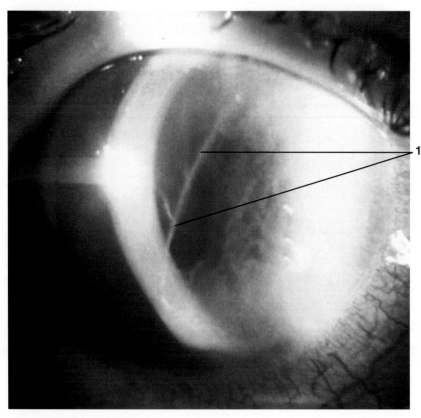

Fig. 10.121 Acute hydrops in keratoglobus. In this case, Descemet's membrane is detached (1). Keratoglobus has been associated with Leber's congenital amaurosis and Ehlers–Danlos syndrome type VI. Some families with both keratoglobus and keratoconus have been reported.

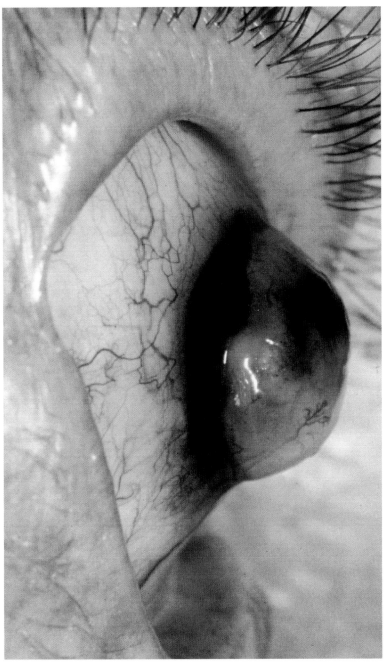

Fig. 10.122 Corneal ectasia caused by long-standing glaucoma and chronic corneal inflammation with thinning.

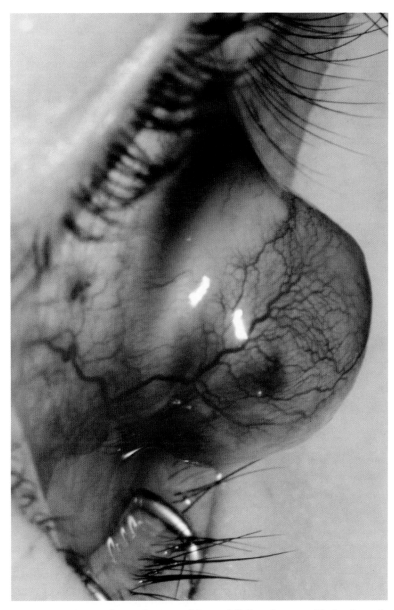

Fig. 10.123 Corneal ectasia caused by a childhood corneal infection of unknown etiology. In both Figs 10.122 and 10.123, the corneas are scarred and vascularized, distinguishing them from keratoconus, pellucid marginal degeneration, and keratoglobus.

Iridocorneal Endothelial Syndrome

The iridocorneal endothelial (ICE) syndrome is not inherited and is almost always unilateral. It occurs more often in females, and has its onset between the ages of 30 and 50 years. ICE is an acronym for iris-nevus (Cogan–Reese) syndrome, Chandler's syndrome, and essential iris atrophy.

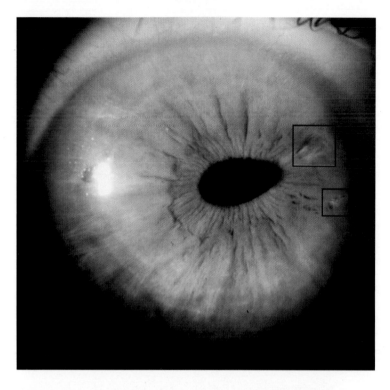

Fig. 10.124 Chandler's syndrome. Areas of iris atrophy are highlighted in the two boxes. The pupil is drawn toward the areas of iris atrophy. Histopathologic examination of this disorder shows abnormal endothelial cells that migrate across the trabecular meshwork and onto the iris. This abnormal endothelial cell proliferation can cause corneal edema, peripheral anterior synechiae with glaucoma, and traction and atrophy of the iris.

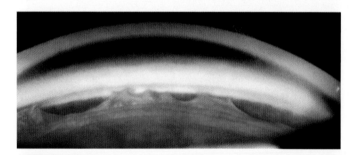

Fig. 10.125 Chandler's syndrome; gonioscopy. Broad bands of peripheral anterior synechiae are seen.

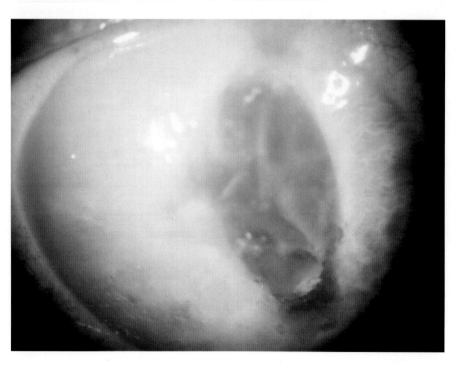

Fig. 10.126 Chandler's syndrome. This advanced case has extensive corneal edema. The pupil is irregular, and there is ectropion uvea.

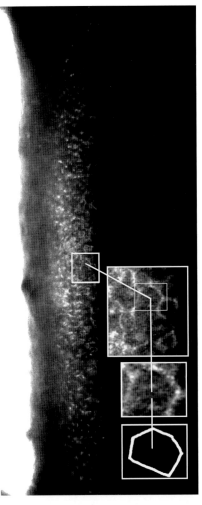

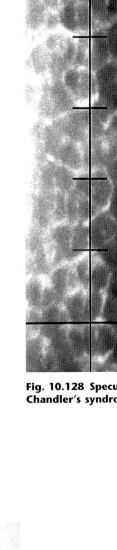

Fig. 10.128 Specular photomicroscopy (high magnification) of Chandler's syndrome. There is a loss of the normal hexagonal cell shape.

Fig. 10.127 Specular photomicroscopy (low magnification) of Chandler's syndrome. The endothelial cells are markedly abnormal. Insets show progressively more magnified views and a schematic of endothelial cells. The dark areas between cells are not cornea guttata but represent undulations in the endothelial surface, with some areas in focus and some out of focus.

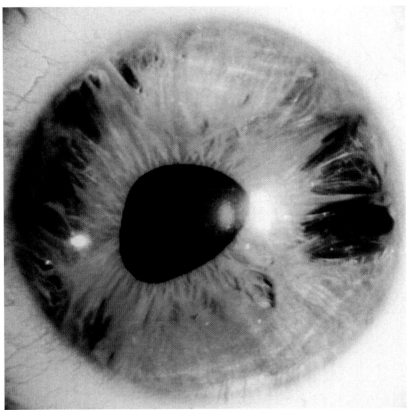

Fig. 10.129 Essential iris atrophy. The peripheral iris is atrophic, and there are areas of absent tissue. The pupil is drawn toward the areas of maximal iris atrophy.

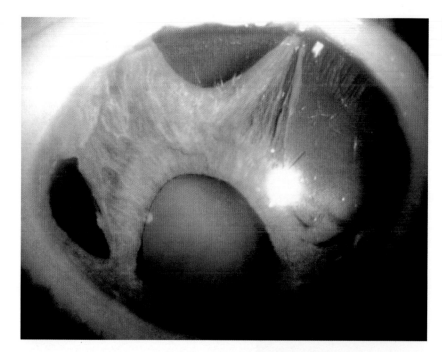

Fig. 10.130 Essential iris atrophy, advanced case. Large portions of the iris are atrophic or absent. Ectropion uvea is present inferiorly.

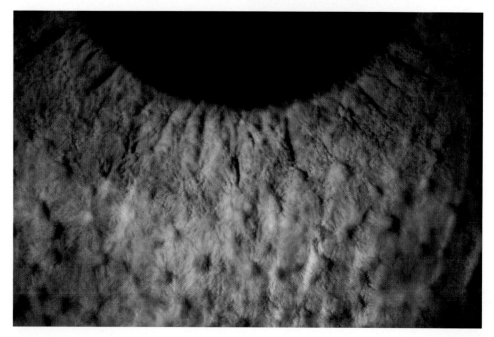

Fig. 10.131 Iris-nevus (Cogan–Reese) syndrome. There are multiple, fine, brown nodules on the iris surface.

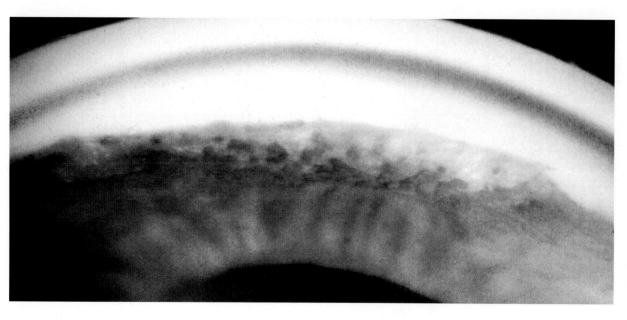

Fig. 10.132 Gonioscopic view of iris-nevus (Cogan–Reese) syndrome. Multiple brown iris nodules are seen on the peripheral iris. There is a broad band of peripheral anterior synechiae.

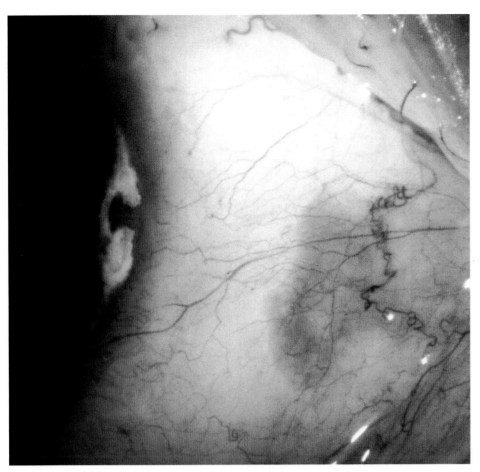

Fig. 10.133 Vogt's limbal girdle type I. This is actually a mild form of limbal calcific band keratopathy. It is usually irregular and slightly elevated, and may contain small "Swiss cheese" holes. There is a clear area separating the lesion from the limbus. The patient also has a calcified scleral plaque.

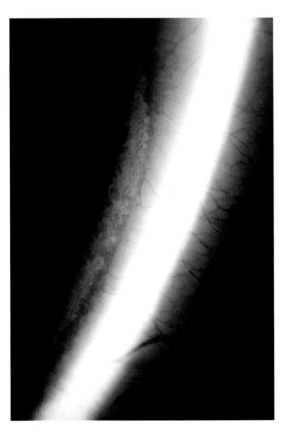

Fig. 10.134 Vogt's limbal girdle type II. Similar to the lesion in Fig. 10.133, this occurs in the interpalpebral zone. There is a vertical chalk-like band of material in the superficial cornea. Several conical protrusions point toward the pupil. The lesion is continuous with the limbus. Histologically, this is a region of elastoid degeneration. This lesion is often associated with pinguecula.

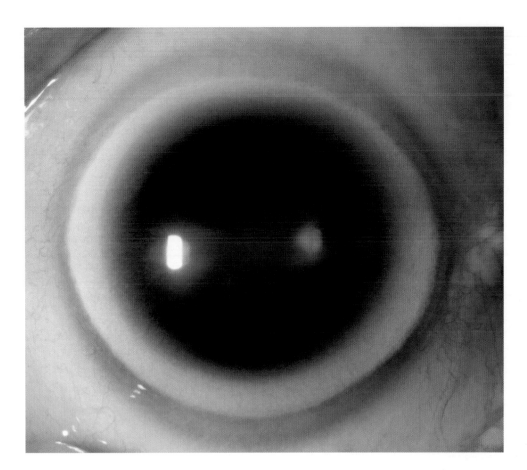

Fig. 10.135 Advanced arcus senilis. This lesion is composed of lipid, and there is a characteristic clear zone between the limbus and outer edge of the lesion. The central edge of the lesion has an irregular border, compared with the peripheral edge.

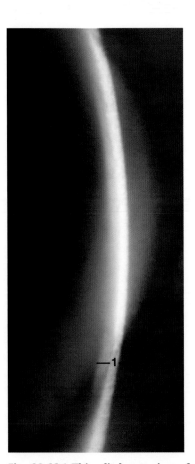

Fig. 10.136 Thin slit-beam view of arcus senilis. Posteriorly, there is a peripheral wedge of lipid (1).

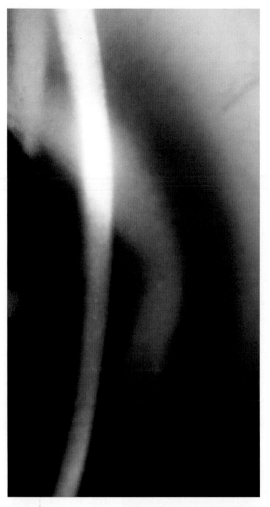

Fig. 10.137 Arcus juvenilis. Peripheral lipid deposition in a young patient often signifies a systemic lipid abnormality. Serum lipid profiles should be obtained.

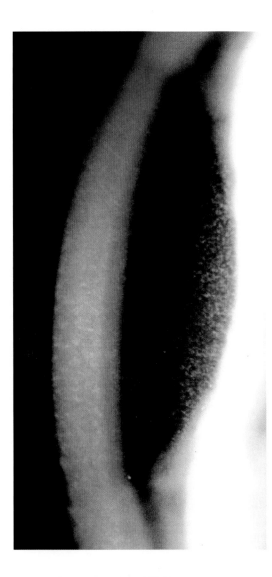

Fig. 10.138 Cornea farinata. This represents an accumulation of fine, white, dust-like particles in the deep corneal stroma. In this case, they are best seen in retro-illumination to the left of the pupillary margin. The deposits are bilateral and not visually significant. They should not be mistaken for cornea guttata (see Fig. 10.83). The term cornea farinata is derived from the word farina, which means "flour."

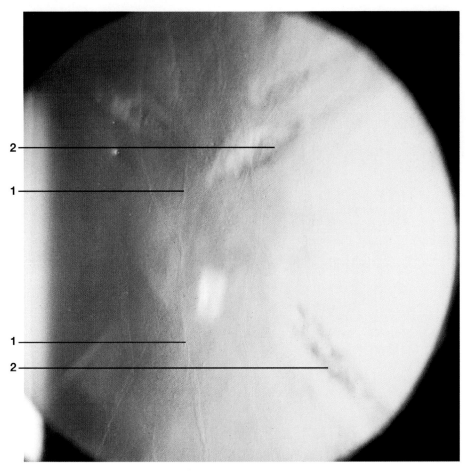

Fig. 10.139 Glass striae (1). These are vertical striations in the deep corneal stroma or Descemet's membrane. They are seen in older patients and tend to be more common in patients with diabetes. They are best seen on retro-illumination and appear as fine twisted strands, some of which have a double-walled configuration. This patient also has cortical spoking from a cataract (2).

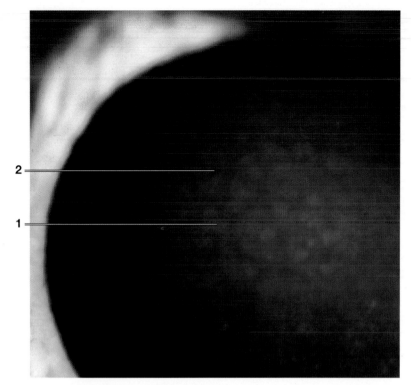

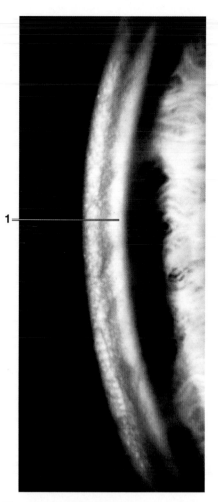

Fig. 10.140 Posterior crocodile shagreen. There are polygonal opacities (1) in the deep corneal stroma separated by relatively clear areas (2). The disorder is bilateral, seen late in life, and not visually significant. Electron microscopy of one case showed an irregular arrangement of the collagen lamellae. There is no heritable pattern, but this condition is clinically identical to central cloudy dystrophy of François, which occurs in an autosomal dominant pattern.

Fig. 10.141 Thin slit-beam view of posterior crocodile shagreen. Opacification is most dense posteriorly (1).

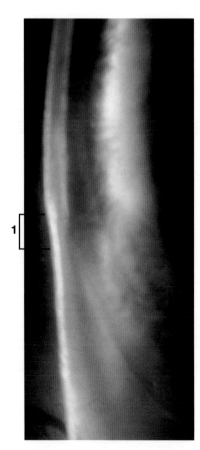

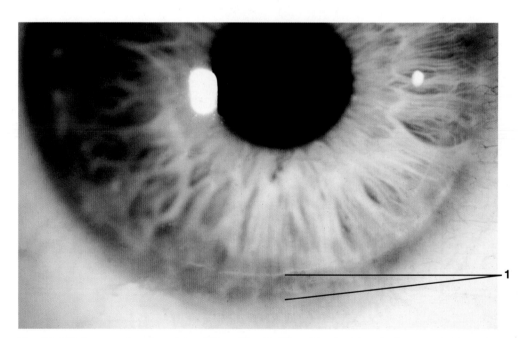

Fig. 10.143 Furrow degeneration, diffuse illumination (1). Occasionally, fine superficial vessels extend into the area of thinning, but this is not associated with acute inflammation.

Fig. 10.142 Furrow degeneration. This is a peripheral thinning of the cornea (1) near the limbus.

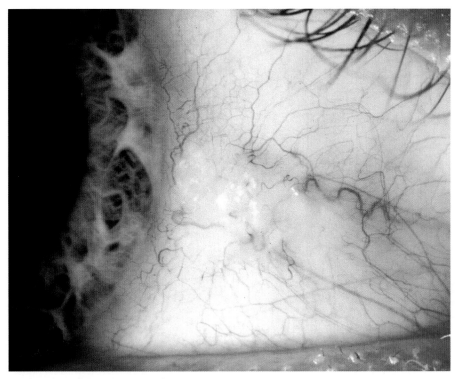

Fig. 10.144 Pinguecula. These elevated, fleshy, conjunctival masses are located in the interpalpebral region, most commonly on the nasal side. They are yellow or light brown, and are associated with chronic actinic exposure, repeated trauma, and dry and windy conditions. Histologically, they are composed of abnormal collagen bundles with staining characteristics similar to those of elastic tissue. The condition is termed elastotic degeneration, but the tissue is not actually composed of elastin.

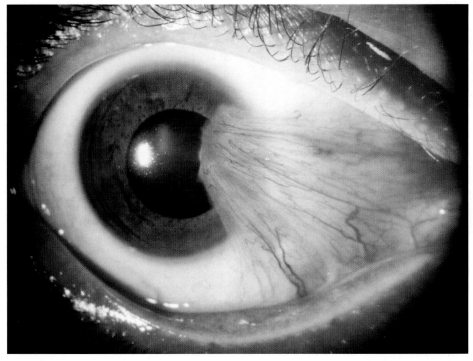

Fig. 10.145 Pterygium. These fibrovascular growths extend from the conjunctiva onto the cornea. They are almost always preceded by pinguecula and, like pinguecula, are associated with chronic actinic exposure, trauma, and dry and windy conditions. There is destruction of Bowman's membrane in the cornea, and for this reason there is residual corneal scarring when these growths are removed. The histopathology, like that of pinguecula, shows elastotic degeneration.

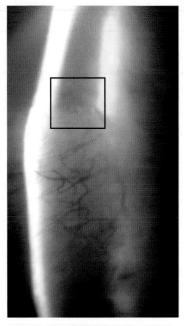

Fig. 10.146 Pterygium with a Stocker line (box).

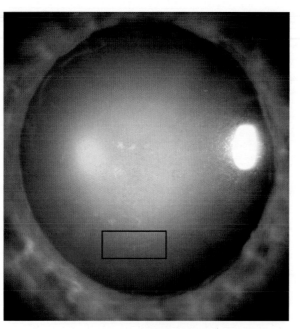

Fig. 10.147 Hudson–Stähli line at the junction of the upper two-thirds and lower one-third of the cornea (box).

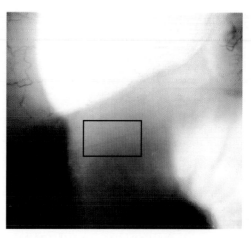

Fig. 10.148 Filtering bleb with Ferry line (box); white light.

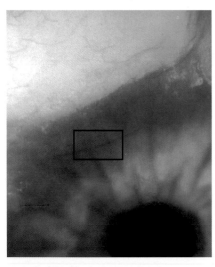

Fig. 10.149 Filtering bleb with Ferry line (box); blue light.

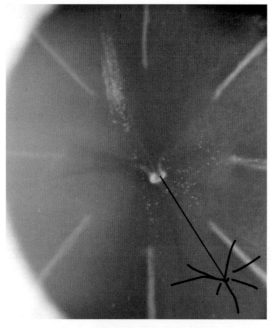

Fig. 10.150 Iron lines associated with radial keratotomy.

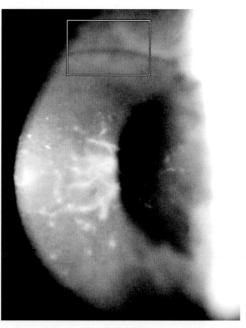

Fig. 10.151 Iron in keratoconus (Fleischer ring) (box).

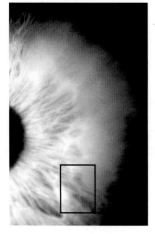

Fig. 10.152 Iron line in Salzmann's nodular degeneration (box).

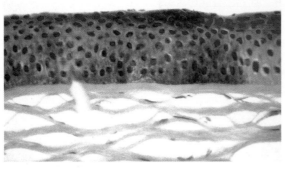

Fig. 10.153 Prussian blue stain demonstrating iron in the epithelium.

Iron lines appear as faint brown deposits in the corneal epithelium. Sometimes they are best seen with the cobalt blue light. Iron deposits occur in areas of irregular tear distribution. Histologically, the iron is seen in the epithelium, especially the basal layer.

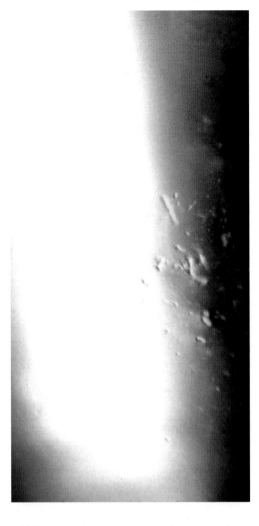

Fig. 10.154 Polymorphic amyloid degeneration. This age-related change of the cornea is usually bilateral and does not affect vision. In the deep corneal stroma, there are small polygonal gray–white opacities and lines that are refractile with indirect illumination. The opacities themselves appear similar to those seen in lattice dystrophy; however, they are usually less extensive, are located in the deepest level of the stroma, and are not associated with any of the sequelae of lattice dystrophy. These deposits are not associated with any systemic disorder of amyloid deposition.

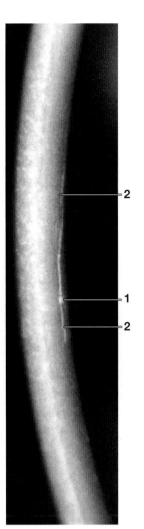

Fig. 10.155 Polymorphic amyloid degeneration. An amyloid deposit (1) and Descemet's fold (2) caused by pressure from the deposit are shown.

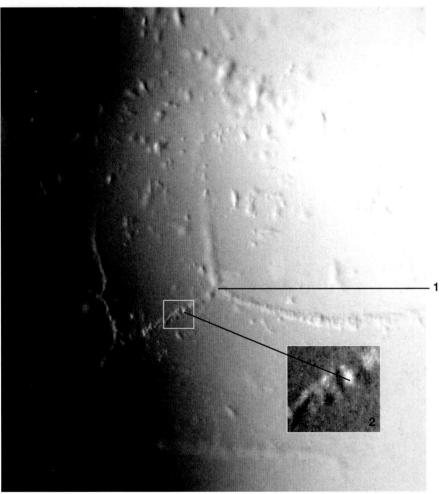

Fig. 10.156 Polymorphic amyloid degeneration. This can appear similar to lattice dystrophy with branching lines (1) composed of smaller nodules (inset [2]).

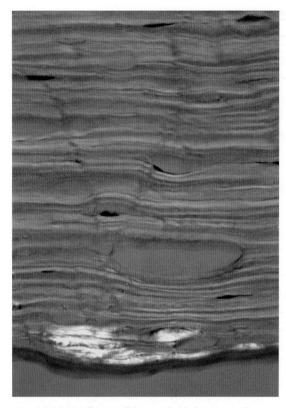

Fig. 10.157 Polymorphic amyloid degeneration.
Fusiform extracellular amyloid material is seen in the very deep stroma (birefringence of Congo red stain).

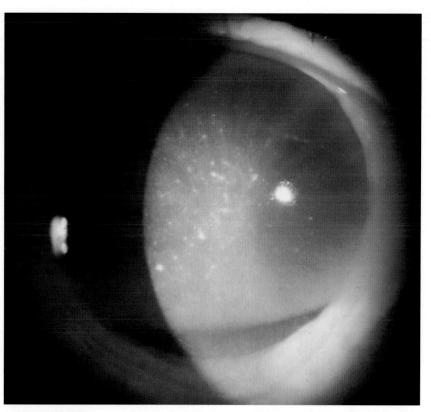

Fig. 10.158 Calcific band keratopathy. Characteristically this occurs in the interpalpebral region. Calcium deposits in this region result from localized elevations of pH favoring calcium precipitation and increased evaporation, which increases the local concentration of calcium. This condition may be idiopathic but is usually associated with localized ocular inflammatory processes or systemic hypercalcemia.

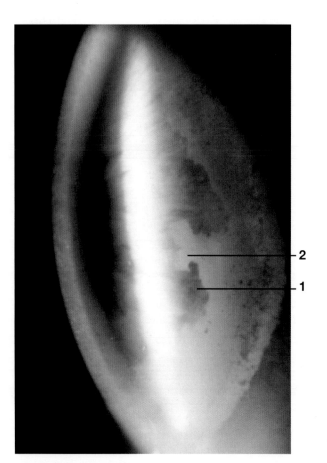

Fig. 10.159 Same patient as in Fig. 10.158 after chelation with EDTA.
The area where calcium was removed is shown (1). Calcium remnants are seen in the peripheral cornea (2). The small holes represent areas where corneal nerves penetrate through Bowman's layer to the superficial epithelium.

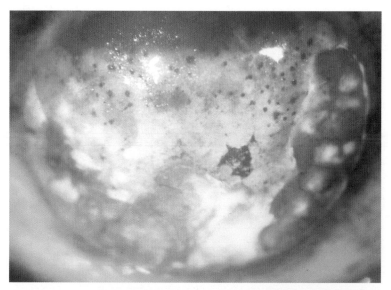

Fig. 10.160 Calcific degeneration. Calcium deposition in the cornea is associated with chronic vascularization or inflammation. Histopathologically, the calcium may be associated with a fibrovascular pannus or may occur deep in the corneal stroma, as opposed to calcific band keratopathy in which the calcium deposition is confined to the region of Bowman's membrane (see Fig. 10.162).

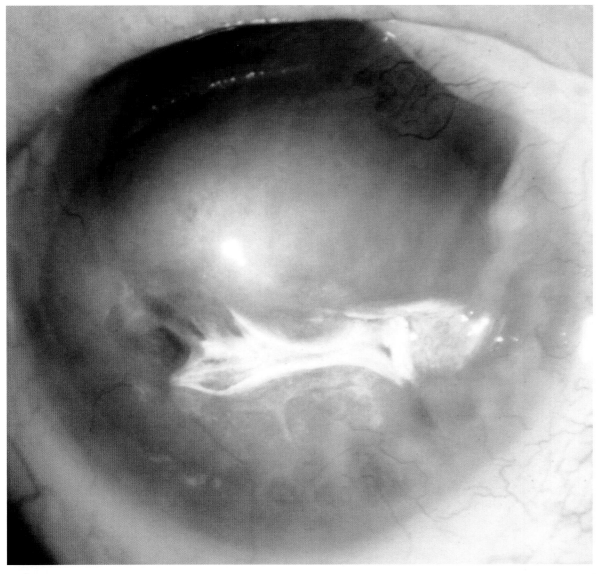

Fig. 10.161 Calcific degeneration. This patient had severe glaucoma and chronic corneal edema from aphakic bullous keratopathy. Histopathologic examination showed calcium associated with a fibrovascular pannus.

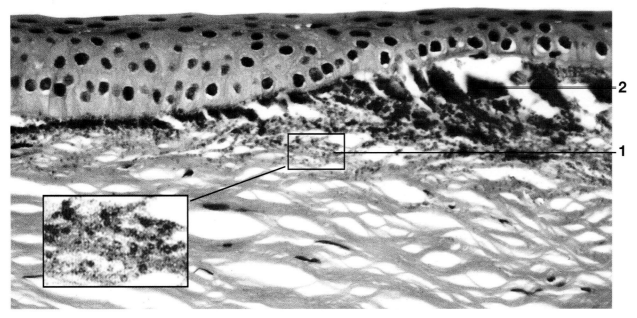

Fig. 10.162 Histopathology of calcific band keratopathy. Basophilic stippling from calcium diffusely replaces Bowman's membrane (1) with larger pieces of calcium (2) in localized accumulations.

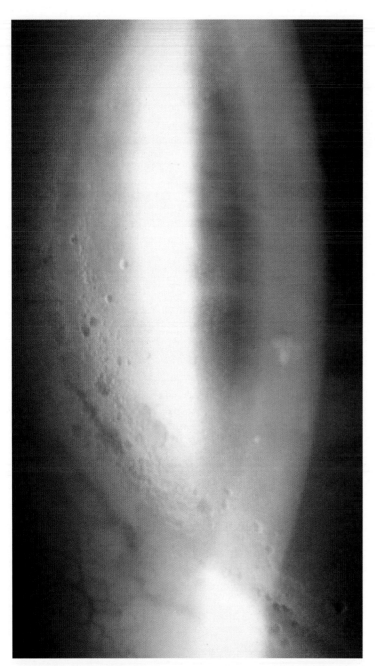

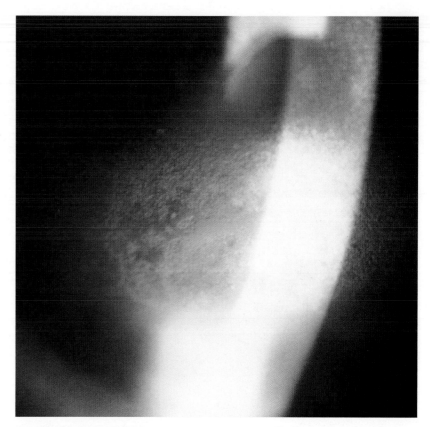

Fig. 10.164 Spheroidal degeneration, advanced. The brownish-yellow deposits are more confluent and are located in the central cornea in this case. Spheroidal degeneration characteristically occurs in the interpalpebral zones and is associated with chronic actinic exposure and dry and windy conditions.

Fig. 10.163 Spheroidal degeneration, mild. There are multiple golden-brown spherules in the superficial cornea.

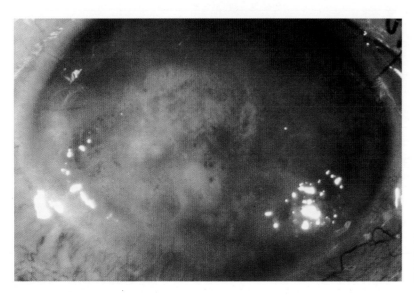

Fig. 10.165 Spheroidal degeneration, band. Similar to band keratopathy, spheroidal degeneration may also be associated with chronic localized ocular inflammation. In this case the inflammation and scarring was due to syphilitic keratitis.

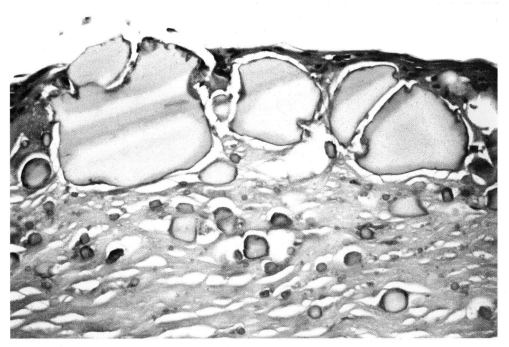

Fig. 10.166 Histopathology of spheroidal degeneration. Extracellular deposits of globular, faintly basophilic material are noted in the superficial stroma and Bowman's layer. The globules are irregularly shaped with well demarcated borders. This condition is similar to calcific band keratopathy except that the deposits are more homogeneous and not stippled.

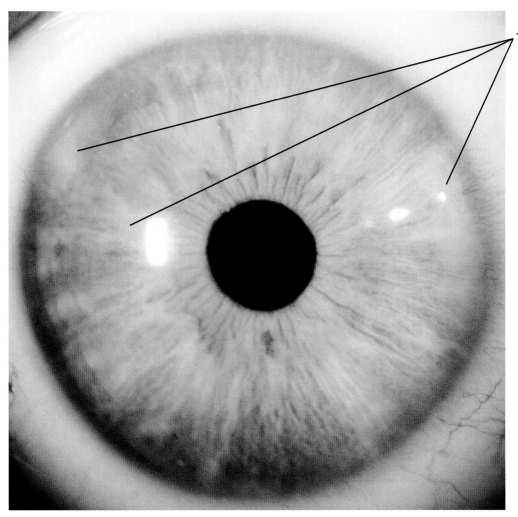

Fig. 10.167 Salzmann's nodular degenerations. These elevated bluish-white superficial nodules (1) are more common in females and most commonly occur in the fifth decade of life or later. The condition may be associated with localized corneal inflammation. Histopathology shows subepithelial hyaline nodules that replace Bowman's layer.

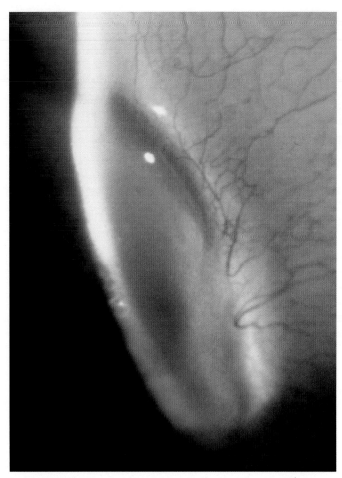

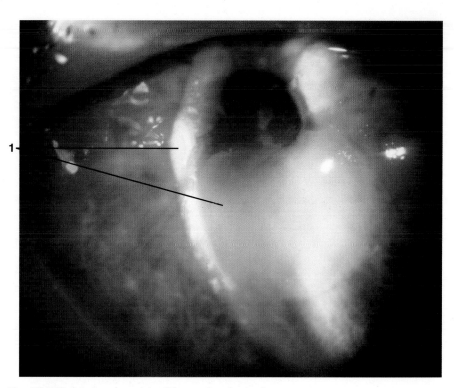

Fig. 10.169 Salzmann's nodules (1) near the visual axis.

Fig. 10.168 Peripheral Salzmann's nodule showing characteristic elevation.

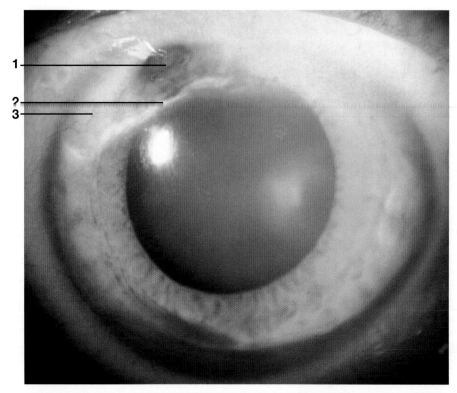

Fig. 10.170 Terrien's marginal degeneration. This slowly progressive marginal thinning of the cornea is more common in males and can occur in all age groups, including children. In contrast to other causes of marginal corneal thinning such as Mooren's ulcer, there is no pain, there are very minor or no episodes of acute inflammation, and the corneal epithelium remains intact. The thinning usually begins superiorly (1) and is associated with a fine line of lipid deposition (2) at the edge of fine superficial vessels (3).

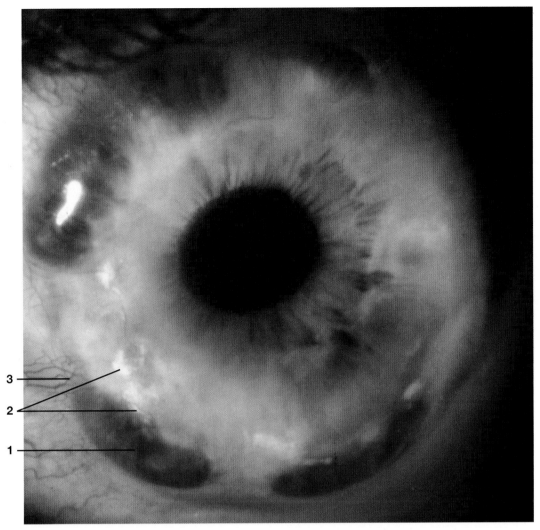

Fig. 10.171 Terrien's marginal degeneration. With time, the thinning spreads circumferentially, as seen in this example. The cornea becomes extremely thin (1) and may bulge anteriorly. There is lipid deposition (2) and superficial vascularization (3).

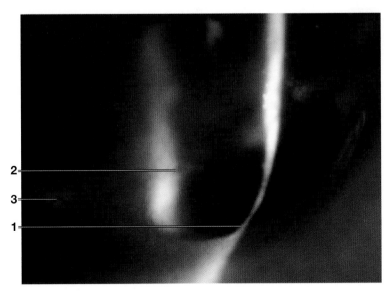

Fig. 10.172 Thin slit-beam view of Terrien's marginal degeneration. The cornea is extremely thin (1) and bulges anteriorly. The epithelium overlying the thin cornea is intact. Minor ocular trauma may result in ocular perforation. Lipid deposition (2) and superficial vascularization (3) are also seen.

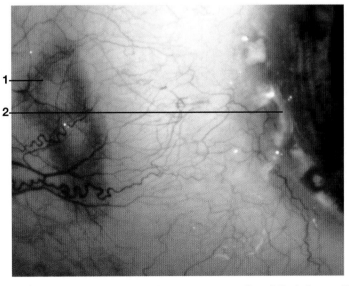

Fig. 10.173 Calcified scleral plaques. Occasionally, calcified plaques (1) are seen in older patients. This patient also has Vogt's limbic girdle type I (2), which represents mild calcific band keratopathy (see Fig. 10.133).

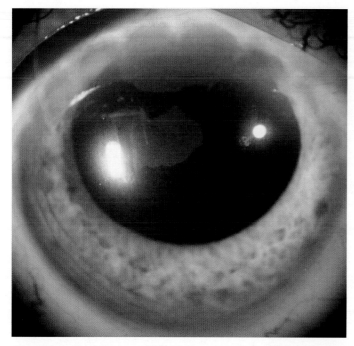

Fig. 10.174 Posterior proliferative endothelial pigmentation in a patient after cataract surgery. These membranes may grow and change shape with time.

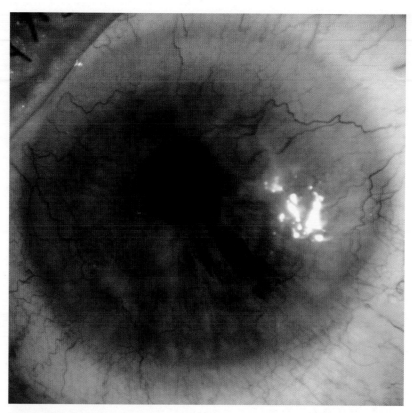

Fig. 10.175 Aniridia. This congenital disorder is associated with glaucoma, cataracts, ectopia lentis, and foveal hypoplasia. These patients may have superficial corneal vascularization and severe corneal scarring. Penetrating keratoplasty is often complicated by poor epithelial healing, recurrence of superficial vascularization, and scarring in the graft. The term aniridia is a misnomer, as all of these patients have some iris tissue present (sometimes only histologically) and in some cases the iris may be only mildly abnormal (as seen here).

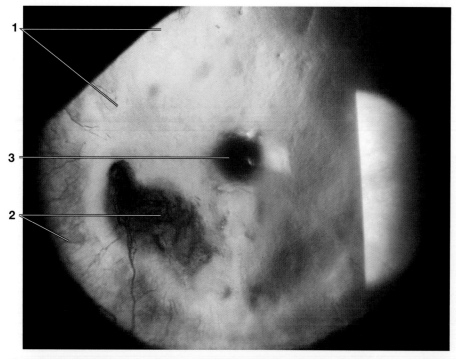

Fig. 10.176 Aniridia seen in retinal retro-illumination. In this patient with aniridia, there is no visible iris tissue (1). Scar tissue and pannus with vascularization (2) are present. There is a small central cataract (3).

Chapter 11

Corneal Infections

There are four basic classes of organisms responsible for infectious keratitis: bacterial, viral, fungal, and parasitic. Whenever possible, the exact diagnosis should be established by direct examination of corneal material and/or culture techniques. However, the clinical appearance of some of these disorders can establish a definitive diagnosis (e.g., herpes simplex epithelial keratitis) or guide treatment until the exact diagnosis is known.

Microbiology

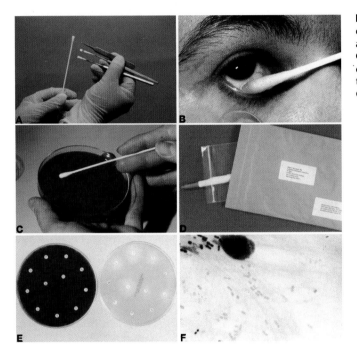

Fig. 11.1 Corneal specimen collection. A, Different instruments can be used to collect corneal specimens. Because corneal infiltrates are often small, care must be taken to obtain an adequate specimen. **B,** A conjunctival culture can be obtained with a cotton-tipped applicator. **C,** The specimen is inoculated directly onto a culture plate. **D,** The specimen can be brought directly to the laboratory or transported through the mail. **E,** Antibiotic sensitivity testing with the disk diffusion method. **F,** This Gram-stained specimen from corneal tissue shows Gram-negative diplobacilli (*Moraxella*).

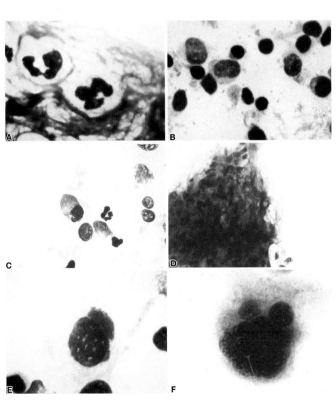

Fig. 11.2 Giemsa stain cytology. A, Polymorphonuclear cells; **B,** mononuclear and epithelial cells; **C,** plasma cell in center; **D,** *Acanthamoeba* cyst in center; **E,** dark purple chlamydial inclusion caps peripheral to nucleus of epithelial cell; **F,** corneal multinucleated epithelial cell from herpes simplex virus (HSV) keratitis.

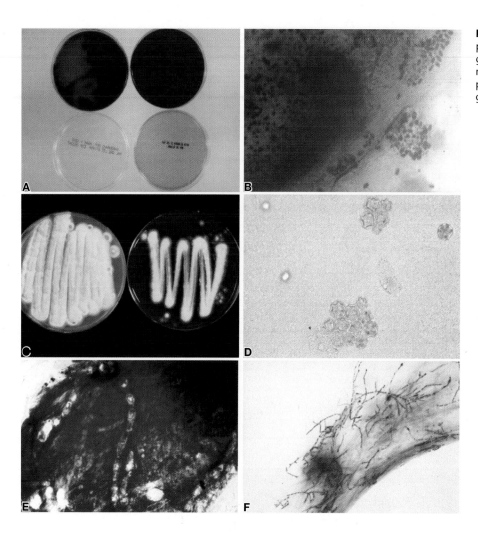

Fig. 11.3 Bacterial laboratory diagnosis. A, Routine culture agar plates; **B,** *Microsporidia* spores from stained corneal specimen; **C,** mold growing on agar plates; **D,** *Acanthamoeba* hexagonal cysts on non-nutrient agar with *Enterobacter aerogenes* overlay; **E,** *Candida albicans* pseudohyphae on giemsa-stained corneal specimen; **F,** *Actinomyces* on giemsa-stained corneal tissue.

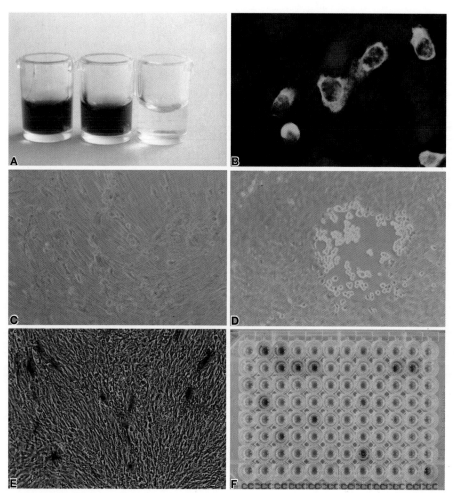

Fig. 11.4 Laboratory diagnosis of viral infection. A, In the Adenoclone test, the presence of andenovirus antigen produces a blue color change in the reaction well. **B,** In the shell vial test, infected cells are stained with monoclonal antibodies conjugated with fluorescein isothiocyanate that appears apple-green using a fluorescent microscope. **C,** When adenovirus is inoculated onto A549 monolayer cells, cell rounding is seen. Adenovirus is confirmed with the Adenoclone test. **D,** When HSV is inoculated onto A549 monolayer cells, cell rounding is seen. HSV is confirmed with an antigen test. **E,** In the enzyme-linked virus-induced system (ELVIS) test, the presence of HSV is indicated by a blue color within the cells. **F,** A positive enzyme-linked immunosorbent assay (ELISA) for chlamydial DNA after polymerase chain reaction (PCR) amplification is seen.

Bacterial Infections

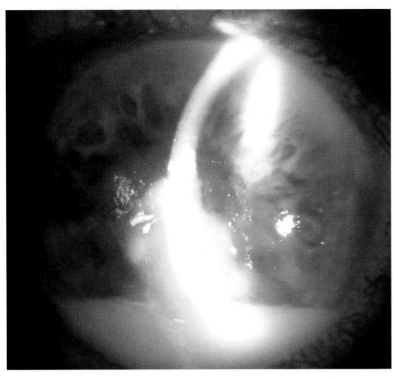

Fig. 11.5 Acute bacterial keratitis. This infection is associated with symptoms of pain, redness, and decreased vision. Here there is a central corneal ulcer caused by *Staphylococcus aureus* and an anterior chamber reaction severe enough to produce a hypopyon.

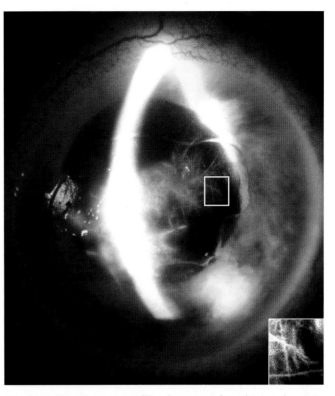

Fig. 11.6 Infectious crystalline keratopathy. This is a descriptive term for a keratitis that has a crystalline appearance in the stroma (inset). The most common bacterial organisms implicated are the *Streptococcus viridans* group (specifically, nutritionally variant streptococci). In this case the causative organism was *Enterococcus faecalis*. Fungal keratitis and calcium deposits can have a similar appearance. The crystalline appearance results from the pattern of the organism within the corneal stroma and a lack of any host inflammatory response (an abundance of white cells would obscure the pattern.). The nutritionally variant streptococci may be difficult to culture on routine media, and the clinical response to antibiotics may not correlate with in vitro sensitivities. Infectious crystalline keratopathy occurs more commonly in patients with corneal grafts (see Fig. 20.29).

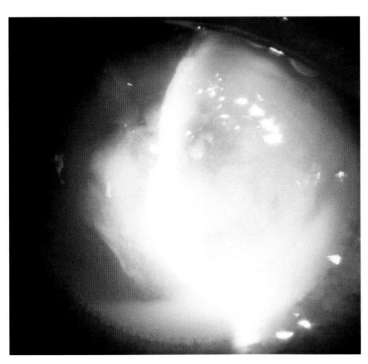

Fig. 11.7 Pseudomonas keratitis in a soft contact lens wearer. There is extensive tissue destruction and a layered hypopyon.

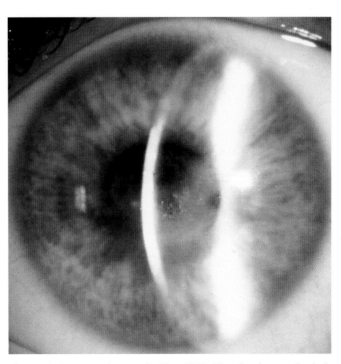

Fig. 11.8 Same patient as in Fig. 11.7. The ulcer has resolved after treatment with fortified antibiotics, and there is corneal scarring.

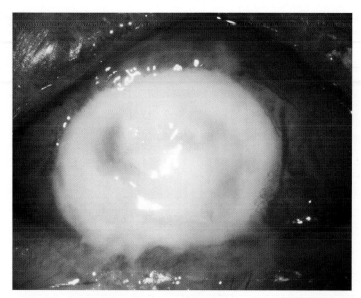

Fig. 11.9 Severe bacterial keratitis with infectious scleritis caused by Pseudomonas organisms. *Pseudomonas* infections can be associated with a large degree of tissue destruction because of enzymes and exotoxins released from the organisms and a vigorous host inflammatory response. The prognosis with scleral extension is extremely poor.

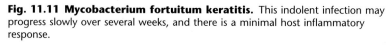

Fig. 11.10 Mycobacterium keratitis. These infections usually arise after trauma or surgical intervention. This patient had dirt kicked into his eye. The periphery of the infiltrate has a characteristic "frosted glass" appearance (inset).

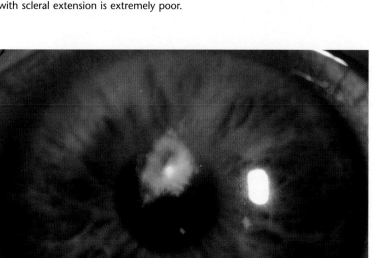

Fig. 11.11 Mycobacterium fortuitum keratitis. This indolent infection may progress slowly over several weeks, and there is a minimal host inflammatory response.

Herpes Simplex Keratitis

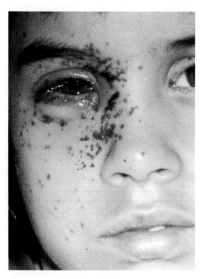

Fig. 11.12 Primary herpes simplex infection of the facial skin. There are multiple vesicular lesions, some of which are crusted over. A blepharoconjunctivitis is present in the right eye.

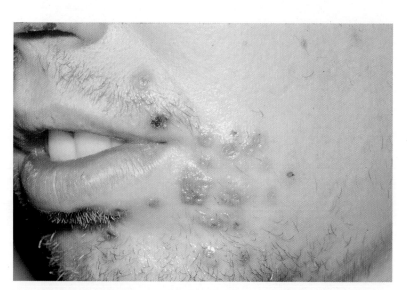

Fig. 11.13 Recurrent herpes simplex vesicles around the mouth. These lesions are usually painless and resolve in 2–3 weeks without scarring.

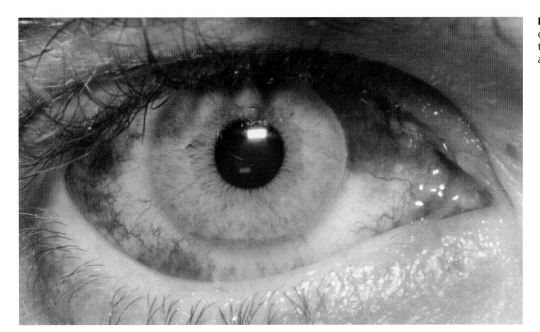

Fig. 11.14 Same patient as in Fig. 11.13. Note the diffuse conjunctivitis. With primary herpes infections, there may be a follicular response and preauricular adenopathy.

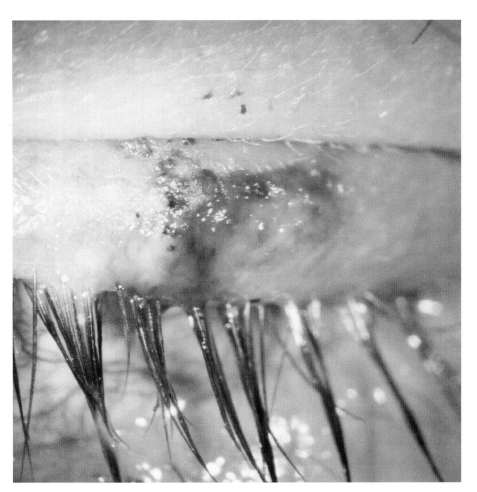

Fig. 11.15 Magnified view of herpes blepharitis. An ulcerative lesion is present on the skin.

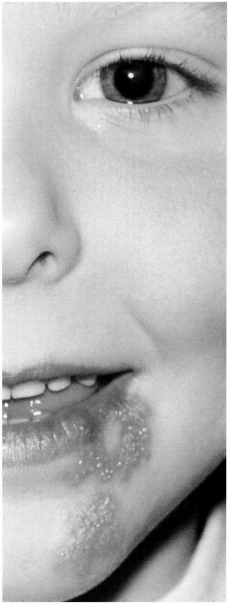

Fig. 11.16 Herpes simplex infection of the skin with conjunctivitis. A corneal scar is present from previous infections.

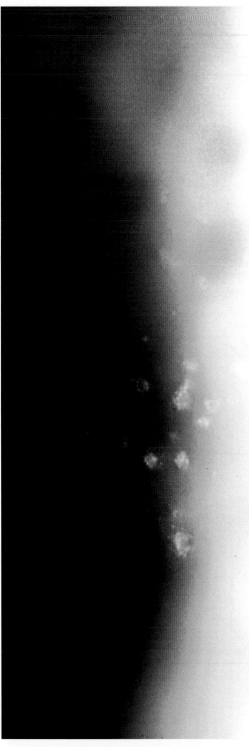

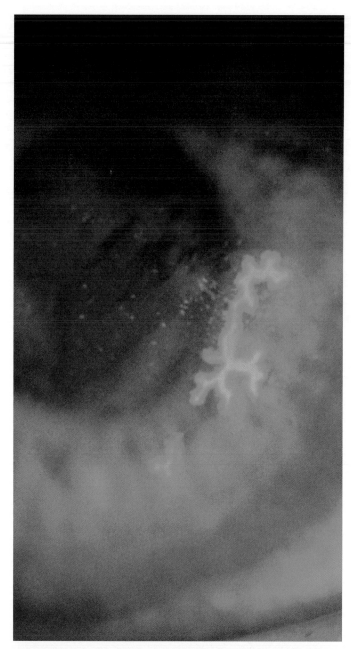

Fig. 11.18 Same patient as in Fig. 11.17, 1 week later with a typical dendrite. The epithelial defect stains with fluorescein. The peripheral cells lining the dendrite are often raised and contain active virus. These cells stain with rose bengal. When the dendrite resolves, scarring occurs.

Fig. 11.17 Earliest stage of epithelial keratitis. Small punctate vesicular lesions can be seen in the epithelium. These coalesce into plaques that eventually enlarge to form dendrites. It is rare to see this early stage.

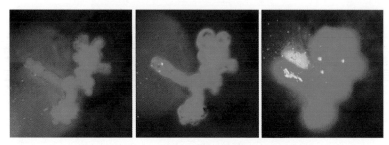

Fig. 11.19 Herpes simplex dendritic ulcer fluorescein staining with time. Immediate view (left) shows the true ulcer. After 1 minute (middle) the stain spreads slightly. In 3 minutes (right) the stain moves into the surrounding epithelium giving a false impression of the size of the ulcer.

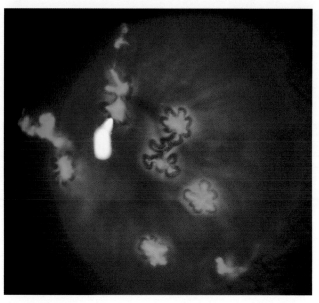

Fig. 11.20 Herpes simplex keratitis with multiple epithelial dendrites.

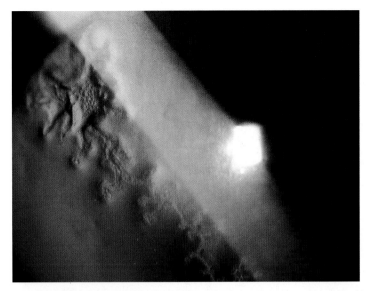

Fig. 11.21 Herpes simplex keratitis. The opened portion of the dendrite is seen in the upper left (geographic ulcer); the remaining closed portion (dendritic ulcer) is also seen. Notable is that herpes extends beneath the epithelium and into the stroma. When these ulcers heal, a scar forms.

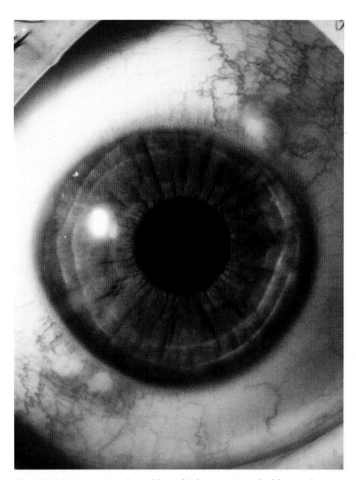

Fig. 11.24 Herpes simplex with multiple conjunctival phlyctenules.

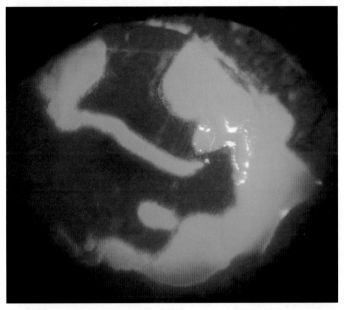

Fig. 11.22 Herpes simplex keratitis with a large geographic ulcer. These ulcers take longer to heal than dendritic ulcers.

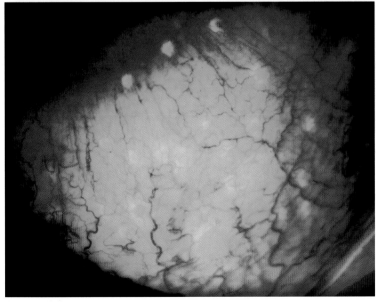

Fig. 11.23 Herpes simplex conjunctival ulcers.

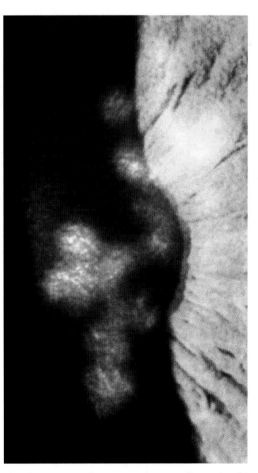

Fig. 11.25 Anterior stromal scars. "Footprints" in a pattern of herpetic ulceration indicate previous herpetic infection.

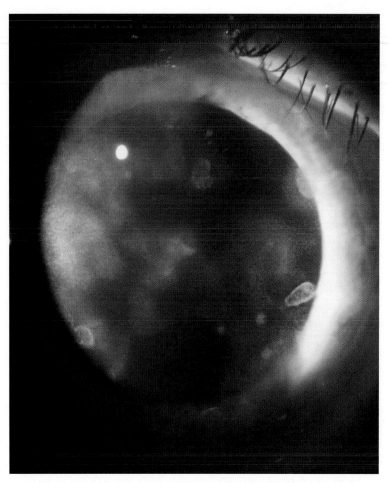

Fig. 11.26 Herpes simplex scars with typical "ground glass" appearance.

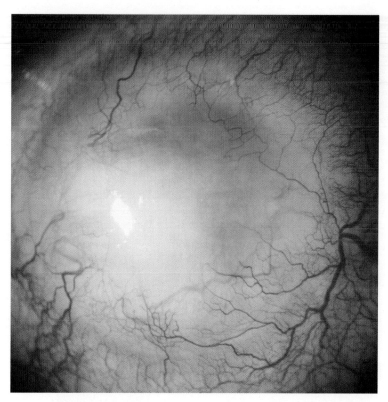

Fig. 11.27 Herpes simplex. Advanced scarring and vascularization are seen.

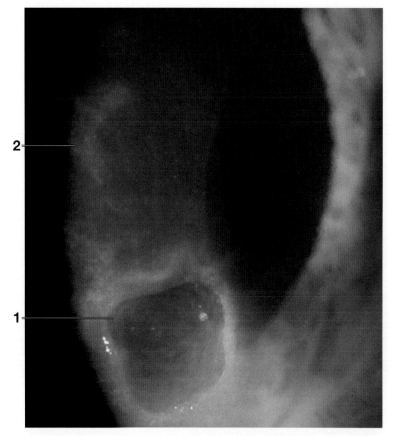

2 —

1 —

Fig. 11.28 Neurotrophic (metaherpetic) ulcer (1). These ulcers are usually round, oblong, or square, and have a characteristic broad, rolled-up, epithelial edge. Anterior stromal scarring—evidence of a previous infection with herpes simplex virus—is seen (2).

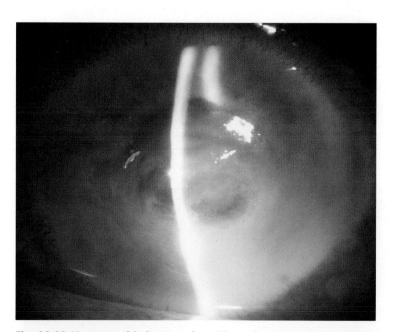

Fig. 11.29 Neurotrophic herpes ulcer. These ulcers occur in eyes with long-standing herpetic disease and are caused by corneal anesthesia rather than active viral infection. Typically, these ulcers are in the lower half of the cornea.

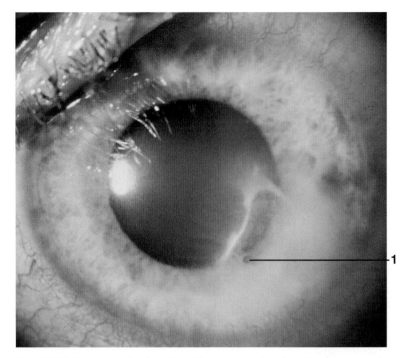

Fig. 11.30 Herpes simplex keratitis with corneal perforation (1).

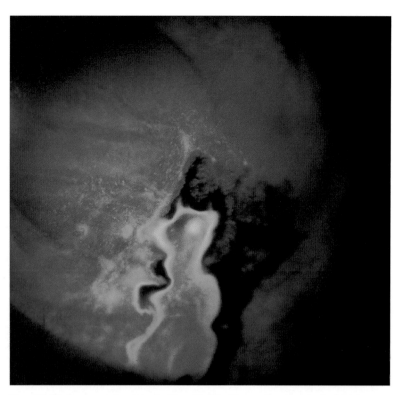

Fig. 11.31 Same patient as in Fig. 11.30. The perforation site is Seidel positive.

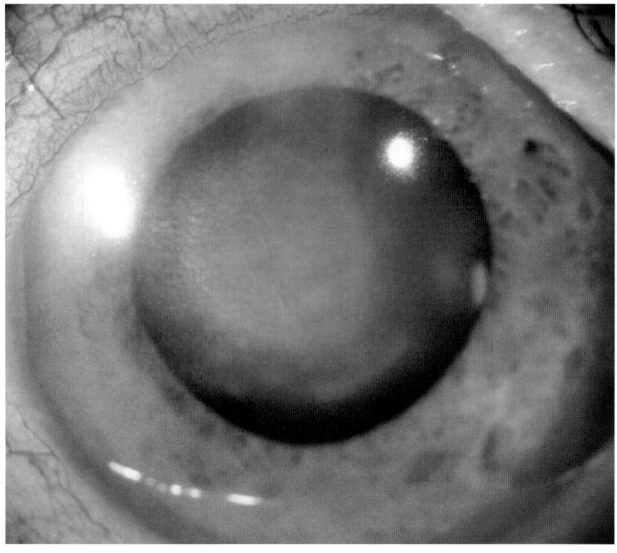

Fig. 11.32 Herpes simplex disciform keratitis. There is a circular area of corneal edema. Although not seen here, keratic precipitates may be seen on the corneal endothelium, and there may be a low-grade iritis. The intraocular pressure is often raised.

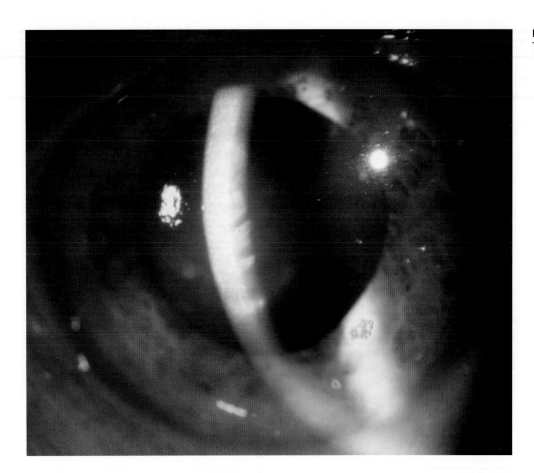

Fig. 11.33 Slit-beam view of disciform keratitis. There is central corneal edema.

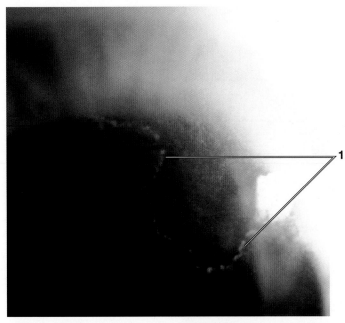

Fig. 11.34 Herpes simplex linear endotheliitis. This rare condition progresses similarly to a corneal allograft rejection. A line of keratic precipitates (1) begins near the limbus and progresses centrally. The cornea is edematous between the advancing line and the limbus. In some patients the condition is bilateral, and may follow cataract surgery. Untreated, this condition may result in permanent corneal decompensation.

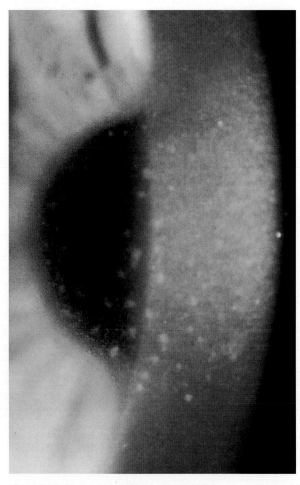

Fig. 11.35 Herpes simplex keratouveitis. In contrast to disciform keratitis, there is diffuse corneal edema and the uveitis is more pronounced. A hypopyon may occur.

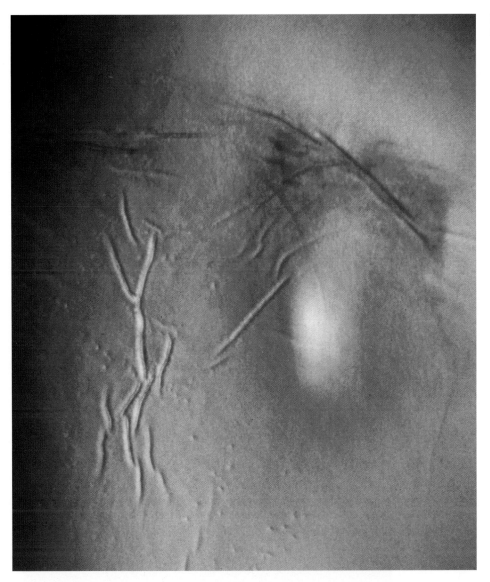

Fig. 11.36 Herpes simplex. Areas of Descemet's proliferation are evident.

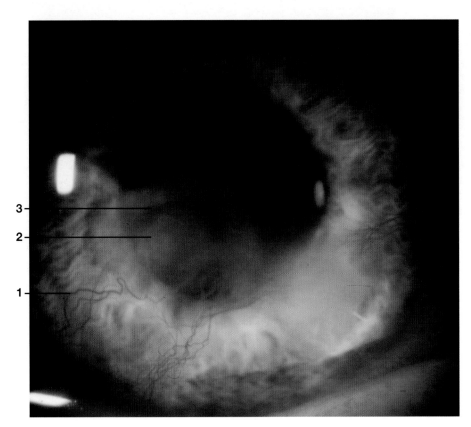

Fig. 11.37 Herpes simplex interstitial keratitis. This is characterized by stromal infiltration and vascularization with an intact epithelium. Here there is vascularization (1) and scarring (2) of the corneal stroma, with a line of iron (3) in the epithelium.

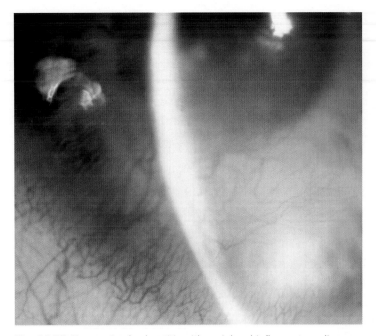

Fig. 11.38 Herpes simplex keratitis with peripheral inflammatory disease.

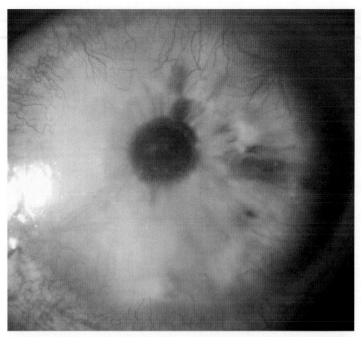

Fig. 11.39 Chronic keratouveitis caused by herpes simplex virus. Keratic precipitates are seen centrally, and there is diffuse corneal haze with stromal vascularization.

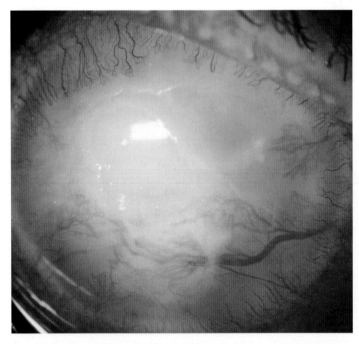

Fig. 11.40 Necrotizing herpes simplex keratitis. Necrotizing infections are characterized by ulceration with tissue loss. This is one of the most serious forms of keratitis because tissue loss can lead to perforation. It is not known whether this form of keratitis results from active viral infection of the stroma or an immunologic reaction to viral antigens.

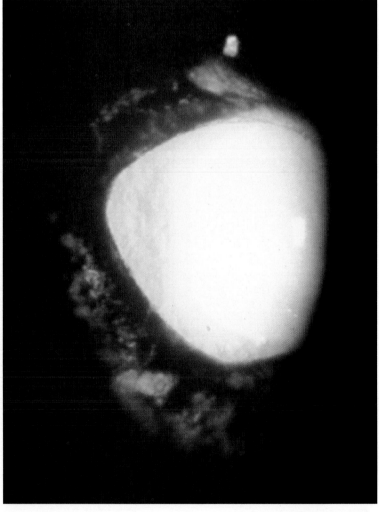

Fig. 11.41 Diffuse iris atrophy caused by recurrent herpes simplex keratouveitis.

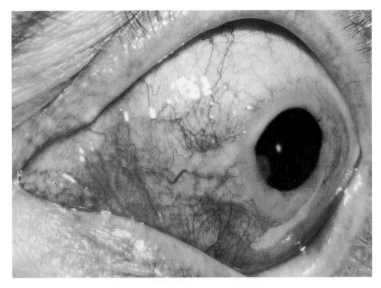

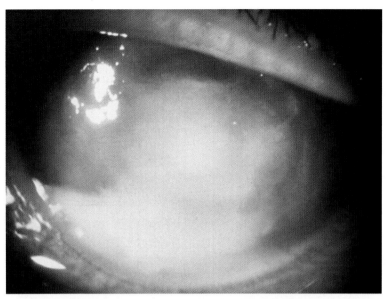

Fig. 11.42 Herpes simplex scleritis. There is diffuse injection of the conjunctiva and deep episcleral vessels, and the inflammation extends into the sclera. This condition is characterized by severe pain and is often difficult to treat.

Fig. 11.43 Chronic herpes simplex keratitis with secondary bacterial infection. Eyes with this disorder are more susceptible to secondary infection. Here there is an extensive corneal ulcer caused by *Moraxella* organisms.

Herpes Zoster Keratitis

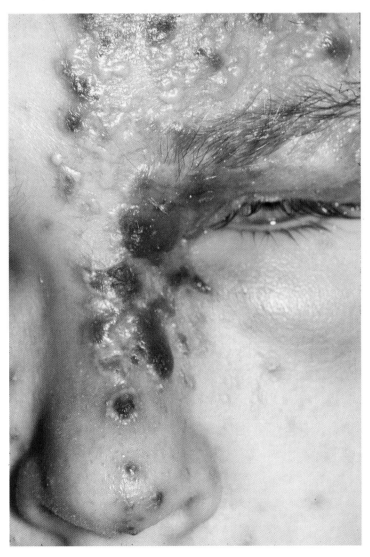

Fig. 11.44 Herpes zoster keratitis. This patient has vesicular and crusted lesions from herpes zoster infection in the distribution of the first division of the fifth cranial nerve. If the tip of the nose is involved (as in this case), it is likely that there is ocular involvement, as both regions are supplied by the nasociliary nerve (Hutchinson's sign).

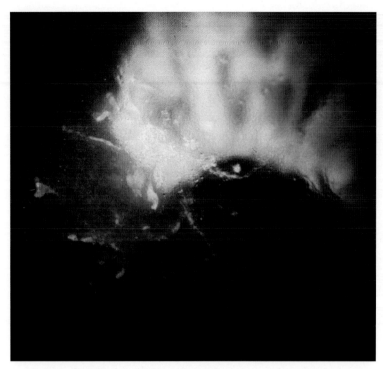

Fig. 11.45 Epithelial dendrites from herpes zoster infection. In contrast to the dendrites seen in herpes simplex infection, these lesions are elevated and appear as mucous plaques stuck on the epithelium. In addition, these dendrites are coarser and do not have the terminal bulbs seen in herpes simplex.

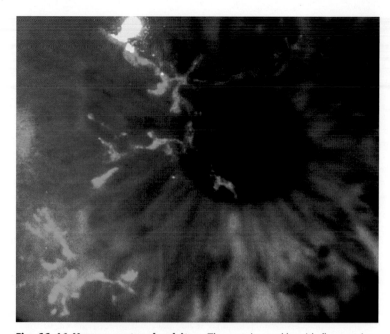

Fig. 11.46 Herpes zoster dendrites. These stain weakly with fluorescein.

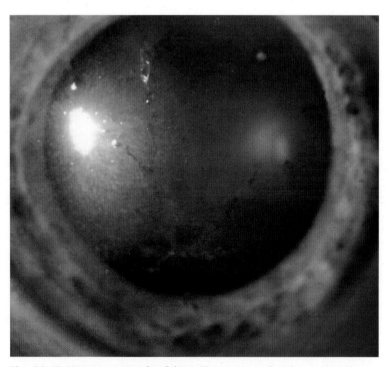

Fig. 11.47 Herpes zoster dendrites. These stain well with rose bengal.

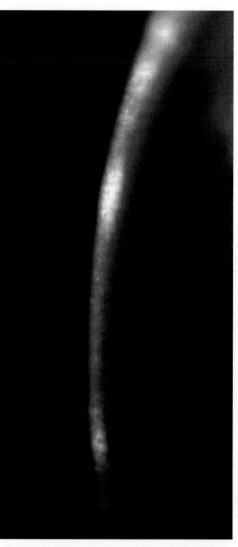

Fig. 11.48 Subepithelial infiltrates in herpes zoster ophthalmicus. These infiltrates probably represent an immunologic reaction to viral proteins. Similar to the subepithelial infiltrates in epidemic keratoconjunctivitis, these occur 10–14 days after the onset of active disease and respond to treatment with topical corticosteroids. They may recur many months to years after active infection.

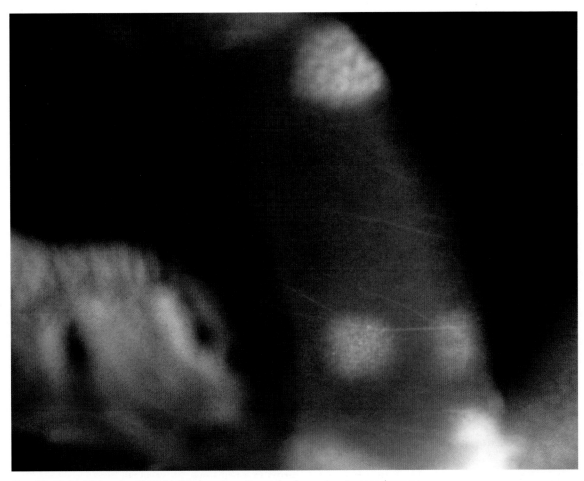

Fig. 11.49 Multiple subepithelial infiltrates along the path of prominent corneal nerves.

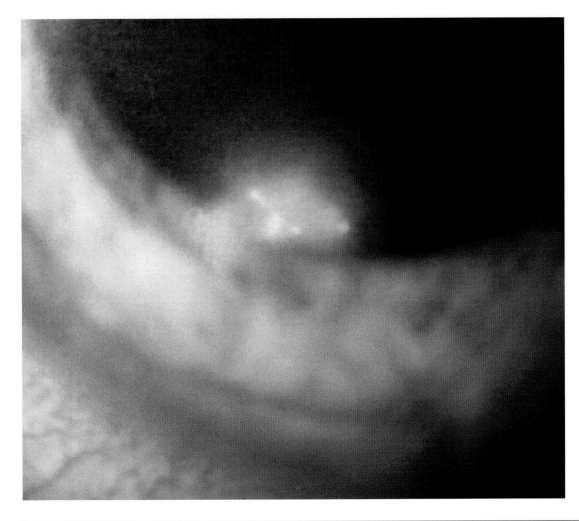

Fig. 11.50 Herpes zoster. Some patients develop a stromal infiltrate. This patient has an infiltrate near the limbus.

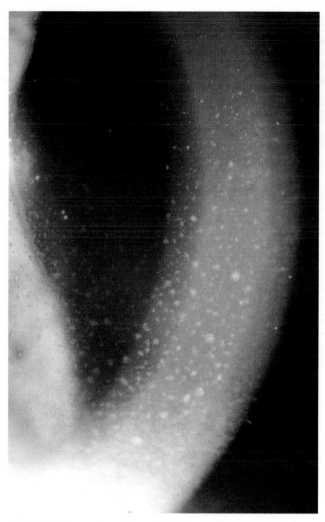

Fig. 11.51 Large keratic precipitates in herpes zoster uveitis. This uveitis may begin with the initial herpes attack and can persist or recur for years after the initial episode. At least half of the patients with zoster uveitis have increased intraocular pressure, which in some cases can lead to severe glaucoma. Patients may need to be maintained chronically on low-dose topical corticosteroids to prevent reactivation.

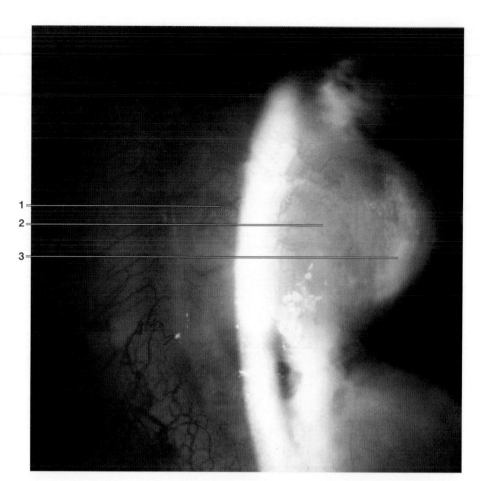

Fig. 11.52 Herpes zoster keratitis in a right eye. Although not limited to previous herpes zoster infection, the findings in this patient should alert the examiner to that possibility. There is a combination of temporal location, vascularization (1), scarring (2), and lipid deposition (3).

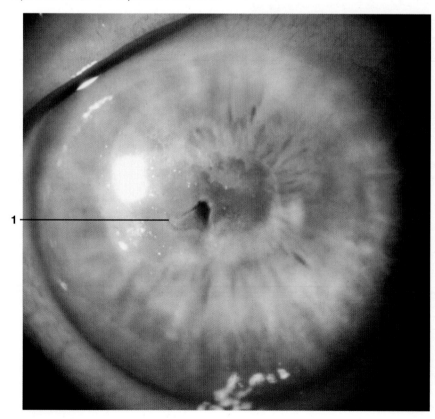

Fig. 11.53 Diffuse corneal scarring from herpes zoster ophthalmicus. Scarring may result from inflammatory disease of the corneal stroma or chronic surface problems. This eye has a small central epithelial defect (1). Surface problems may be caused by many factors, including corneal anesthesia, dry eye, lagophthalmos, entropion, and ectropion.

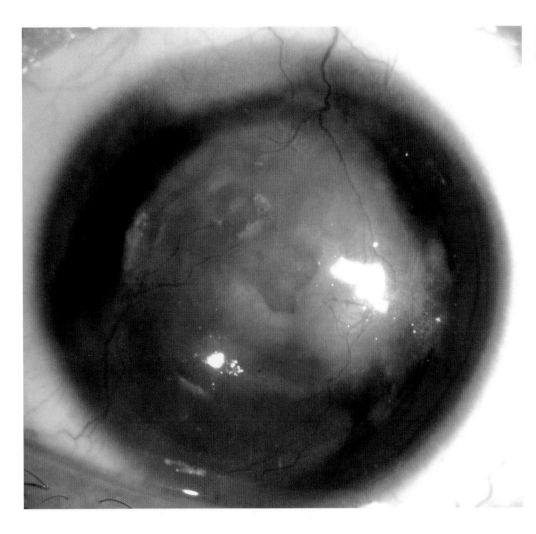

Fig. 11.54 Herpes zoster keratitis, old scar. Chronic inflammation leads to severe scarring and vascularization of the cornea.

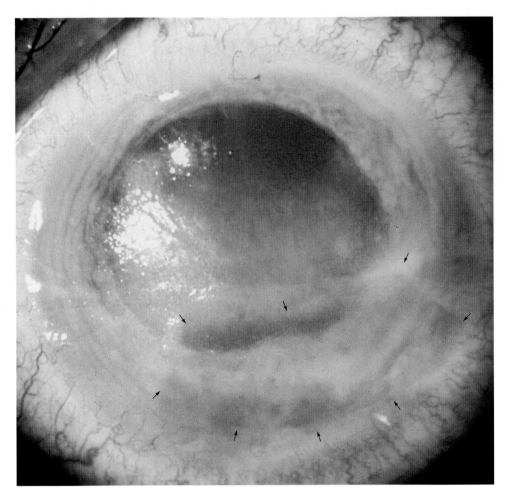

Fig. 11.55 Herpes zoster ophthalmicus with a neurotrophic ulcer. The lesion (arrows) is characteristically oval, has broad, gray epithelial edges, and is usually located in the lower half of the cornea. If untreated, these lesions often progress to perforation. Treatment includes increasing corneal lubrication and coverage of the lesion with a tarsorrhaphy or, in extreme cases, a conjunctival flap. Topical corticosteroids are not indicated.

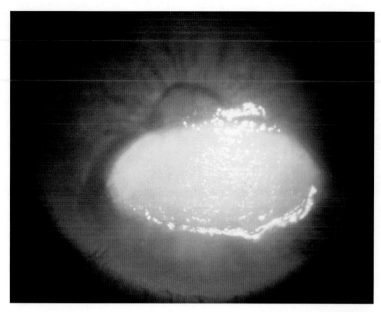

Fig. 11.56 Herpes zoster ophthalmicus with an indolent corneal ulcer. The ulcer is shallow, with fairly discrete edges and a dense, very level base. Predisposing factors include corneal anesthesia, dry eye, and lid abnormalities.

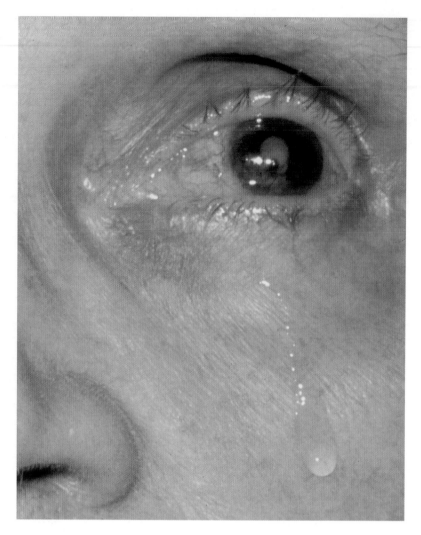

Fig. 11.58 Corneal perforation from a chronic herpes zoster neurotrophic ulcer. There is an aqueous tear on the patient's cheek.

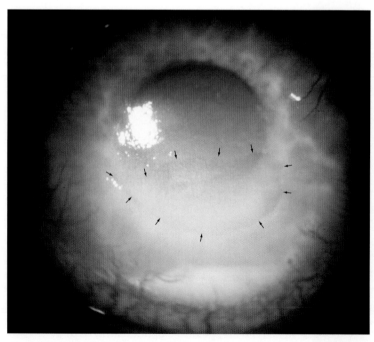

Fig. 11.57 Neurotrophic ulcer (arrows) after a herpes zoster infection. This patient has a hypopyon; although this is not infectious, it is prudent to obtain routine cultures and treat with antibiotics until the diagnosis is certain.

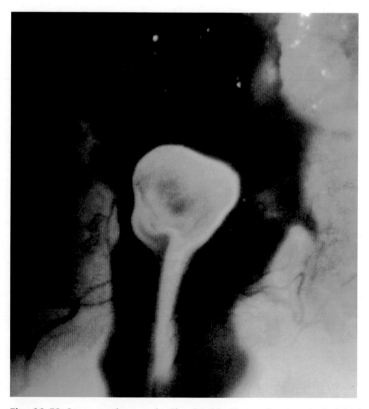

Fig. 11.59 Same patient as in Fig. 11.58. The perforation site is Seidel positive.

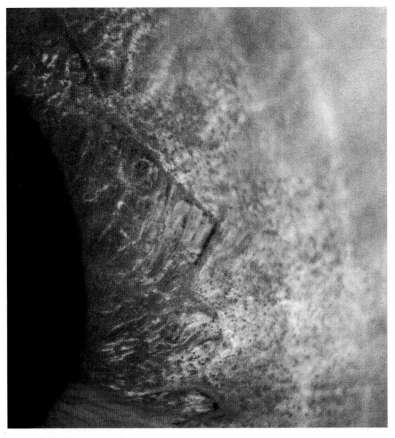

Fig. 11.60 Sectoral iris atrophy in herpes zoster. This finding is attributed to a localized vasculitis.

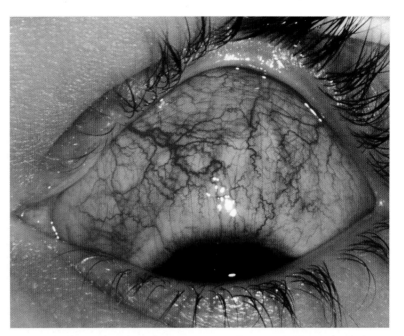

Fig. 11.61 Herpes zoster scleritis 2 weeks after the initial episode of herpes zoster infection. This process was localized to the superior sclera. Like other forms of scleritis, it is extremely painful.

Fungal Keratitis

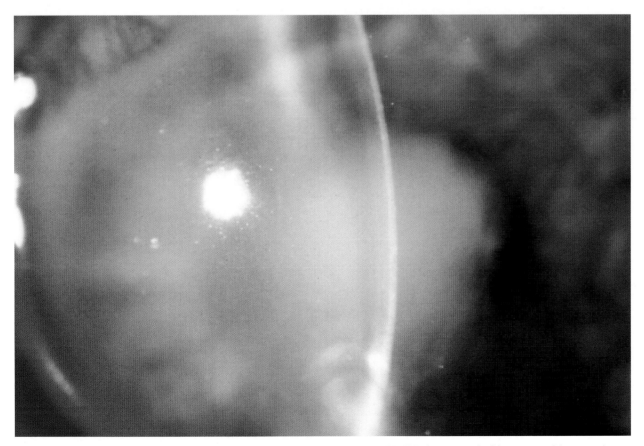

Fig. 11.62 Candida keratitis. This case resulted in an anterior chamber "puff ball." The patient had been treated for several weeks with intensive topical corticosteroids for an unexplained keratitis.

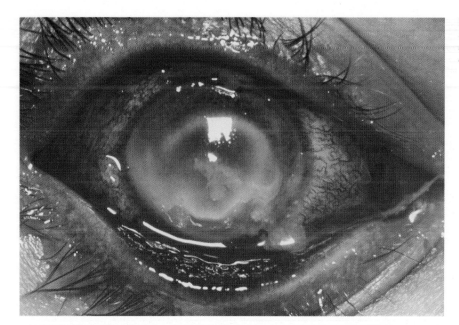

Fig. 11.63 Fungal keratitis. Infection with filamentous fungi is usually associated with outdoor trauma, particularly from vegetable matter. This is a case of an *Aspergillus* corneal ulcer. There is a ring infiltrate, and the edges of the infiltrate have a feathery appearance.

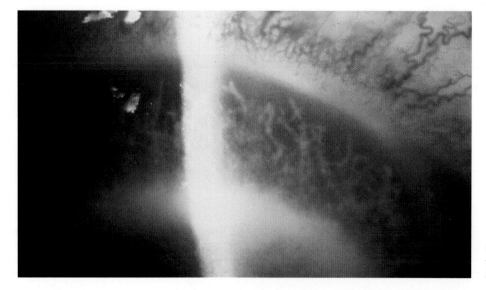

Fig. 11.64 Fungal keratitis. This is a higher magnification of the infiltrate in an *Aspergillus* corneal ulcer. The edges are indistinct and have filamentary extensions.

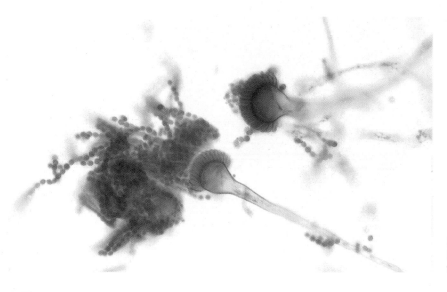

Fig. 11.65 Aspergillus infection, shown by lactophenol cotton blue stain. Septate hyphae with phialides are seen on top of swollen vesicles. The phialides produce chains of round conidia spores.

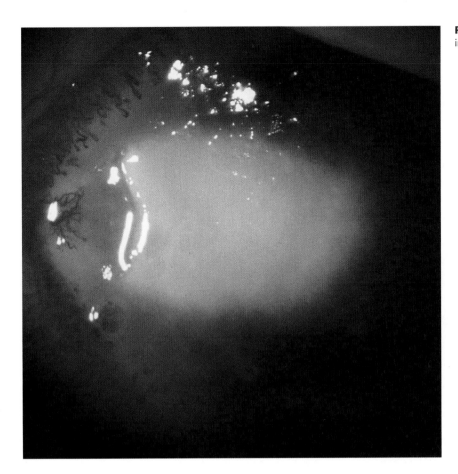

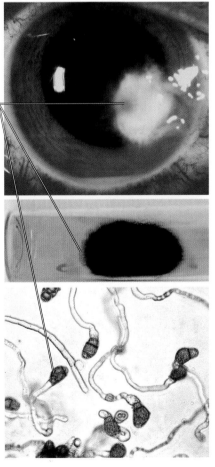

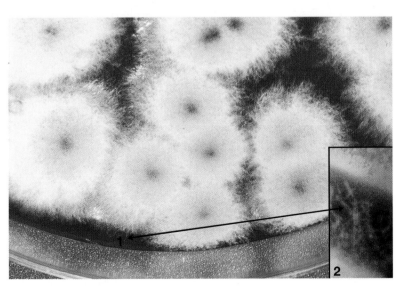

Fig. 11.66 Fusarium infection of the cornea. There is a dense stromal infiltrate with indistinct margins.

Fig. 11.67 Filamentous growth on blood agar from a patient with Fusarium keratitis. The growth on the agar plate (1) is similar to that on the cornea (2) of the patient in Fig. 11.64.

Fig. 11.68 Curvularia keratitis. *Curvularia* is a dematiaceous fungus (with a brown or black coloration). Brown pigmentation (1) is seen in the patient (top), the Sabouraud's culture (middle), and the slide preparation (bottom).

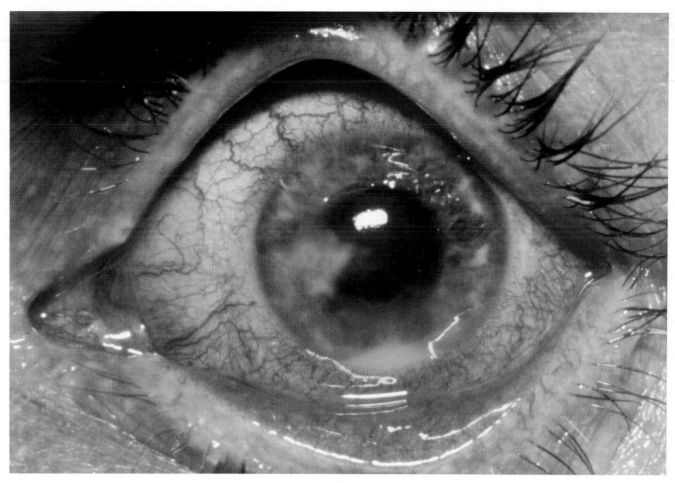

Fig. 11.69 Fungal keratitis. This deep ulcer with hypopyon was caused by *Cephalosporium* infection. It did not respond to medical treatment.

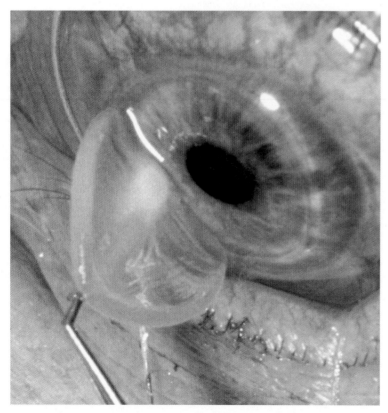

Fig. 11.70 Same patient as in Fig. 11.69 during penetrating keratoplasty. The deep infiltrate can be seen on the posterior cornea. There is fibrin overlying the lens.

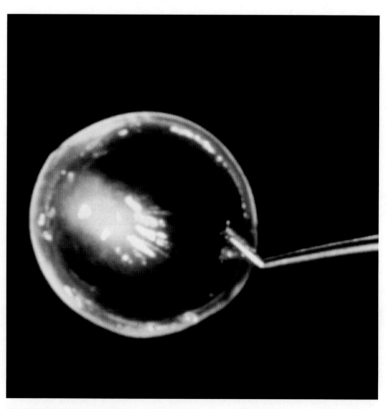

Fig. 11.71 Same patient as in Figs 11.69 and 11.70. The excised host button with fungal infiltrate is shown.

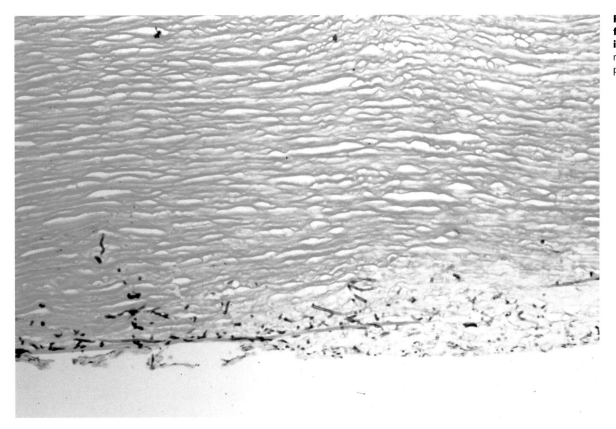

Fig. 11.72 Histopathology of fungal keratitis in same patient as in Figs 11.69–11.71. Hyphae with right-angled branching pattern are seen penetrating the deep posterior cornea.

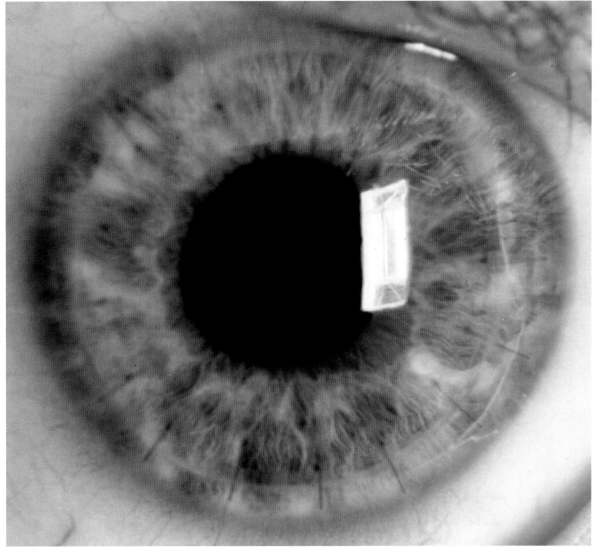

Fig. 11.73 Same patient as in Figs 11.69–11.72. There is a clear graft 1 year after penetrating keratoplasty.

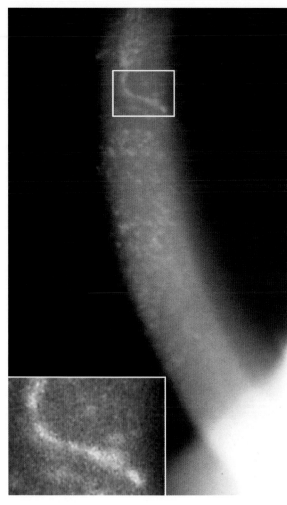

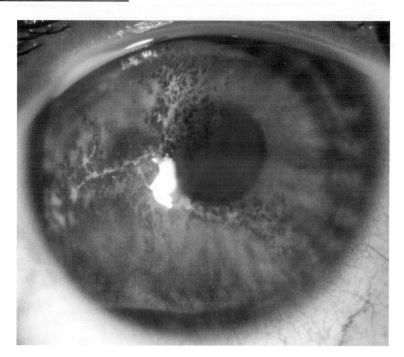

Fig. 11.75 *Acanthamoeba* keratitis. Fluorescein staining shows a dendritic pattern similar to that of herpes simplex keratitis. In contrast to the dendrites seen in herpes simplex infection, these lesions are more irregularly shaped and do not have terminal bulbs. At this stage, *Acanthamoeba* keratitis is often misdiagnosed as herpes simplex keratitis. Similar to herpes simplex keratitis, it may have a waxing and waning course, and may respond favorably to topical corticosteroids.

Fig. 11.74 *Acanthamoeba* keratitis. This occurs most commonly in the setting of contact lens wearers who use tap water in their care regimen; however, it can occur with non-contact lens-related trauma. This patient was diagnosed with *Acanthamoeba* keratitis 2 weeks after the onset of symptoms. In the earliest stages there is a diffuse epitheliopathy with multiple intraepithelial linear infiltrates (inset). These linear infiltrates often form dendritic patterns. The diagnosis of *Acanthamoeba* keratitis must be made early, as in this patient, because the prognosis is markedly improved with early detection.

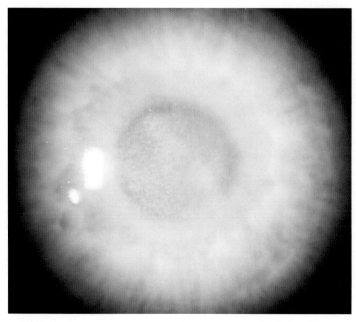

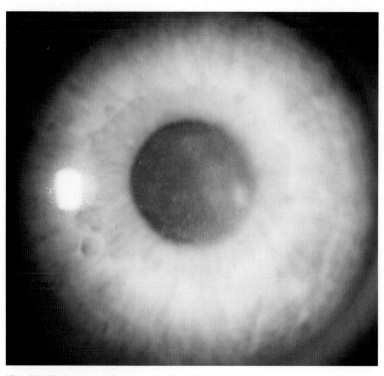

Fig. 11.76 *Acanthamoeba* keratitis with diffuse stromal infiltration.

Fig. 11.77 Same patient as in Fig. 11.76. This is the appearance of the eye after 5 months of treatment.

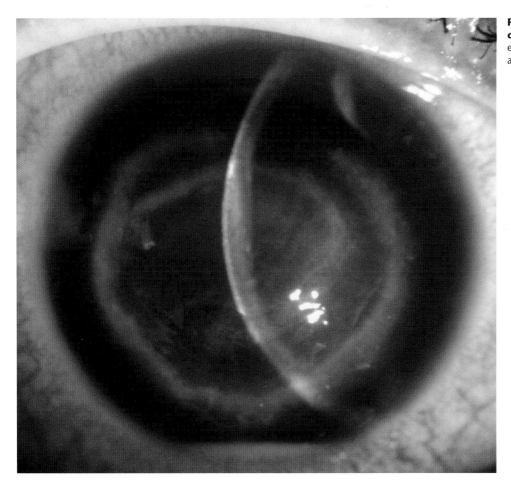

Fig. 11.78 Acanthamoeba keratitis with a characteristic ring infiltrate. The central cornea is edematous and there is a layered hypopyon. A ring infiltrate is a late finding in *Acanthamoeba* keratitis.

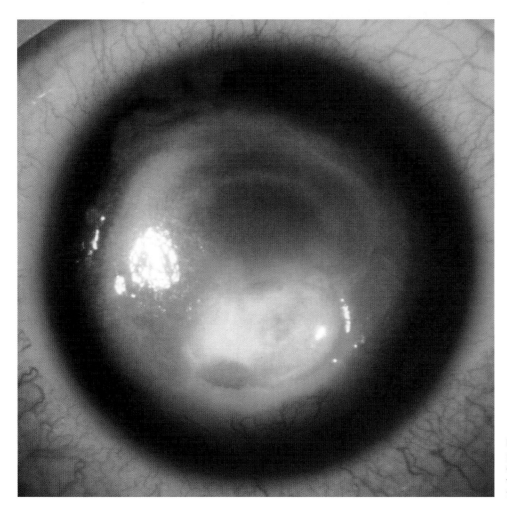

Fig. 11.79 Same patient as in Fig. 11.78. The disease progressed despite 4 months of treatment. This patient eventually required a penetrating keratoplasty. The blood vessels on the inferior cornea suggest a chronic process, as these vessels take weeks to form.

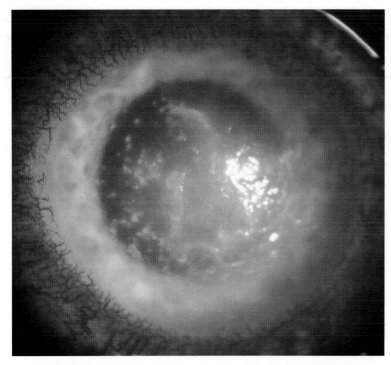

Fig. 11.80 Diffuse *Acanthamoeba* **keratitis with scleritis.** Severe pain usually occurs with both scleritis and keratitis. Early epithelial involvement does not produce severe pain.

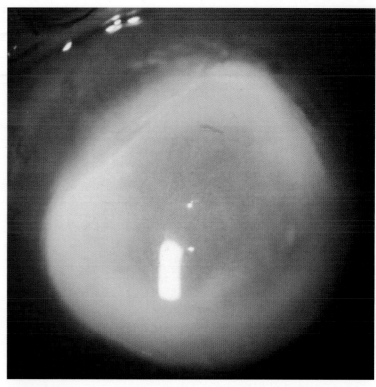

Fig. 11.81 Severe case of *Acanthamoeba* **keratitis, unresponsive to treatment.** This case was complicated by topical anesthetic abuse.

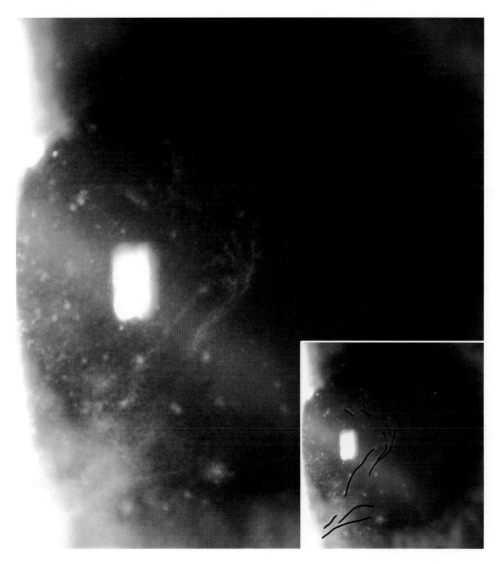

Fig. 11.82 *Acanthamoeba* **keratitis with radial neuritis.** This finding may precede advanced stromal keratitis and is highly suggestive of *Acanthamoeba* infection. It usually begins centrally and progresses peripherally toward the limbus. The inset is a minification of the entire figure. The black lines were drawn to emphasize the pattern of infiltration.

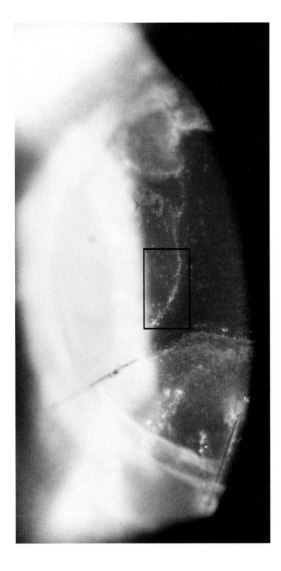

Fig. 11.83 *Acanthamoeba* keratitis. This patient presented with irregular epithelial lines (box) 6 months after penetrating keratoplasty for *Acanthamoeba* infection. Initially these lines were felt to be an epithelial rejection; however, when they failed to respond to topical corticosteroids, a scraping confirmed the diagnosis of recurrent *Acanthamoeba* infection in the graft.

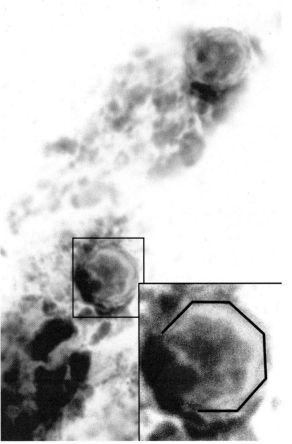

Fig. 11.84 Polygonal *Acanthamoeba* cysts with large nuclei and dark nucleoli. The cysts have a hexagonal shape (inset). When the *Acanthamoeba* infection is in the epithelium (see Figs 11.74, 11.75, and 11.83), a superficial scraping of the involved areas often yields cysts that are readily visible with hematoxylin and eosin or Gram stain. Once the organism is in the corneal stroma, it can be difficult to recover without a corneal biopsy. Culture on a non-nutrient agar plate overlaid with *Escherichia coli* bacteria can establish the diagnosis definitively.

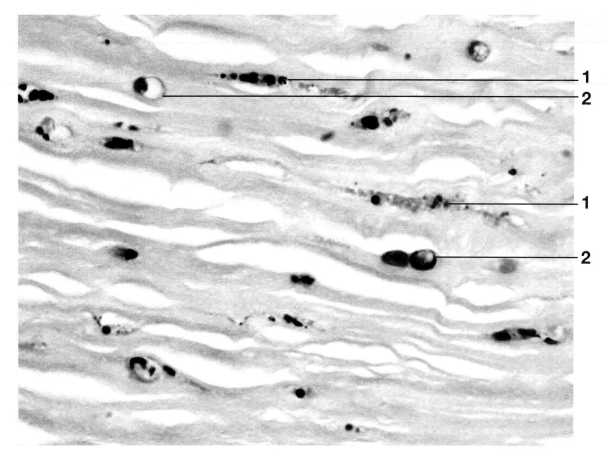

Fig. 11.85 *Acanthamoeba* **hematoxylin and eosin (H&E) stain.** Trophozoites (1) and cysts (2) are seen on this H&E-stained section.

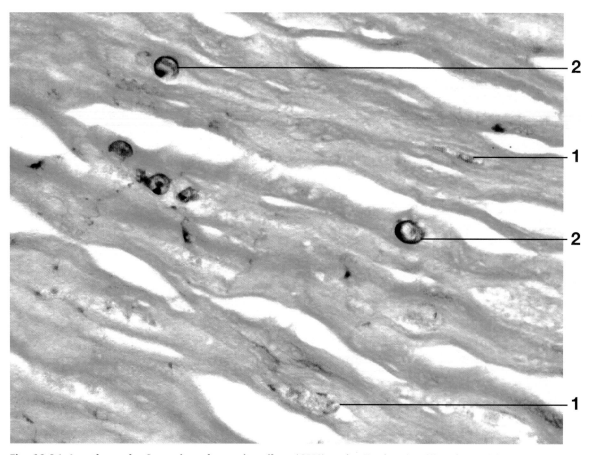

Fig. 11.86 *Acanthamoeba* **Gomori methenamine silver (GMS) stain.** Trophozoites (1) and cysts (2) are seen on this GMS-stained section.

Chapter 12

Interstitial Keratitis

Interstitial keratitis is a non-necrotizing inflammation of the corneal stroma often associated with vascularization. There may be stromal infiltrates or stromal edema. Historically, the most common etiology for interstitial keratitis was syphilis; however, with improved prenatal screening, this cause of interstitial keratitis has become exceedingly rare.

Syphilitic Interstitial Keratitis

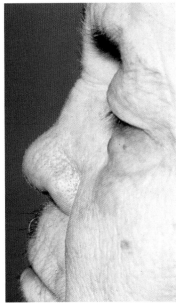

Fig. 12.1

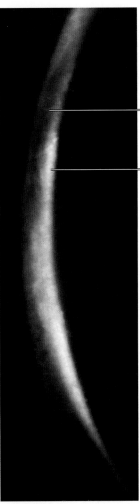

Fig. 12.2

Figs 12.1 and 12.2 Fig.12.1 (above left) shows congenital syphilitic facies, with prominence of the maxillary bone and saddle nose deformity. Fig. 12.2 (above right) is an example of inactive interstitial keratitis. Posterior stromal scarring (1) and ghost vessels (2) are seen.

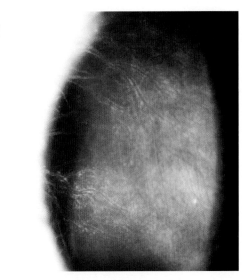

Fig. 12.3 Inactive syphilitic interstitial keratitis. Ghost vessels and diffuse scarring are seen in the cornea. Some of the vessels actually transmit a very small column of blood.

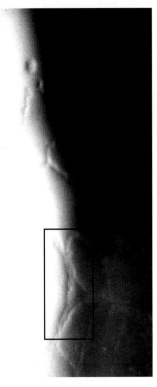

Fig. 12.4 Inactive syphilitic interstitial keratitis. Prior to the use of corticosteroids to treat interstitial keratitis, patients often developed ridges or bands of Descemet's membrane (box).

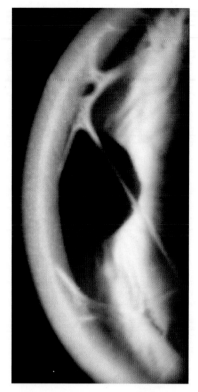

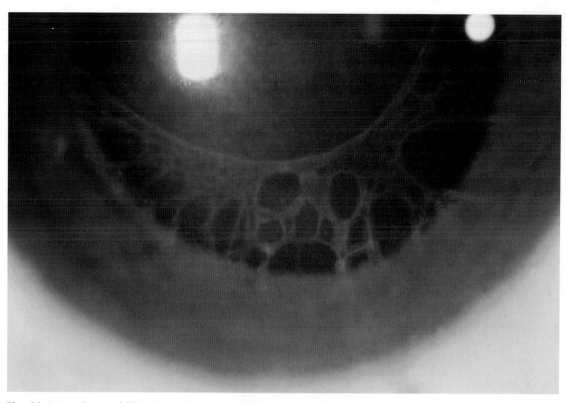

Fig. 12.5 Inactive syphilitic interstitial keratitis. Strands of Descemet's membrane can extend into the anterior chamber, forming a web of interconnecting fibers.

Fig. 12.6 Inactive syphilitic interstitial keratitis. Extensive nets of Descemet's proliferation are seen in diffuse illumination.

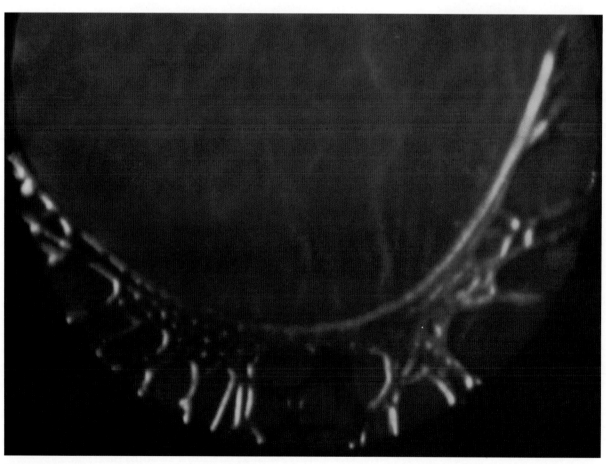

Fig. 12.7 Inactive syphilitic interstitial keratitis. This is the same patient as in Fig. 12.6 with the use of red reflex to demonstrate the thick scrolls of extra basement membrane material.

Nonsyphilitic Interstitial Keratitis

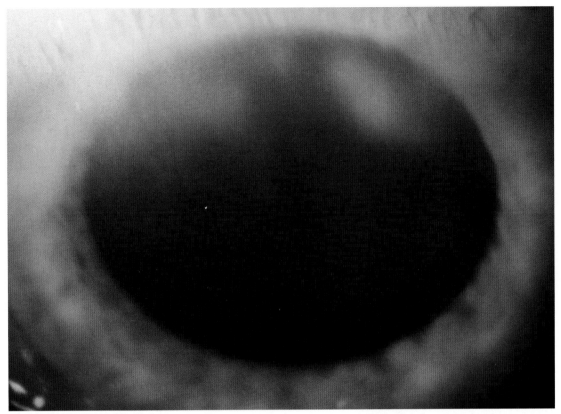

Fig. 12.8 Cogan's syndrome. This consists of interstitial keratitis, vertigo, and hearing loss. The interstitial keratitis usually begins in the peripheral cornea with round, white, stromal opacities. It is important to recognize this diagnosis because early treatment with systemic corticosteroids may prevent permanent hearing loss. Approximately 10% of patients with Cogan's syndrome have evidence of a systemic vasculitis.

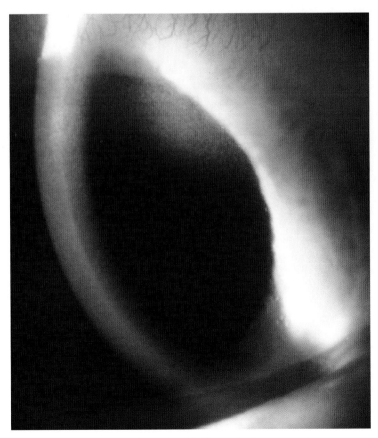

Fig. 12.9 Slit-beam view of peripheral infiltrates in Cogan's syndrome.

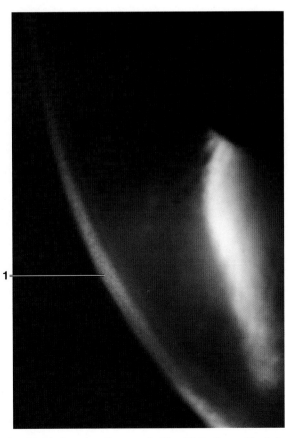

Fig. 12.10 Same patient as in Fig. 12.9, 2 months later. New inflammation is seen inferiorly (1).

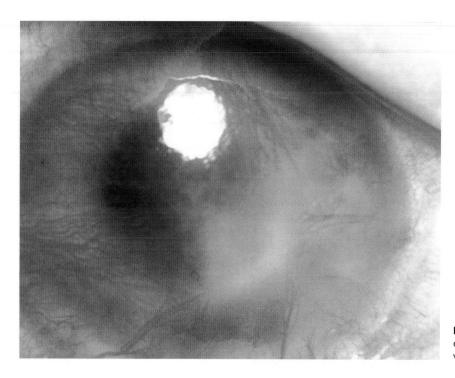

Fig. 12.11 Cogan's syndrome. This patient with a long-standing history of Cogan's disease has active interstitial keratitis with extensive stromal vascularization.

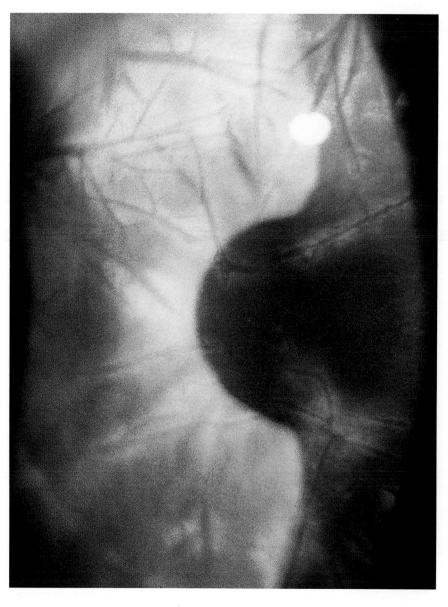

Fig. 12.12 Inactive Cogan's syndrome with stromal scarring and ghost vessels.

Chapter 13

Noninfectious Keratopathy

This chapter discusses noninfectious causes of corneal pathology. Most of these disorders relate to problems with the corneal surface. Some, such as neurotrophic keratopathy, exposure keratopathy, and radiation keratopathy, require aggressive treatment or progressive corneal ulceration may ensue.

Recurrent Erosion Syndrome

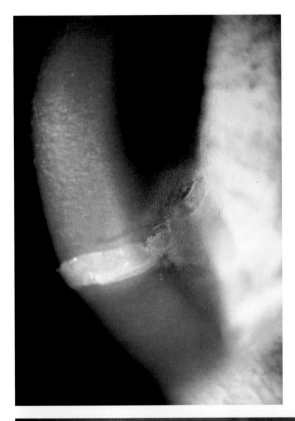

Fig. 13.1 Recurrent erosion syndrome. This is characterized by the sudden onset of ocular pain that often awakens the patient from sleep, although the symptoms can occur at any time. It is associated with a history of prior trauma in the involved eye and may also be accompanied by corneal dystrophy, the two most common being epithelial basement membrane dystrophy and lattice corneal dystrophy. The pathogenesis of traumatic recurrent erosion relates to thickened basement membrane with poor hemidesmosomal attachment to the anterior corneal stroma. In the acute stages the epithelium may be irregular and loose (as seen here), or absent.

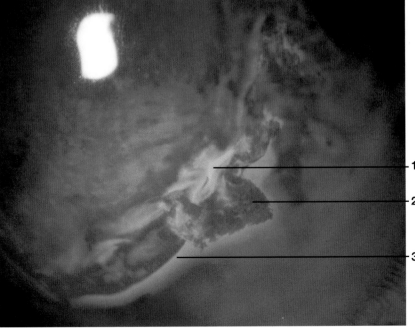

Fig. 13.2 Posttraumatic recurrent erosion in same patient as in Fig. 13.1. Areas of epithelial loss (positive staining) (1), lack of fluorescein over elevated epithelium (negative staining) (2), and pooling of fluorescein (3) are seen.

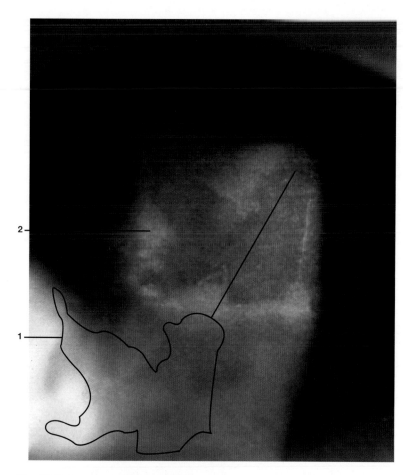

Fig. 13.3 Posttraumatic recurrent erosion. Surrounding the edges of the erosion (1) is a white infiltrate (2). These infiltrates are usually sterile but occasionally may be associated with infections.

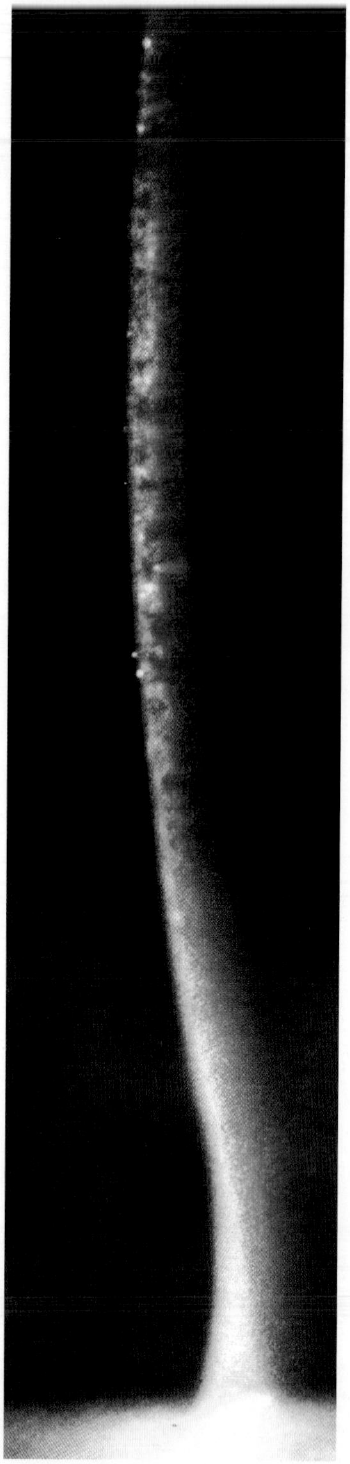

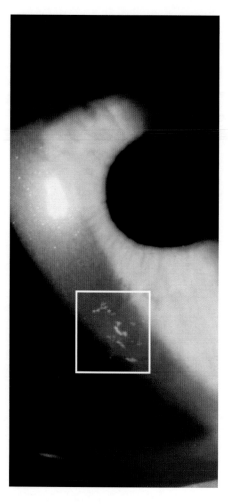

Fig. 13.4 Posttraumatic recurrent erosion. This thin slit-beam view demonstrates anterior stromal haze, which is often associated with chronic recurrent erosions.

Fig. 13.5 Direct view of posttraumatic recurrent erosion with intraepithelial debris (box).

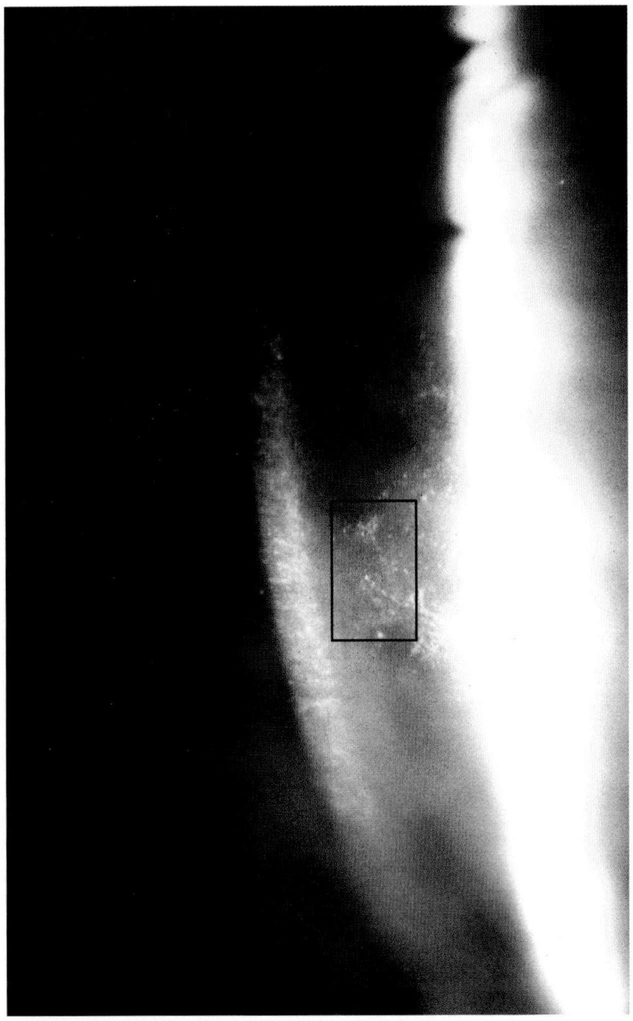

Fig. 13.6 Indirect view of posttraumatic recurrent erosion with intraepithelial debris (box).

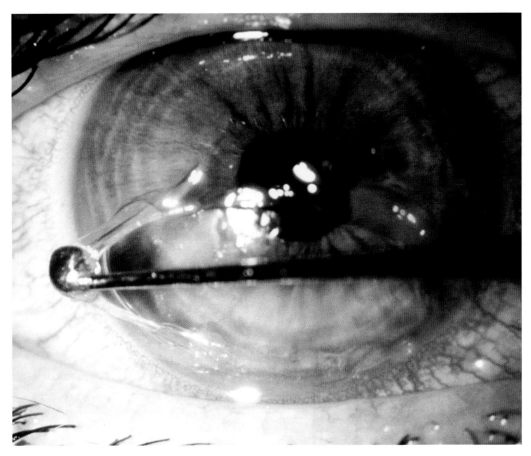

Fig. 13.7 Recurrent erosion syndrome. There is a large area of loose epithelium that extends well beyond the region of the acute erosion. It can sometimes be delineated with a moist cotton swab.

Filamentary Keratitis

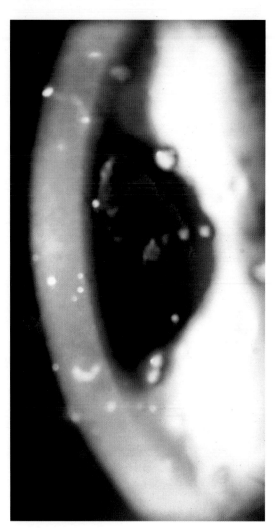

Fig. 13.8 Filamentary keratitis. Filaments are accumulations of mucus attached to loose epithelium. As opposed to free mucus in the tear film, filaments cause a foreign body sensation, remain adherent to the cornea with each blink, and cause a small epithelial defect when removed. Filaments are associated with various conditions, including patching of the eyelids (as seen here), ptosis, dry eye, recurrent erosion, fifth nerve paresis, seventh nerve paresis, chronic bullous keratopathy, superior limbic keratoconjunctivitis, herpes simplex keratitis, and toxicity from topical medications. Administration of 10% acetylcysteine (Mucomyst) dissolves the mucus and may be effective in the treatment of chronic filamentary keratitis.

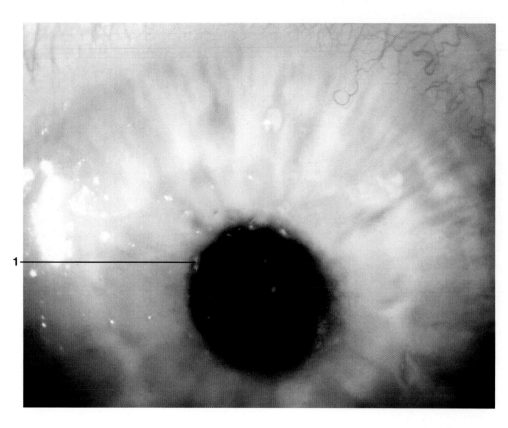

Fig. 13.9 Filamentary keratitis. This patient had a third nerve palsy and resultant ptosis. There are small (micro) filaments (1) on the cornea.

Thygeson's Superficial Punctate Keratitis

Thygeson's superficial punctuate keratitis is a chronic, usually bilateral, disorder characterized by focal epithelial lesions without stromal involvement. It can affect all ages but is more common in children and young adults. Patients complain mainly of foreign body sensation and photophobia. The conjunctiva is uninflamed.

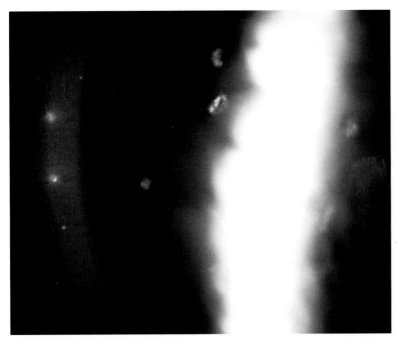

Fig. 13.10 Direct and indirect view of Thygeson's superficial punctate keratitis.

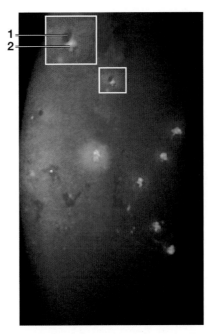

Fig. 13.11 Fluorescein staining of Thygeson's superficial punctate keratitis. Dark areas where fluorescein rolls off elevated edges of lesions (negative staining) (1) and elevated white pearls evident with central fluorescein staining (positive staining) (2) are shown.

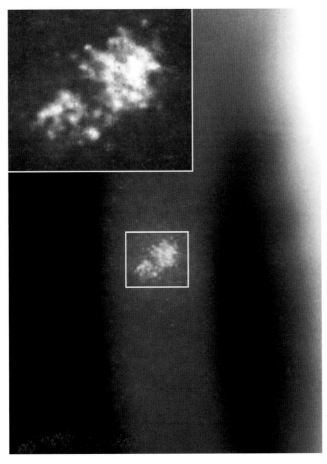

Fig. 13.12 Early Thygeson's superficial punctate keratitis with elevated pearls (inset).

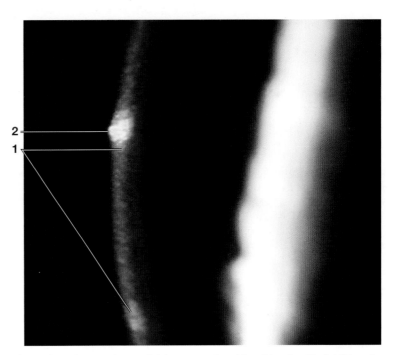

Fig. 13.13 Thygeson's superficial punctate keratitis, with subepithelial (1) and elevated pearly (2) components.

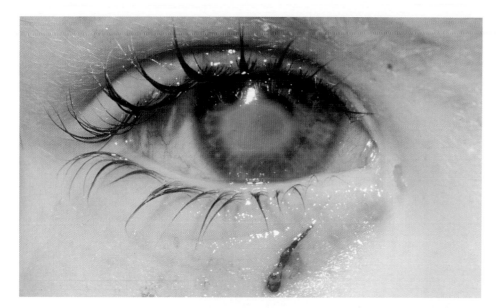

Fig. 13.14 Neurotrophic keratopathy. This is the right eye of a patient with Prader–Willi syndrome and congenital insensitivity to pain. He developed a neurotrophic corneal ulcer in the eye at the age of 2 years. There is an inferior paracentral epithelial defect.

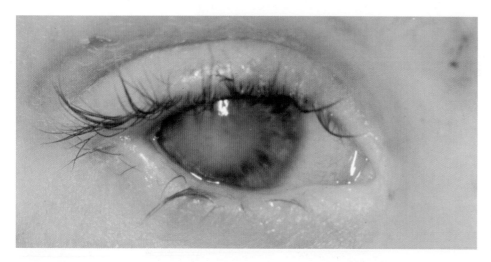

Fig. 13.15 Same patient as in Fig. 13.14, with a corneal scar. The epithelium has healed after treatment with a tarsorrhaphy, punctal occlusion, and aggressive lubrication.

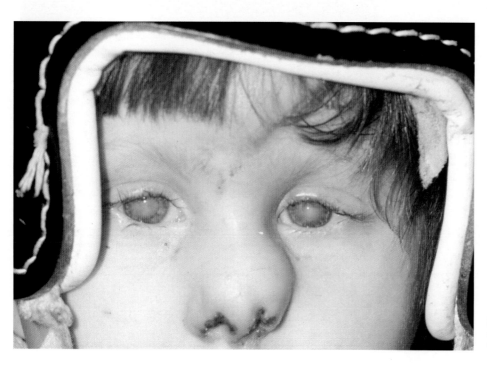

Fig. 13.16 Same patient as in Figs 13.14 and 13.15. There are bilateral corneal scars. The nose deformity is from repetitive trauma. The protective helmet is to prevent skull fractures.

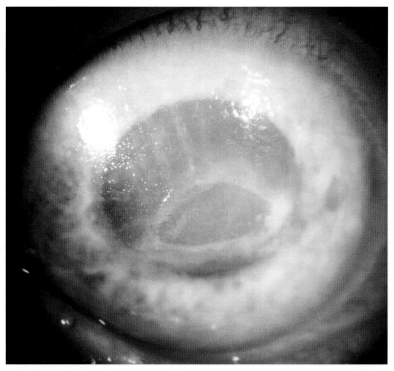

Fig. 13.17 Neurotrophic ulcer after surgical intervention for trigeminal neuralgia. Characteristically, the ulcer is in the inferior paracentral cornea and has thick, rolled, epithelial edges. Tarsorrhaphy is often needed to prevent further ulceration and perforation.

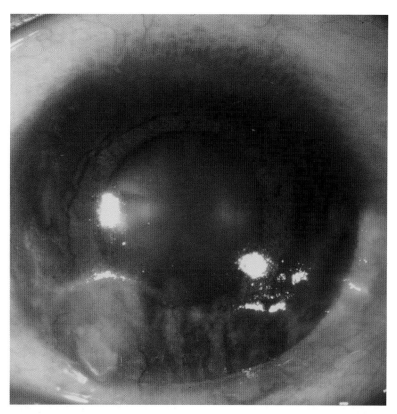

Fig. 13.18 Neurotrophic keratopathy. This patient had a chronic inferior keratitis and corneal thinning. There was absent sensation in the ipsilateral distribution of cranial nerve five, divisions one through three. Neuroimaging disclosed an acoustic neuroma.

Dellen

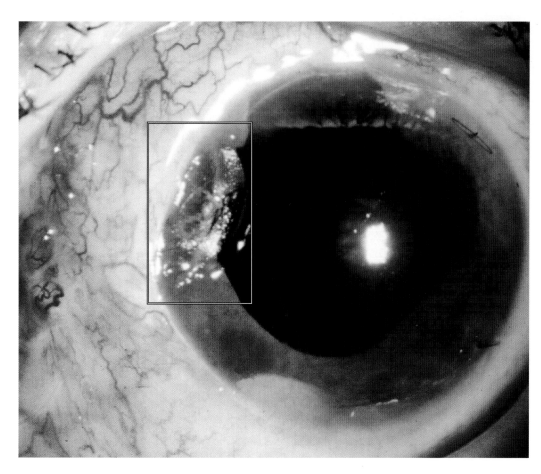

Fig. 13.19 Dellen. These are localized areas of corneal thinning with intact epithelium and lack of corneal infiltration. They occur next to areas of elevated tissue and are caused by localized drying of the cornea. The dellen in the box was caused by an elevation of the conjunctiva after scleral buckle surgery. The lesion resolved when the conjunctival swelling abated.

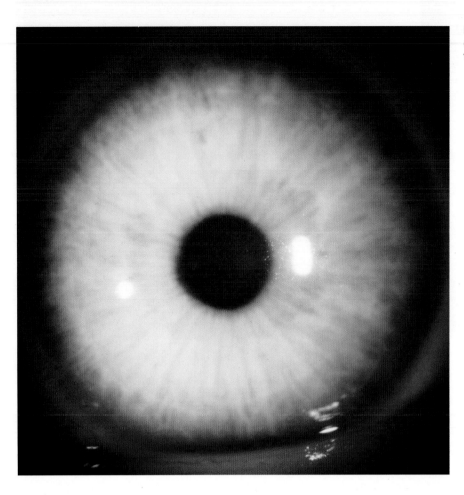

Fig. 13.20 Neurogenic keratopathy. This 34-year-old man noticed decreased vision in his right eye when he went hunting during the winter. This is the appearance of the cornea at room temperature.

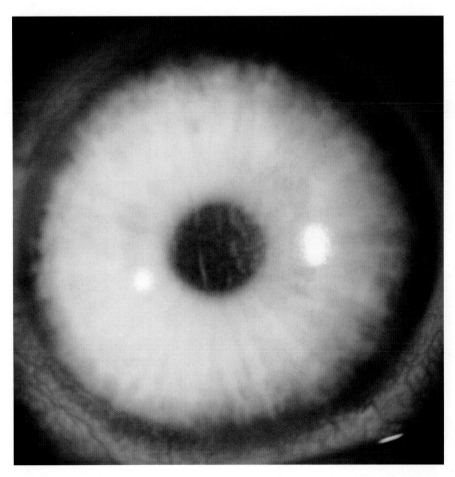

Fig. 13.21 Same patient as in Fig. 13.20. After exposure to a cold environment (a meat freezer), there was diffuse stromal edema with Descemet's folds, as seen here. The etiology was related to trigeminal nerve dysfunction caused by a meningioma.

Exposure Keratopathy

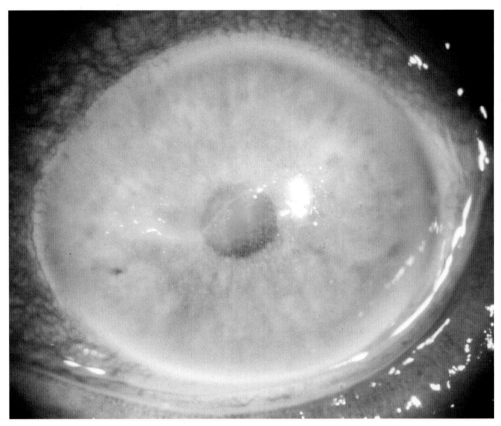

Fig. 13.22 Chronic corneal exposure from thyroid eye disease. Exophthalmos and lid retraction contributed to this complication.

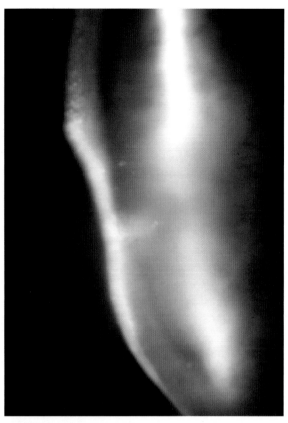

Fig. 13.23 Chronic progressive external ophthalmoplegia. This patient developed exposure keratopathy, thinning, and scarring. Predisposing factors included overcorrection after ptosis surgery and lack of a Bell's phenomena with eyelid closure.

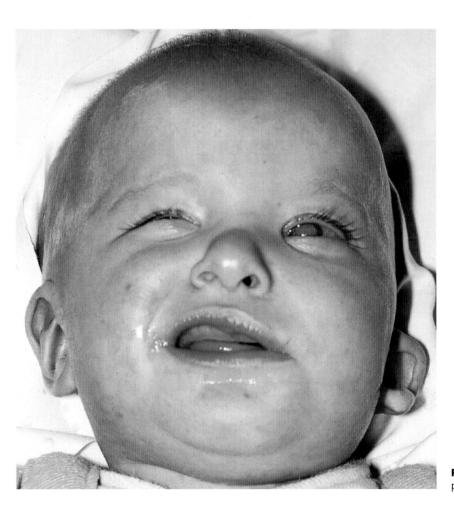

Fig. 13.24 Exposure corneal ulcer in an infant from a left seventh nerve paralysis.

Radiation Keratopathy

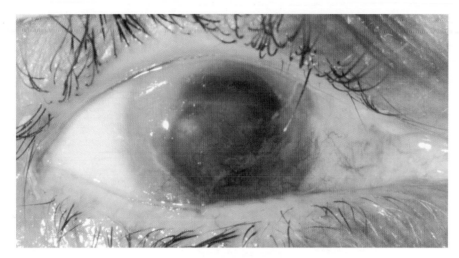

Fig. 13.25 Radiation keratopathy after radiation treatment for a malignant fibrous histiocytoma of the orbit. The cornea is scarred and vascularized. There is mucus in the tear film from an associated dry eye. The patient also had radiation retinopathy.

Toxicity

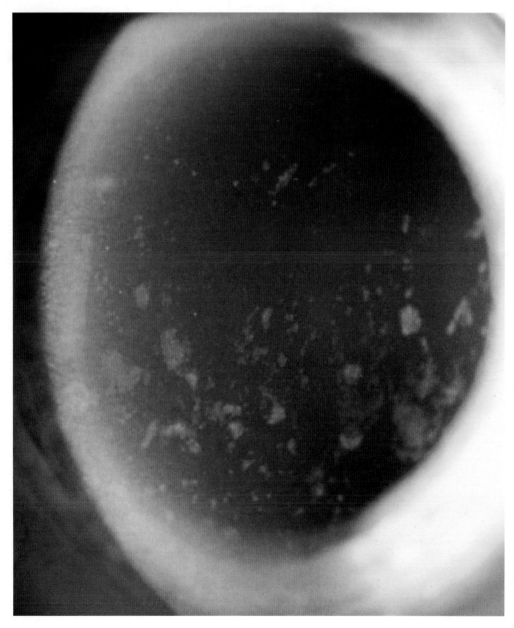

Fig. 13.26 Toxic reaction. It is common to see a diffuse irregular epitheliopathy after instillation of topical anesthetic. The surface is most affected in the interpalpebral region.

Factitious Disease

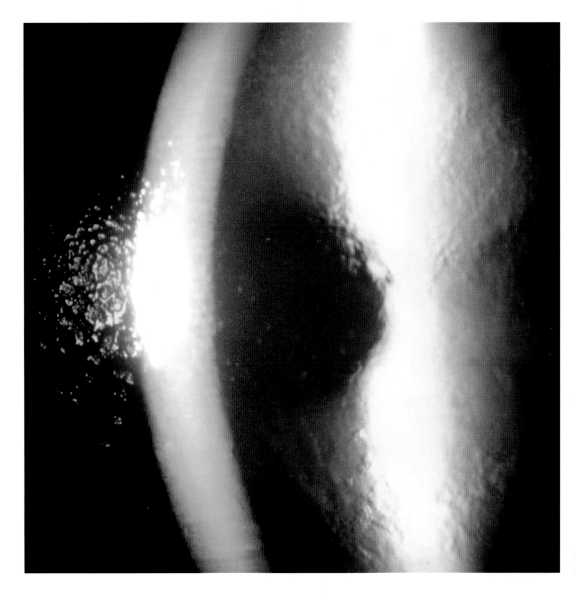

Fig. 13.27 Factitious keratopathy after topical anesthetic abuse.

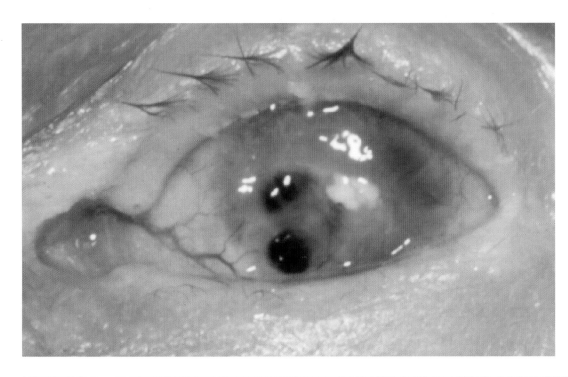

Fig. 13.28 Factitious disease. A retired physician admitted to using topical lidocaine in his left eye. The corneal stroma is necrotic, and there are two areas of perforation with protruding uvea.

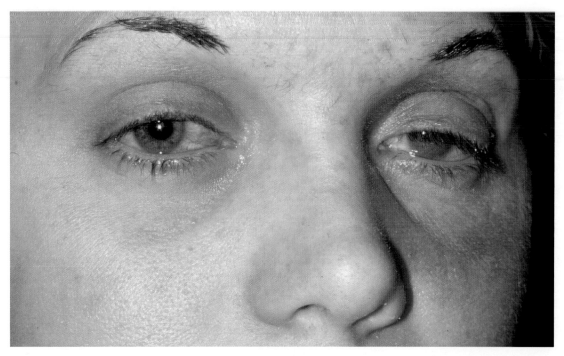

Fig. 13.29 Scarring of the skin, lids, conjunctiva, and cornea. The patient admitted under hypnosis that she was putting caustic chemicals in her eyes.

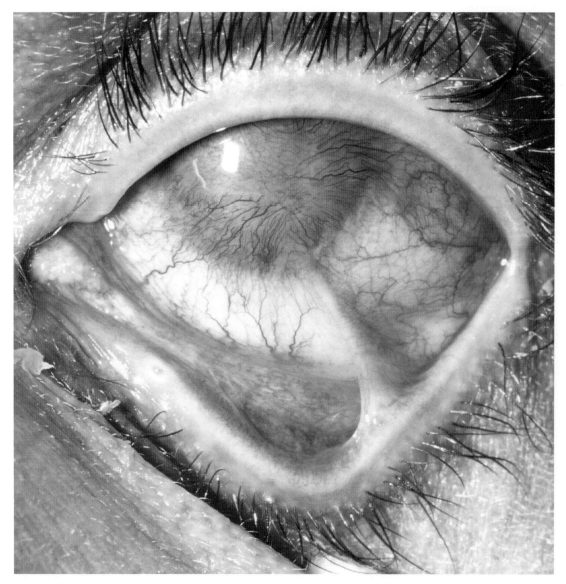

Fig. 13.30 Same patient as in Fig. 13.29. There is extensive conjunctival and corneal scarring.

Chapter 14

Immunologic Disorders of the Cornea

Some immunologic disorders are unique to the cornea, but many are associated with systemic disease. The abundance of collagen and blood vessels in the sclera and corneal limbus predispose the sclera and cornea to manifestations of collagen vascular diseases. Some of these disorders, such as rheumatoid arthritis, affect the cornea after long-standing systemic disease, whereas others, such as Wegener's granulomatosis and polyarteritis nodosa, may have their initial manifestations in the sclera and cornea.

Rheumatoid Arthritis

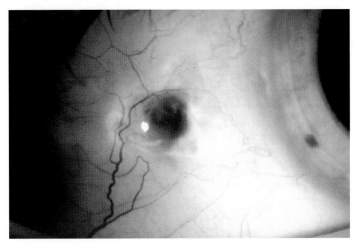

Fig. 14.1 Scleromalacia perforans. This is a slow thinning of the sclera unassociated with pain or episodes of acute inflammation. This patient with rheumatoid arthritis was noted to have an early area of scleromalacia perforans. The sclera is excavated in this region, and the underlying uvea is well seen.

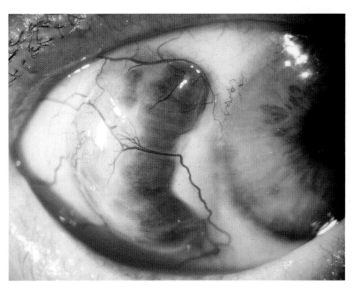

Fig. 14.2 Advanced scleromalacia perforans in rheumatoid arthritis. The sclera is diffusely thin, and uveal tissue protrudes as a staphyloma. Minor trauma can be associated with ocular perforation.

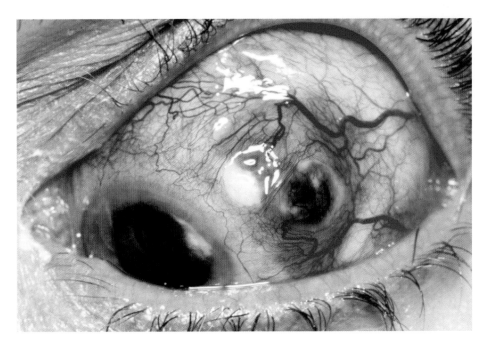

Fig. 14.3 Necrotizing scleritis in rheumatoid arthritis. In contrast to scleromalacia perforans, these lesions are painful and are associated with acute inflammation. Systemic immunosuppression is usually required to treat these patients.

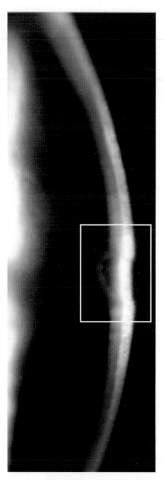

Fig. 14.4 Central corneal ulceration in rheumatoid arthritis. These central ulcers (box) tend to occur in extremely dry eyes and can progress very rapidly to perforation, without significant pain.

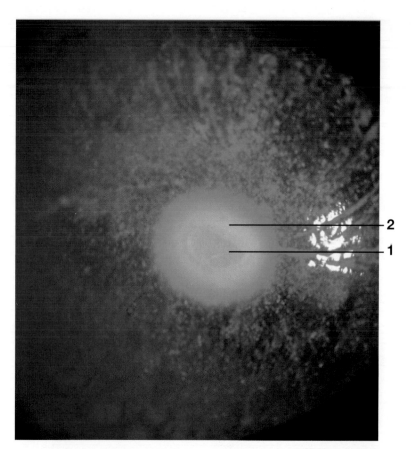

Fig. 14.5 Same patient as in Fig. 14.4. An area of true fluorescein staining devoid of all epithelium (1), and an area of unhealthy epithelium, which soaks up fluorescein and stains less intensely (2), are shown.

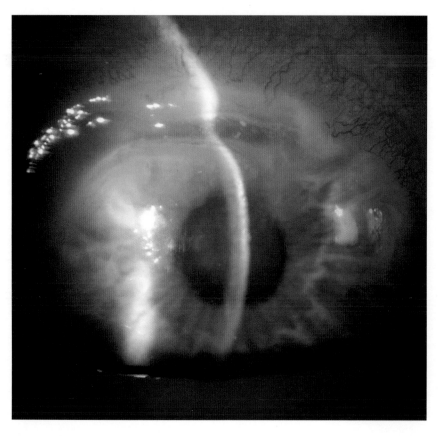

Fig. 14.6 Peripheral corneal ulcer in rheumatoid arthritis. In contrast to the central ulcer just seen, peripheral ulcers in rheumatoid arthritis usually occur at the edge of peripheral corneal vascularization. These eyes tend to be less dry than those with central ulceration, and there is usually an associated scleritis with some degree of pain. In this example, the cornea is thinned superiorly at the edge of a region of corneal vascularization. These ulcers may progress to perforation and often require some form of systemic immunosuppression for treatment.

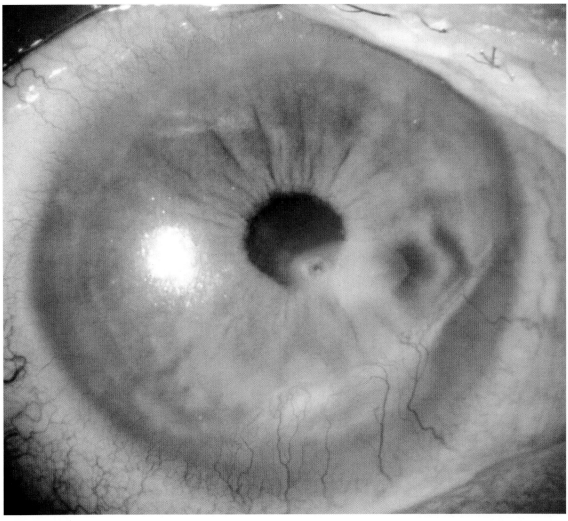

Fig. 14.7 Rheumatoid arthritis. There is peripheral scarring from previous peripheral ulcerations. In addition, there is central ulceration with perforation.

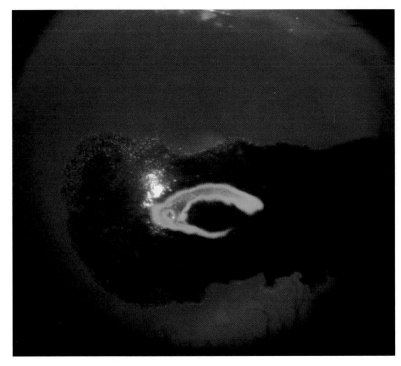

Fig. 14.8 Same patient as in Fig. 14.7. The area of perforation is Seidel positive.

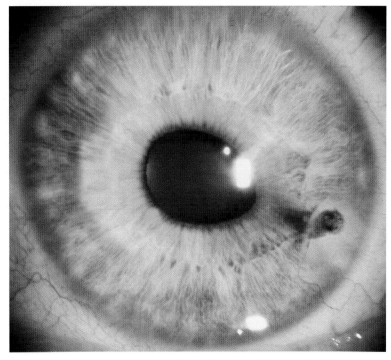

Fig. 14.9 Rheumatoid arthritis. This patient had an old peripheral perforation plugged with iris tissue. The epithelium healed over the iris and a corneal scar formed.

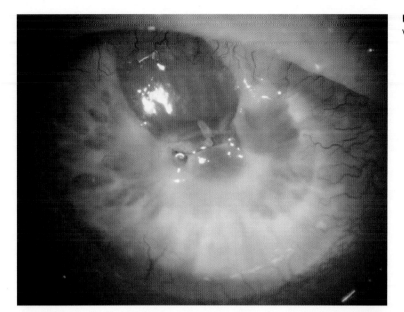

Fig. 14.10 Rheumatoid arthritis. There is extensive melting of the central cornea with perforation.

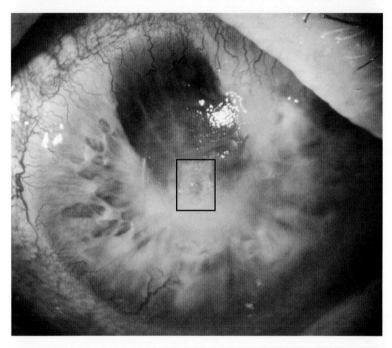

Fig. 14.11 Same patient as in Fig. 14.10, with tissue adhesive closing the perforation site. If epithelium and vascular tissue grow beneath the glue (box) to heal the area of perforation, the glue will become dislodged. If this does not occur, a lamellar or penetrating keratoplasty may be necessary to seal the perforation site.

Nonrheumatoid Collagen Vascular Disease

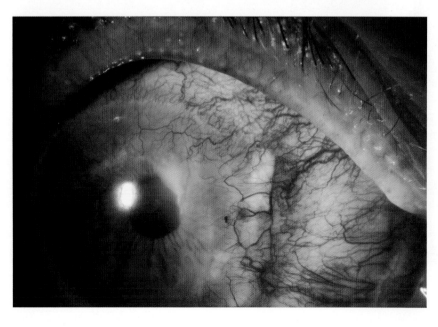

Fig. 14.12 Polyarteritis nodosa. This systemic vasculitis affects small and medium-sized arteries. Anterior segment manifestations include episcleritis, diffuse scleritis, necrotizing scleritis, and peripheral necrotizing keratitis (as seen here). Ocular findings may be the initial manifestation of this disease.

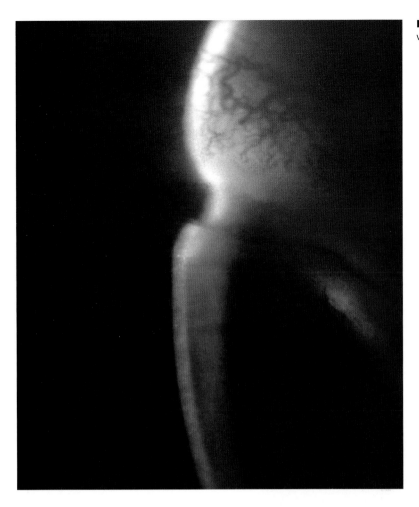

Fig. 14.13 Systemic lupus erythematosus. Marginal corneal ulcer in a patient with systemic lupus erythematosus.

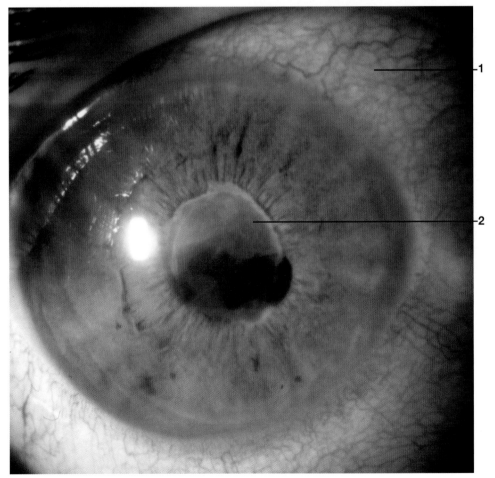

Fig. 14.14 Systemic lupus erythematosus. This patient has scleritis (1) and an associated uveitis with a fibrinous pupillary membrane (2).

Immunologic Disorders of the Cornea **255**

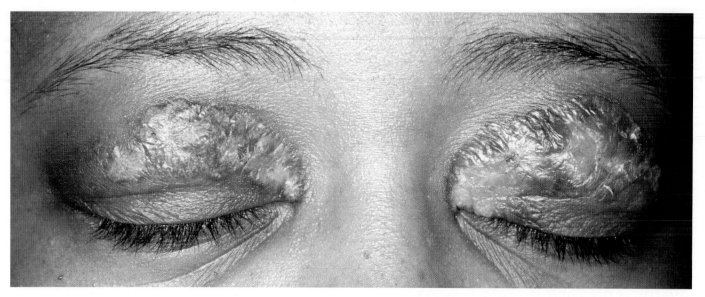

Fig. 14.15 Discoid lupus erythematosus. Eyelid involvement may be the initial manifestation. The lesions are characteristically erythematous, raised plaques with superficial scaling. A small proportion of patients with discoid lupus may progress to systemic lupus, and 20% of patients with systemic lupus may have the skin lesions of discoid lupus.

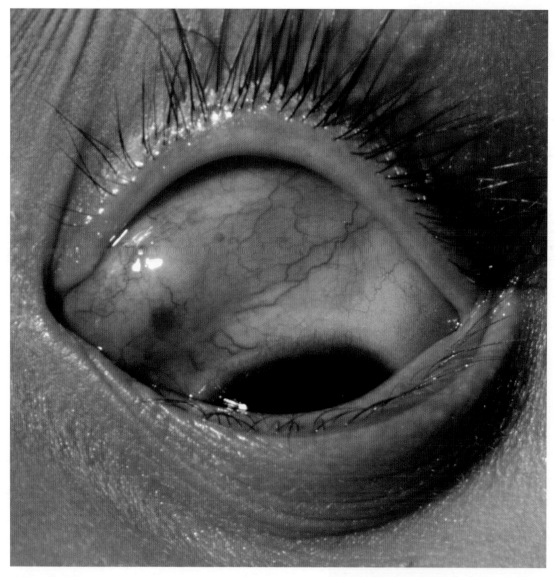

Fig. 14.16 Wegener's granulomatosis. This necrotizing granulomatous reaction frequently involves the upper and lower respiratory tracts and the kidneys. The initial sign in this patient with Wegener's granulomatosis was a conjunctival mass.

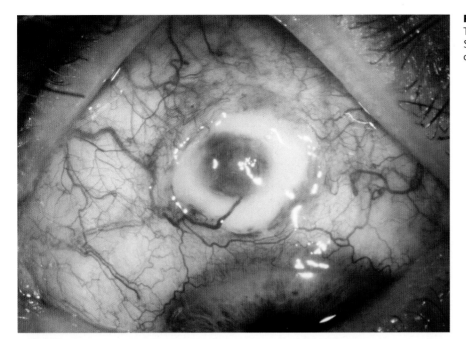

Fig. 14.17 Necrotizing scleritis in Wegener's granulomatosis.
There is central absence of scleral tissue, and the uvea is easily visualized. Surrounding this central area is a ring of avascular, necrotic sclera. The conjunctival epithelium over this area is absent.

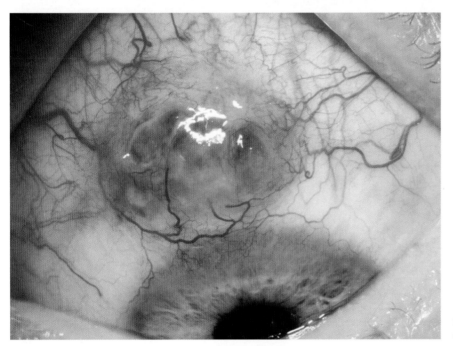

Fig. 14.18 Same patient as in Fig. 14.17, 2 months after treatment with systemic cyclophosphamide.

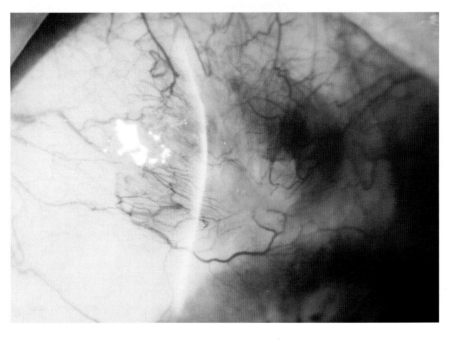

Fig. 14.19 Same patient as in Figs 14.17 and 14.18, 4 months after treatment with systemic cyclophosphamide. The conjunctival epithelium is healed, and the sclera is well vascularized and scarred.

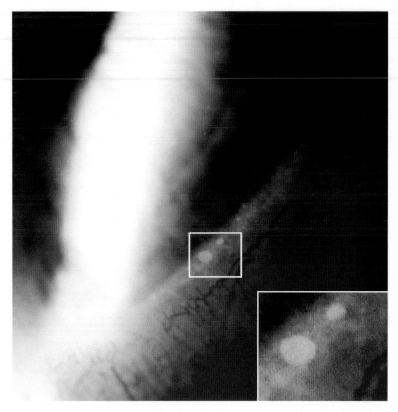

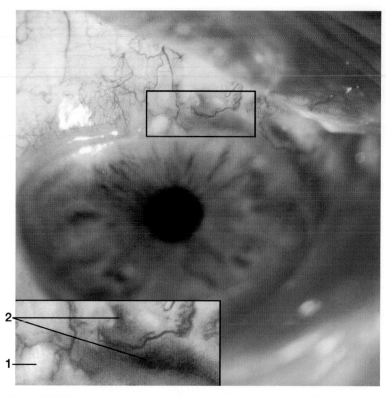

Fig. 14.20 Wegener's granulomatosis. Early peripheral corneal infiltration (inset) in Wegener's granulomatosis.

Fig. 14.21 Wegener's granulomatosis with a limbal ulcer (inset). There is an area of active infiltration (1); the cornea is thinned in this region (2).

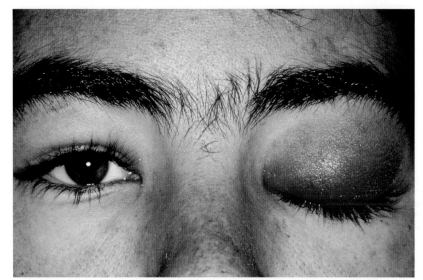

Fig. 14.22 Dermatomyositis. This is an inflammatory disease of skeletal muscles associated with cutaneous lesions. A violaceous discoloration may occur on the upper eyelids (heliotrope rash).

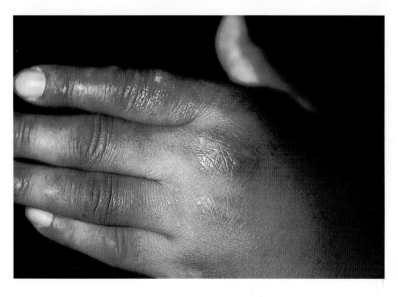

Fig. 14.23 Dermatomyositis. Papules (Gottron's papules) may develop over the joints of the hands.

Staphylococcal Disease

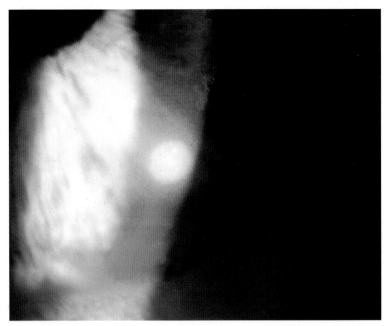

Fig. 14.24 Staphylococcal marginal infiltrate. These infiltrates are hypersensitivity reactions to staphylococcal antigen. Characteristically, there is a clear area between the infiltrate and limbus. Patients often present with ocular pain and redness. These lesions respond well to topical antibiotic-corticosteroid combination drops.

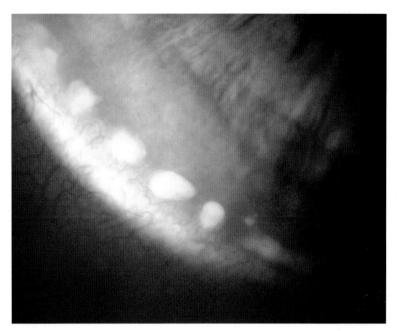

Fig. 14.25 Multiple staphylococcal marginal infiltrates near the limbus.

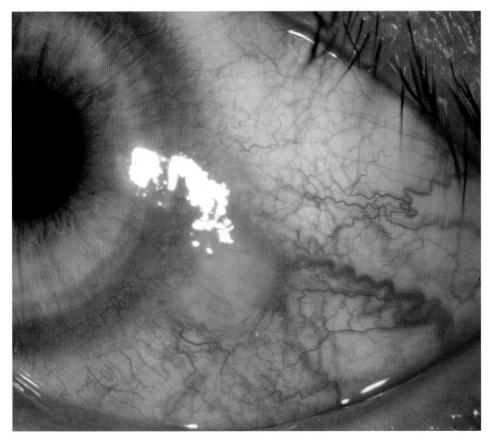

Fig. 14.26 Conjunctival phlyctenule. A phlyctenule is a type IV hypersensitivity reaction usually associated with a response to staphylococcal antigen; however, it can occur in the presence of tuberculosis. The word phlycten means "blister." These lesions start as an elevation of the conjunctiva, progressively become ulcerated, and eventually form a localized scar over a 2-week interval. Mild ocular discomfort can occur, and the symptoms are relieved by topical corticosteroids.

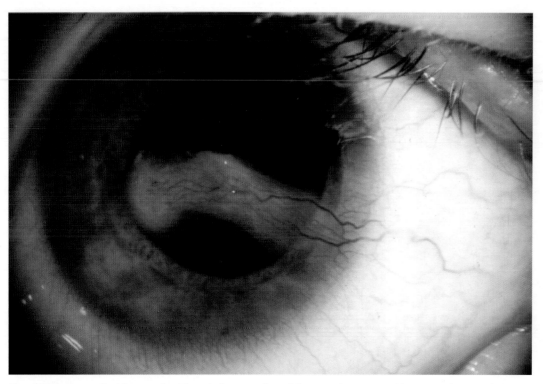

Fig. 14.27 Corneal phlyctenule. These lesions can "march" across the cornea with progressive vascularization and scarring.

Mooren's Ulcer

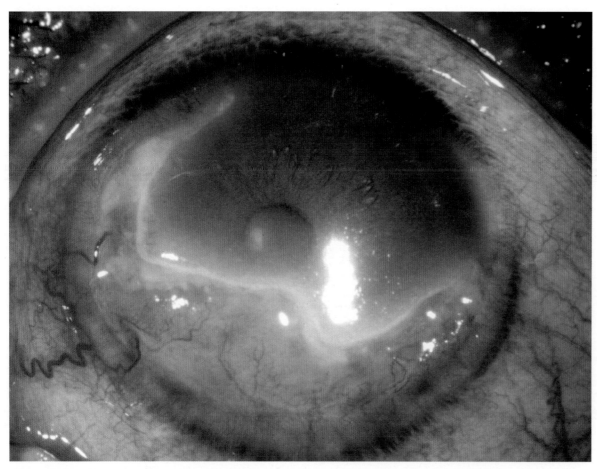

Fig. 14.28 Mooren's ulcer. This condition presents as a necrotizing lesion of the cornea. It is a diagnosis of exclusion, as many other conditions can present somewhat similarly. It is characterized by corneal thinning and ulceration extending inward from the limbus centrally. The epithelium is absent in areas of active ulceration; however, there may be a vascularized pannus leading up to areas of active ulceration. Typically, there is an abrupt transition between involved and uninvolved cornea, with an overhanging edge. The disease can sometimes be characterized by extreme pain.

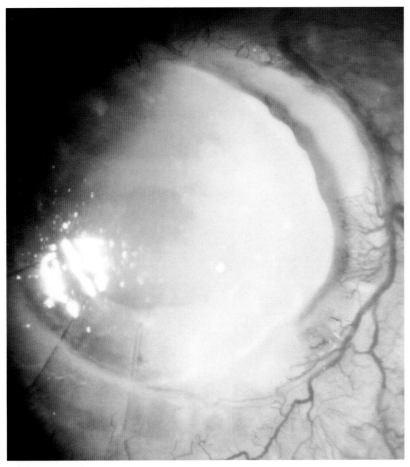

Fig. 14.29 Mooren's ulcer. A penetrating keratoplasty was performed. There was recurrence of Mooren's ulcer in the cornea, with the characteristic overhanging edge between areas of involved and uninvolved cornea.

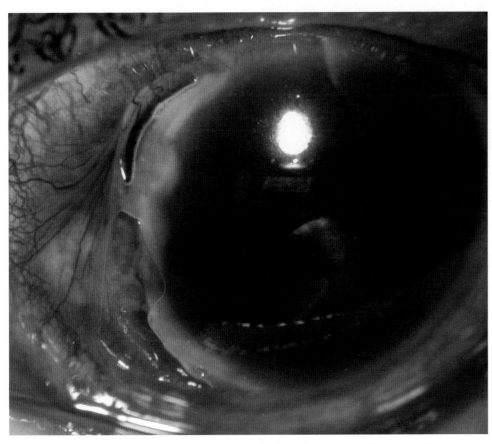

Fig. 14.30 Mooren's ulcer. A severe case of Mooren's ulcer demonstrating the characteristic overhanging edge of corneal tissue.

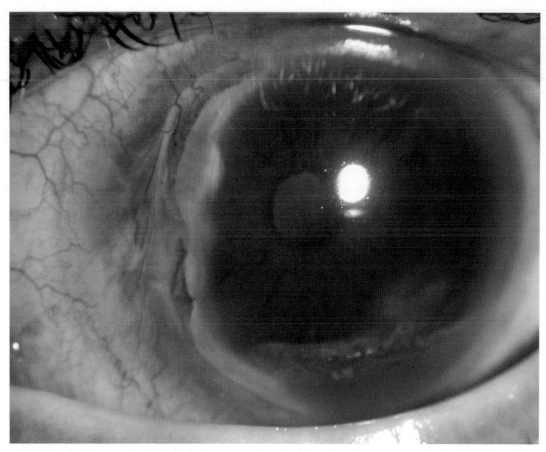

Fig. 14.31 Mooren's ulcer. This is the same patient as in Fig. 14.30, 24 hours after the placement of a bandage soft contact lens and the institution of topical corticosteroid treatment.

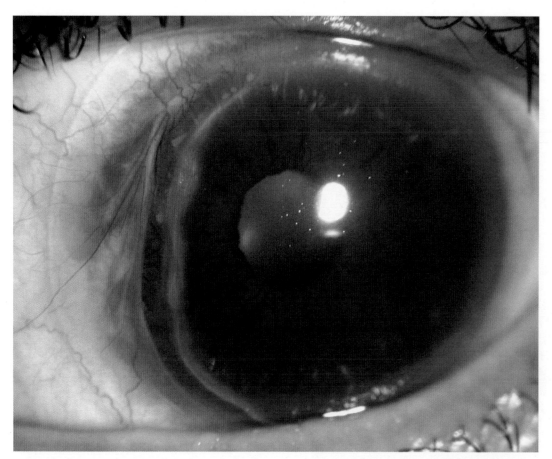

Fig. 14.32 Mooren's ulcer. This is the same patient as seen in Figs 14.30 and 14.31, 2.5 months later. The bandage contact lens is still in place and topical corticosteroids have been discontinued. There is no active inflammation and the ulcer has stabilized.

Chapter 15

Corneal Trauma

Because the cornea is the most powerful refractive element of the eye and one of the most sensitive tissues of the body, even minor injury can produce significant visual and symptomatic problems. Prompt diagnosis and appropriate treatment are essential.

Foreign Body, Mechanical, Thermal, and Radiation Trauma

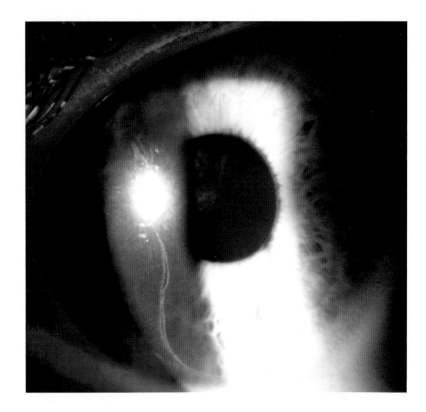

Fig. 15.1 Corneal abrasions. These are common after minor trauma. Here a fingernail injury produced a vertically oriented abrasion.

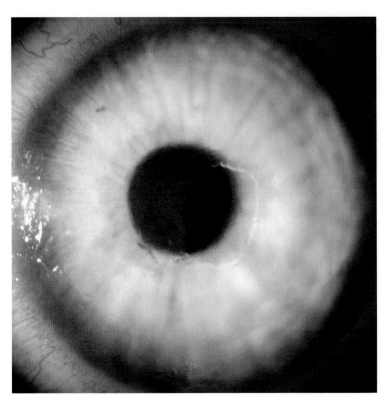

Fig. 15.2 Corneal abrasion after a chemical (detergent) injury. Chemical injuries usually affect the interpalpebral region, as this area is the first to come in contact with the chemical. These defects usually heal rapidly with pressure patching and antibiotic ointments. If a secondary infection is suspected, frequent administration of topical antibiotics rather than pressure patching should be initiated.

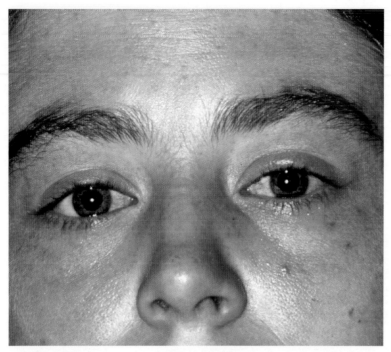

Fig. 15.3 Dermatitis and keratoconjunctivitis from ultraviolet sterilizing operating room equipment. The reaction of the skin is similar to that seen after excessive exposure to sunlight (sunburn).

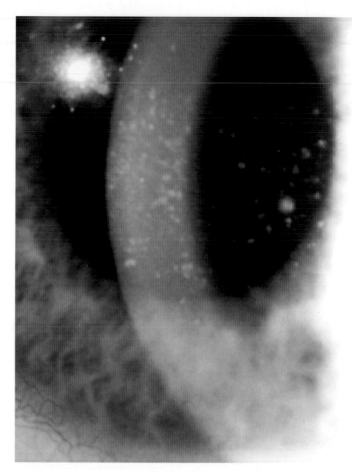

Fig. 15.4 Same patient as in Fig. 15.3. There is a diffuse punctate keratopathy caused by excessive exposure to ultraviolet light. The keratitis begins several hours after exposure and is extremely painful.

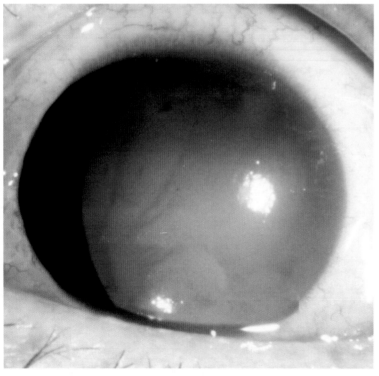

Fig. 15.5 Blunt trauma to the eye from an elastic cord. There was a 360° iridodialysis, and the iris fell en bloc into the vitreous cavity. The lens was dislocated temporally and posteriorly.

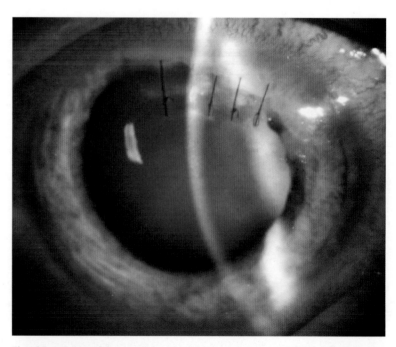

Fig. 15.6 Corneal laceration. This has been re-approximated with 10-0 nylon sutures.

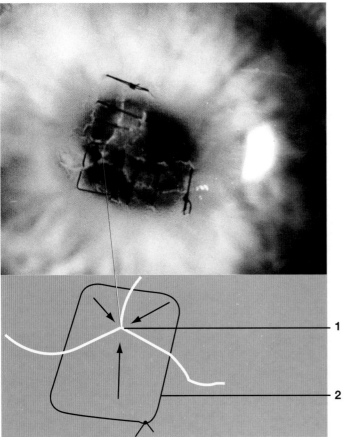

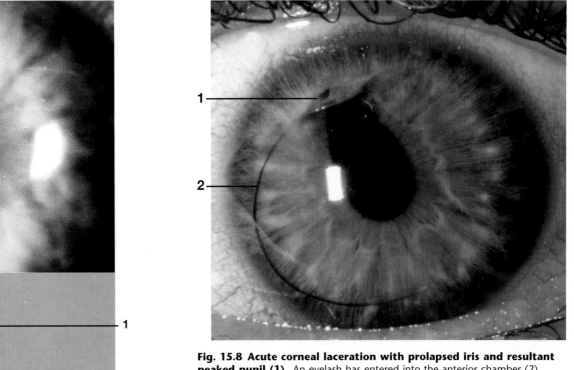

Fig. 15.8 Acute corneal laceration with prolapsed iris and resultant peaked pupil (1). An eyelash has entered into the anterior chamber (2).

Fig. 15.7 Complex corneal laceration repair. There is a stellate laceration (1) repaired by a horizontal mattress or purse-string suture (2), which pulls, in this case, the three triangles of tissue together.

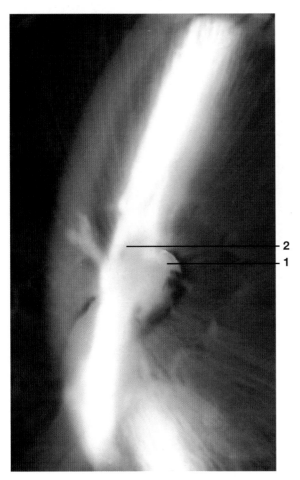

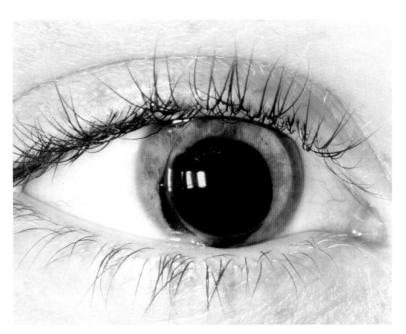

Fig. 15.10 Same patient as in Fig. 15.9. The postoperative appearance after corneal transplant, lensectomy, and vitrectomy is evident. The patient is wearing an aphakic contact lens.

Fig. 15.9 Penetrating corneal trauma. A central white cataract (1) is shown. Lens material and iris adhere to the posterior cornea (2).

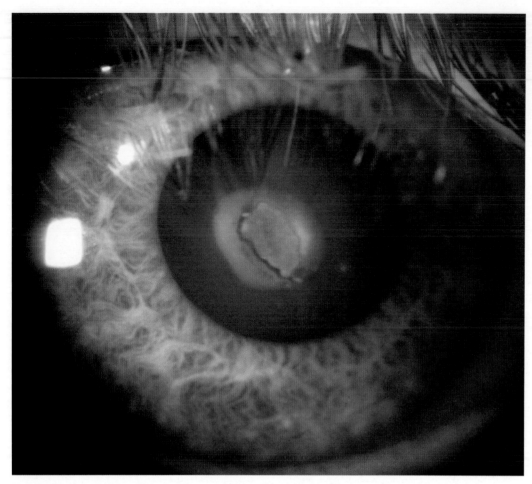

Fig. 15.11 Necrotic corneal perforating wound from a stick injury in a 5-year-old boy.

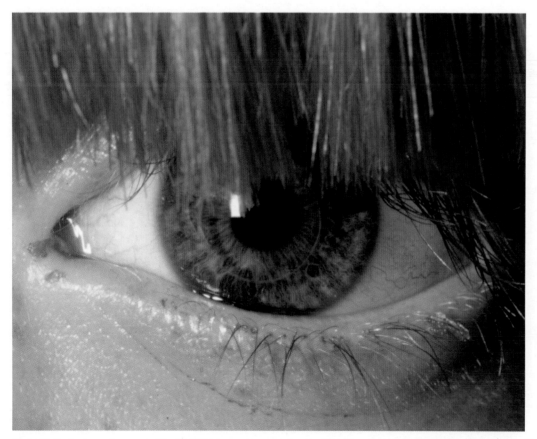

Fig. 15.12 Same patient as in Fig. 15.11, after penetrating keratoplasty.

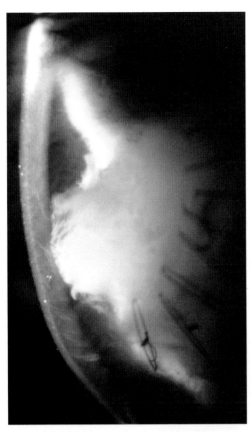

Fig. 15.13 Traumatic cataract and corneal laceration. The lens material is against the corneal endothelium and was removed at a second operation.

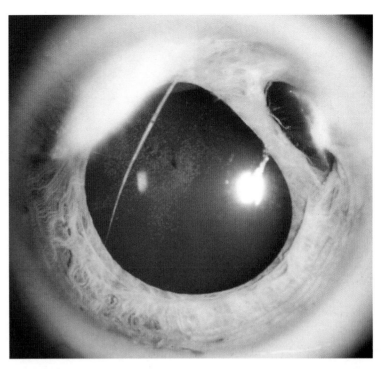

Fig. 15.14 Previous corneal laceration. A scar is seen superiorly. There is a lash in the anterior chamber.

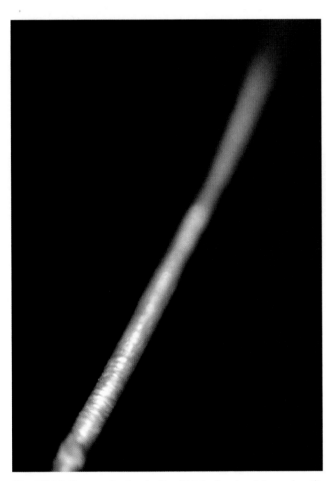

Fig. 15.15 Same patient as in Fig. 15.14, showing intraocular cilia wrapped in Descemet's proliferation.

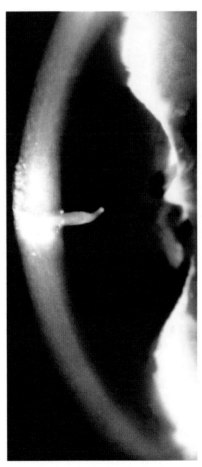

Fig. 15.16 Appearance of the cornea 12 years after a penetrating dart injury. There is a wick of Descemet's proliferation extending from the posterior cornea. A localized traumatic cataract with posterior synechiae is present.

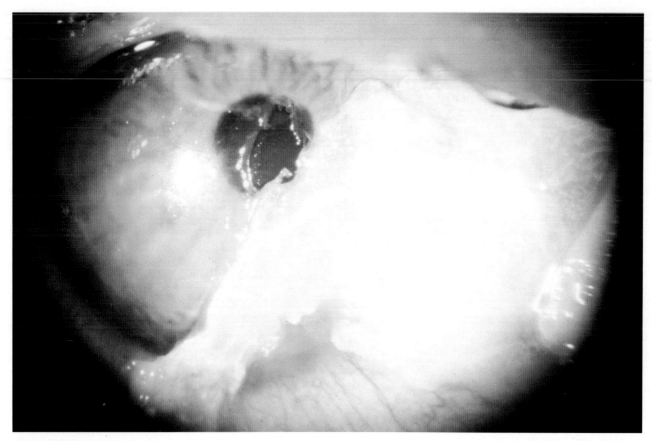

Fig. 15.17 Epoxy glue injury to the cornea. Fortunately, the glue is usually stuck only to the epithelium and does not cause severe scarring.

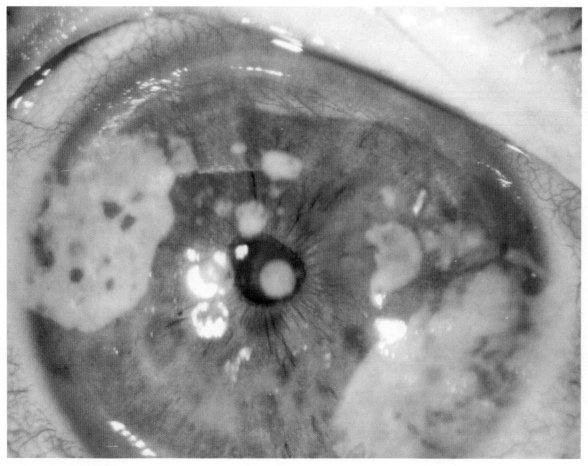

Fig. 15.18 Epoxy glue on the cornea. This is a different patient to that in Fig. 15.17.

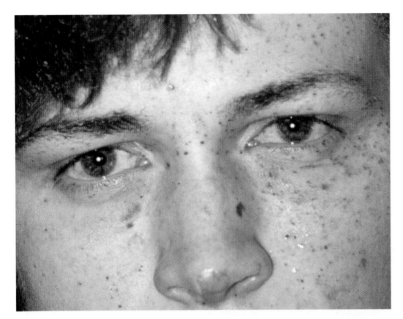

Fig. 15.19 Multiple skin and corneal foreign bodies after a blast injury. The superficial foreign bodies should be removed carefully; deep foreign bodies may need to be left behind.

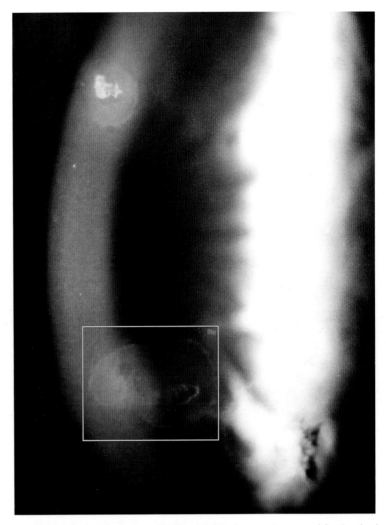

Fig. 15.20 Same patient as in Fig. 15.19. An anterior corneal foreign body has been removed. There is a traumatic endothelial ring (right side of box). The ring is formed from a concussive effect of the foreign body and is composed of swollen endothelial cells and deposits of fibrin and leukocytes on the endothelium. The ring resolved several days after the injury.

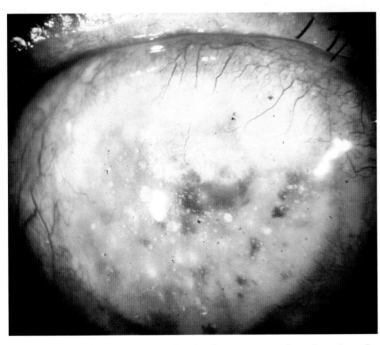

Fig. 15.21 Multiple foreign bodies in the cornea and conjunctiva after an old blast injury. The cornea has diffuse scarring and vascularization.

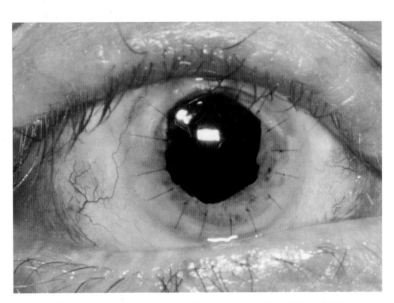

Fig. 15.22 Same patient as in Fig. 15.21, after penetrating keratoplasty.

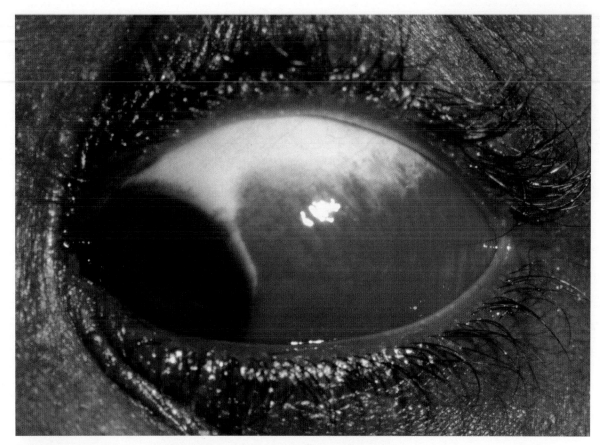

Fig. 15.23 Subconjunctival hemorrhage. Such hemorrhages can occur after trauma, with Valsalva maneuvers or coughing, or from a broken blood vessel caused by hypertension. They are seen more frequently in patients on anticoagulation therapy. Rarely, systemic hematologic disorders can be manifested by subconjunctival hemorrhages. Most commonly, they are spontaneous, with no identifiable cause.

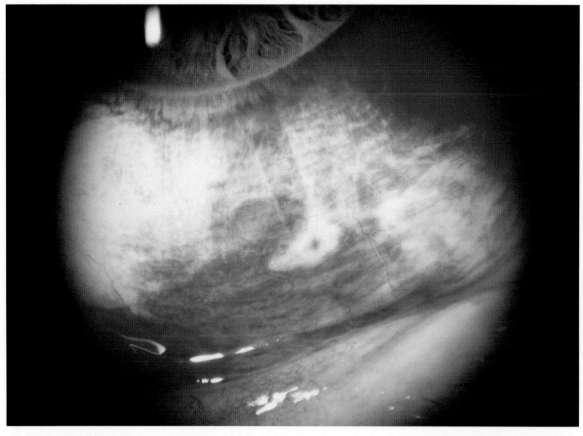

Fig. 15.24 Subconjunctival hemorrhage. As the hemorrhage resolves, it may settle to the most dependent area of the eye and assume a yellow color as the blood is broken down and absorbed.

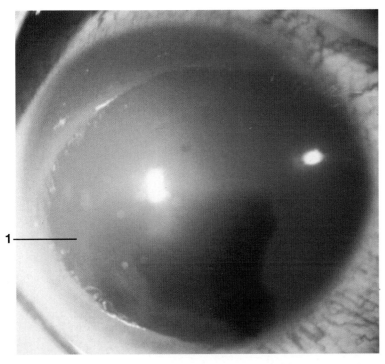

1 —————

Fig. 15.25 Early blood staining in the cornea caused by a traumatic hyphema. This appears as a deep brown discoloration of the posterior cornea (1). Corneal blood staining is an indication for surgical removal of the hyphema.

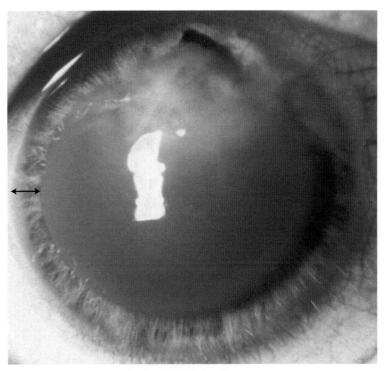

Fig. 15.26 Late corneal blood staining. With time the blood in the cornea becomes yellow. The blood clears over several years, beginning at the limbus and progressing centrally.

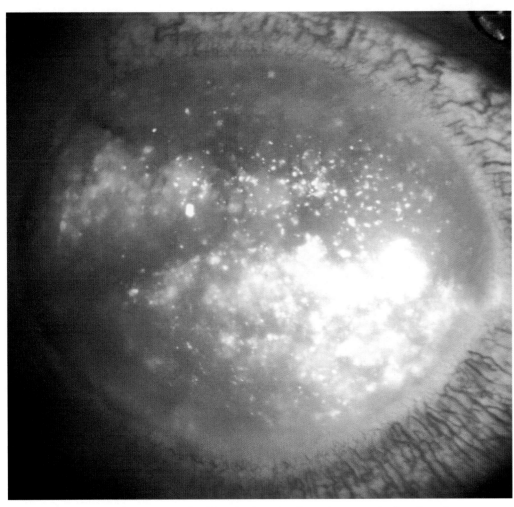

Fig. 15.27 Long-standing intraocular blood. The red cell membranes are broken down into cholesterol. Multiple refractile crystals of cholesterol can form within the eye (cholesterolosis bulbi).

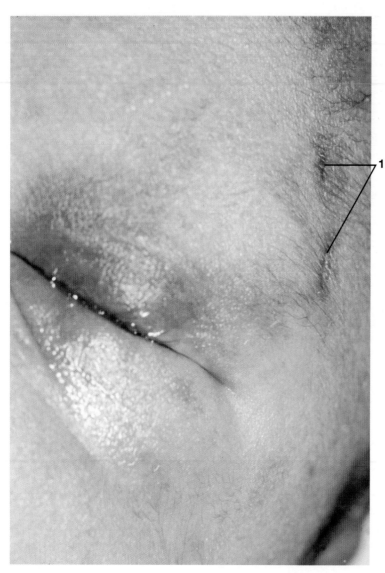

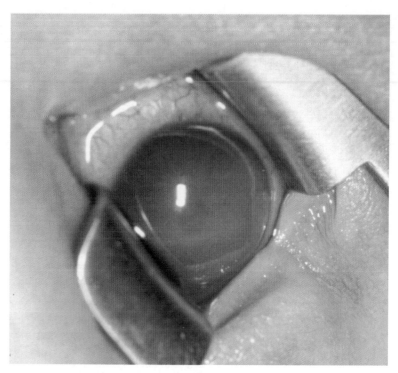

Fig. 15.29 Same patient as in Fig. 15.28. There is acute corneal edema from the forceps injury.

Fig. 15.28 Forceps injury in a 1-day-old infant. There are skin lesions from the forceps (1).

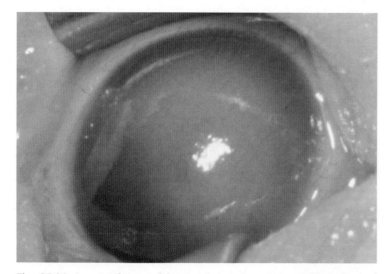

Fig. 15.30 A second case of forceps injury in a 1-day-old infant. Again, there is acute corneal edema.

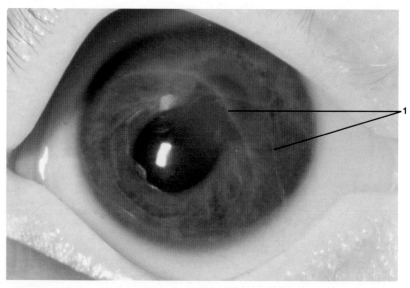

Fig. 15.31 Same patient as in Fig. 15.30, at age 3 months. The central cornea has cleared, and there are vertically oriented breaks in Descemet's membrane (1).

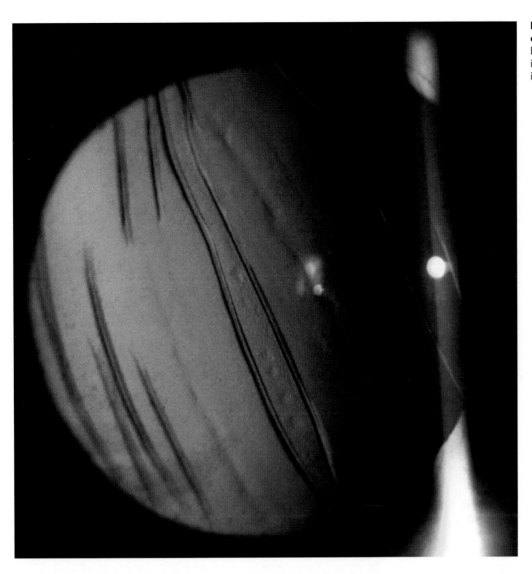

Fig. 15.32 Forceps injury with multiple vertically oriented breaks in Descemet's membrane. The breaks have a railroad track appearance on retro-illumination. Endothelial cells migrate into the area of injury.

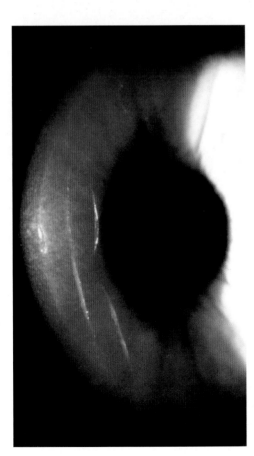

Fig. 15.33 Direct beam view of forceps injury with breaks in Descemet's membrane.

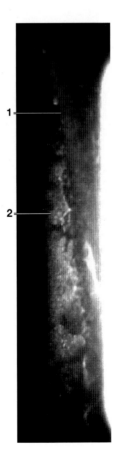

Fig. 15.34 Specular photomicrograph of the patient in Fig. 15.33. There is a rolled-up edge of Descemet's membrane (1). Endothelial cells are enlarged (2) and have migrated from the adjacent tissue into the area of injury.

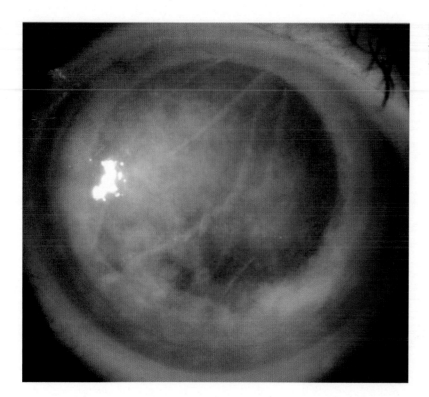

Fig. 15.35 Delayed-onset corneal edema after a forceps injury. This 57-year-old man developed new-onset corneal decompensation and required penetrating keratoplasty. The breaks in Descemet's membrane can be visualized through the corneal edema.

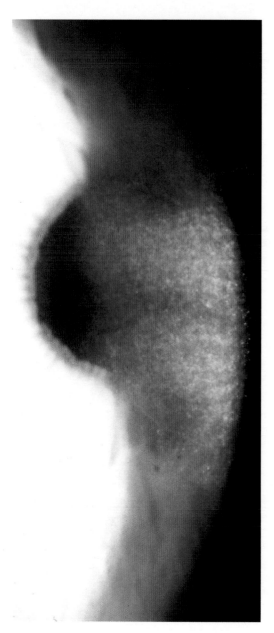

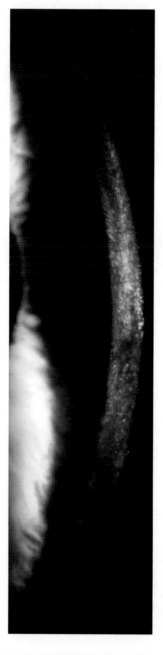

Fig. 15.36 A 27-year-old man was struck by lightning. He developed a broad area of corneal scarring from the injury.

Fig. 15.37 Thin slit-beam view of the patient in Fig. 15.36. There is scarring in all layers of the stroma. Cataracts may also develop after a lightning injury, sometimes many years after the acute event.

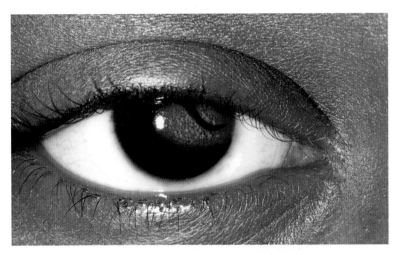

Fig. 15.38 Thermal injury from a curling iron.

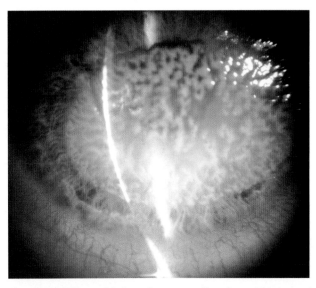

Fig. 15.39 Thermal injury from a curling iron. This is another example of extensive thermal injury to the corneal epithelium from a curling iron.

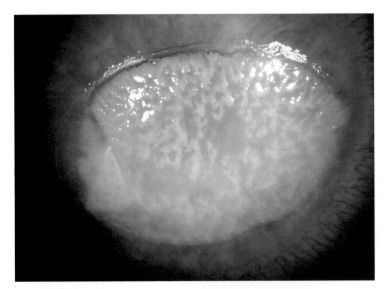

Fig. 15.40 Fluorescein stain of injured area in the same patient as in Fig. 15.39.

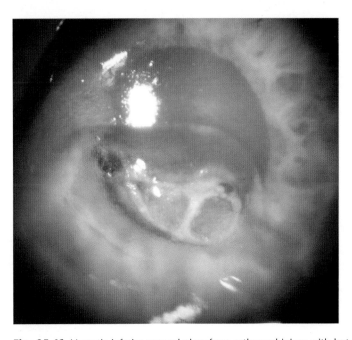

Fig. 15.41 Necrotic inferior corneal ulcer from a thermal injury with hot metal.

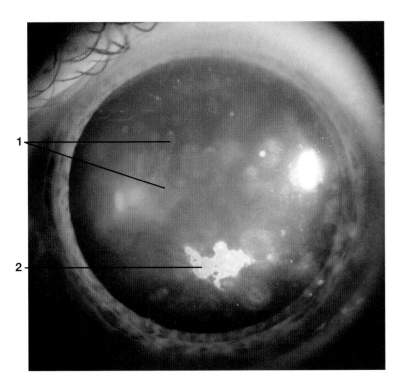

Fig. 15.42 Thermal injury. Argon laser photocoagulation can injure the cornea. In this case, there are extensive corneal scars (1) and calcific degeneration (2).

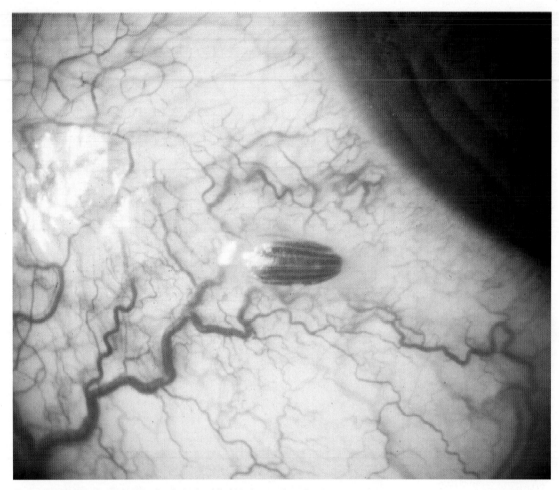

Fig. 15.43 Corn husk foreign body embedded in the conjunctiva.

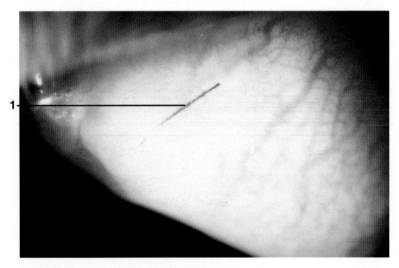

Fig. 15.44 Grasshopper leg (1) embedded in the conjunctiva.

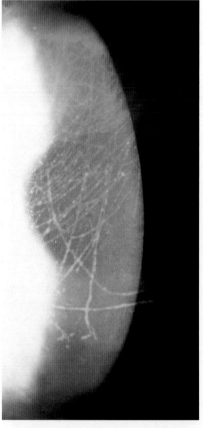

Fig. 15.45 Same patient as in Fig. 15.44. There are multiple vertical epithelial abrasions (from blinking) from the grasshopper leg embedded in the superior tarsal conjunctiva. This pattern of corneal abrasion should always prompt the examiner to evert the lids and look carefully for a foreign body.

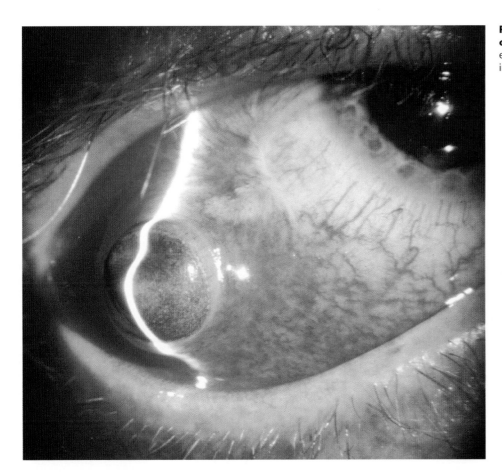

Fig. 15.46 This patient shot an empty shotgun shell casing with a bullet. The casing exploded, and the primer cap embedded in his conjunctiva. There was no deep penetrating injury to the globe.

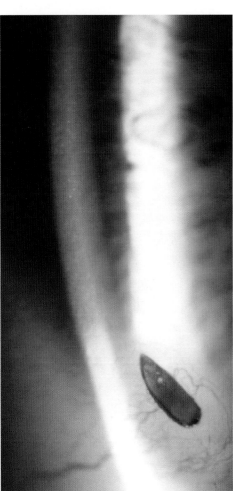

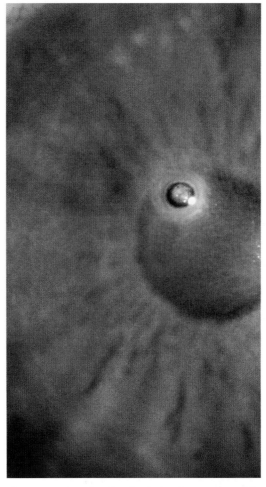

Fig. 15.47 Corn husk foreign body embedded in the cornea. There is no sign of infection in this case, but patients should always be observed carefully for the development of fungal keratitis after injury with vegetable matter.

Fig. 15.48 Iron foreign body in the cornea with an early rust ring. The foreign body and rust ring can be gently removed with a hypodermic needle or small forceps. Care should be taken not to penetrate deep into the stroma because this may cause unnecessary scarring. This was particularly necessary here, as the foreign body is near the visual axis.

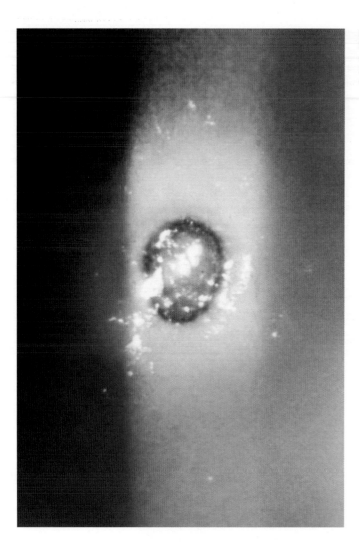

Fig. 15.49 Rust ring with surrounding infiltrate several days after the iron foreign body had been removed. There was a toxic inflammatory response to the rust ring that resolved when the ring was removed. Patients with foreign bodies may develop infectious keratitis and should be treated with antibiotics until the epithelial defect and inflammation have resolved.

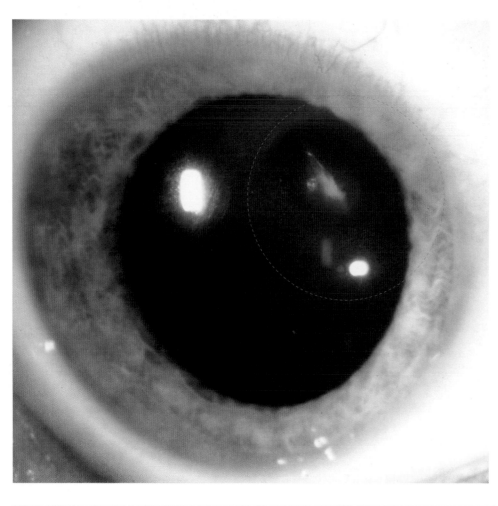

Fig. 15.50 Iron foreign body. In this patient an iron foreign body penetrated deep into the corneal stroma and was not initially removed. This is the appearance of the eye several years after the injury. There is an intrastromal rust ring (dotted circle). The iron foreign body was removed surgically.

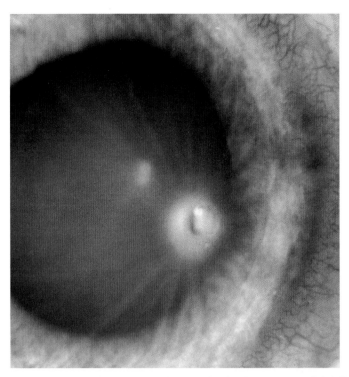

Fig. 15.51 Deep iron corneal foreign body that was not initially removed. Necrosis of the surrounding tissue resulted in a perforation. There are corneal striae surrounding the foreign body, suggesting low pressure as a result of leaking aqueous.

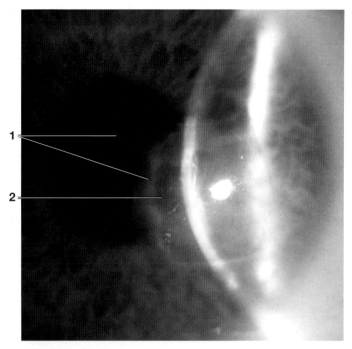

Fig. 15.52 Same patient as in Fig. 15.51 after a freehand lamellar keratoplasty. The scar is in the visual axis (1), and the edge of the graft encroaches on the visual axis (2).

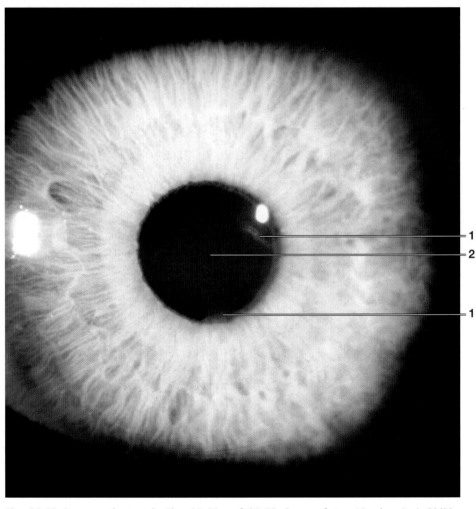

Fig. 15.53 Same patient as in Figs 15.51 and 15.52, 2 years later. Visual acuity is 20/20. There is some scarring in the visual axis (1); however, most of the visual axis remains clear (2).

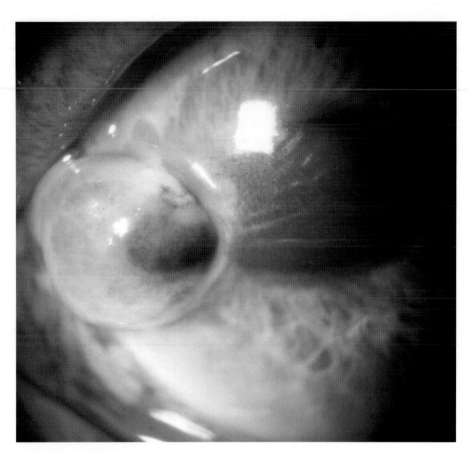

Fig. 15.54 Perforated staphyloma from an old corneal foreign body.

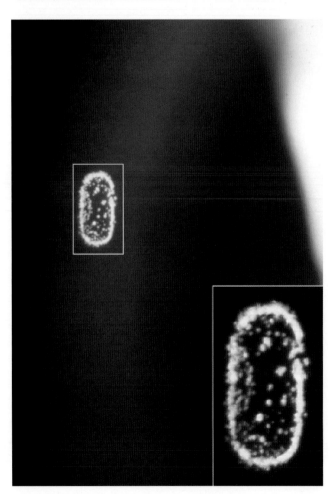

Fig. 15.55 Coat's white ring. This is composed of iron and probably develops when a rust ring from an iron foreign body is not entirely removed. It is located in the superficial cornea. Inside the ring are small white opacities (inset).

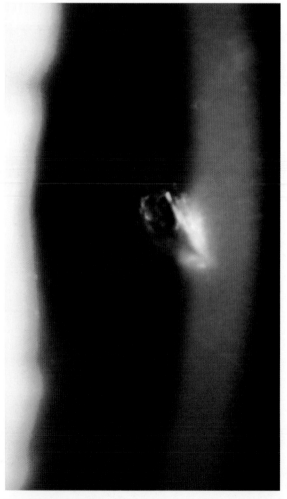

Fig. 15.56 Old glass foreign body in the corneal stroma with an associated scar. Glass is inert, and deep glass foreign bodies can be left in the stroma if their removal is difficult and could potentially cause more corneal damage.

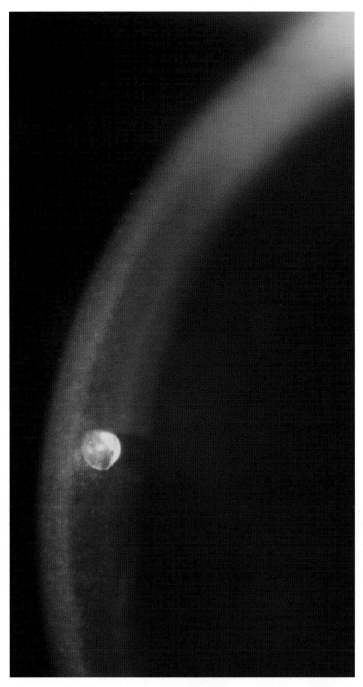

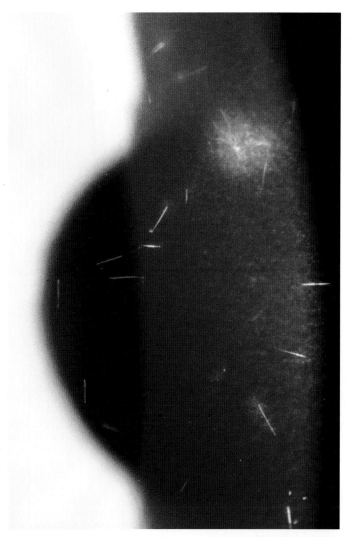

Fig. 15.58 Tarantula hairs in the cornea. A 22-year-old man rubbed his left eye after playing with his pet tarantula. He immediately experienced redness, burning, and a foreign body sensation. Slit-lamp examination showed multiple tarantula hairs in the corneal stroma. Some of the anterior tarantula hairs had associated subepithelial infiltrates. (One of these is seen superiorly.)

Fig. 15.57 Old corneal foreign body from an explosion injury. Similar to the glass foreign body seen in Fig. 15.56, aggressive attempts at removal are not necessary.

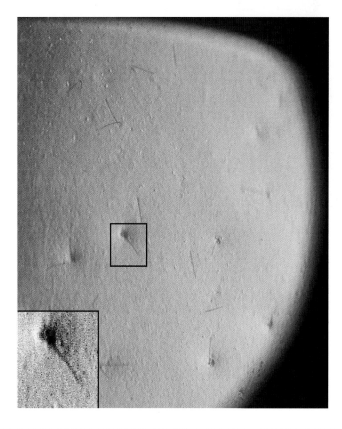

Fig. 15.59 Same patient as in Fig. 15.58. The red reflex view highlights the tarantula hairs. An individual hair is seen in the inset. These hairs have many barbs (similar to fish hooks) and can penetrate deep into the corneal stroma and anterior chamber. There is one reported case of tarantula hairs penetrating through the sclera and causing a peripheral choroiditis. The hairs cannot be removed, and treatment is symptomatic with topical corticosteroids.

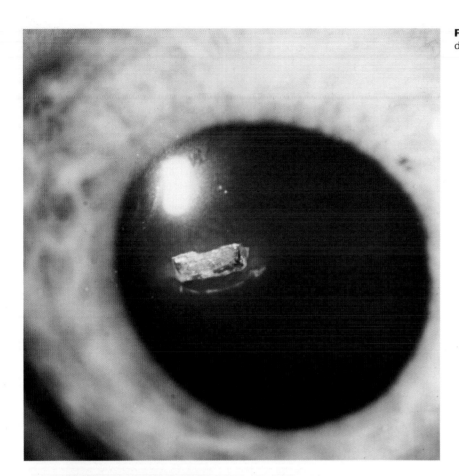

Fig. 15.60 Vegetable foreign matter in the corneal stroma. The depth of penetration cannot be appreciated in this view.

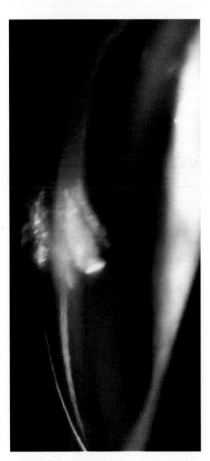

Fig. 15.61 Same patient as in Fig. 15.60. Gonioscopy shows that the foreign body penetrates the cornea and is surrounded by an inflammatory reaction.

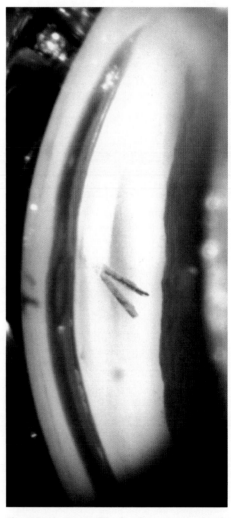

Fig. 15.62 Vegetable foreign matter in the corneal stroma. Penetrating injury from vegetable foreign matter is seen by gonioscopy in another patient.

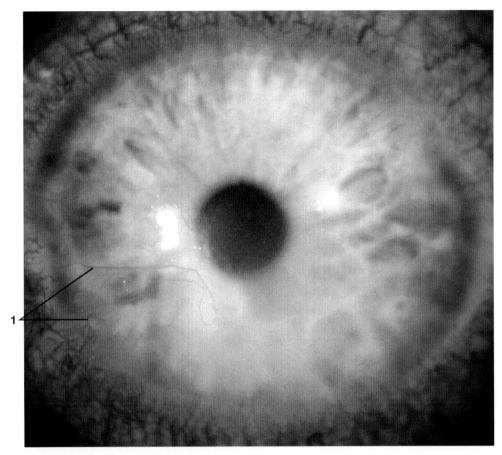

Fig. 15.63 Intraocular glass foreign body. Corneal edema may develop from a retained intraocular foreign body. Here there was an intraocular glass foreign body in the angle that could be appreciated only by gonioscopy. There is vascularization (1) from chronic corneal edema. Unexplained inferior corneal edema should raise suspicion about a foreign body in the inferior anterior chamber angle.

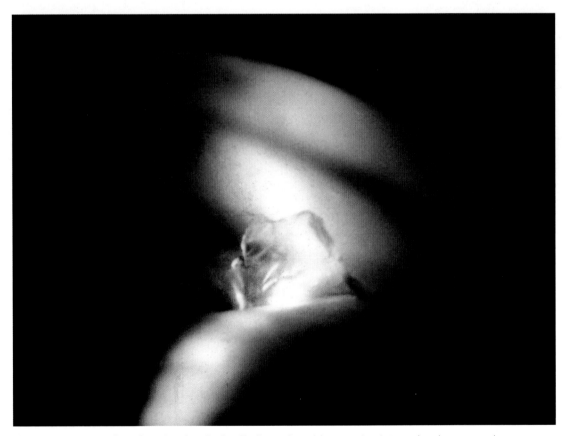

Fig. 15.64 Intraocular glass foreign body. Similar patient demonstrating intraocular glass as seen by gonioscopy.

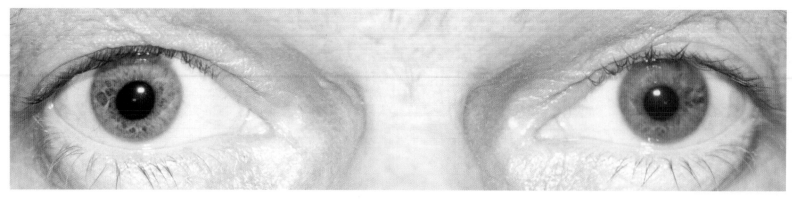

Fig. 15.65 Intraocular iron foreign body. An intraocular iron foreign body in the left eye caused heterochromia in this patient.

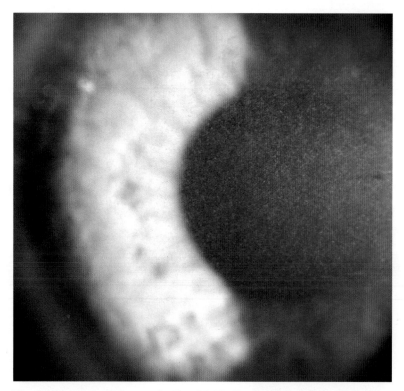

Fig. 15.66 Same patient as in Fig. 15.65. There are brown deposits in the deep corneal stroma from the iron foreign body.

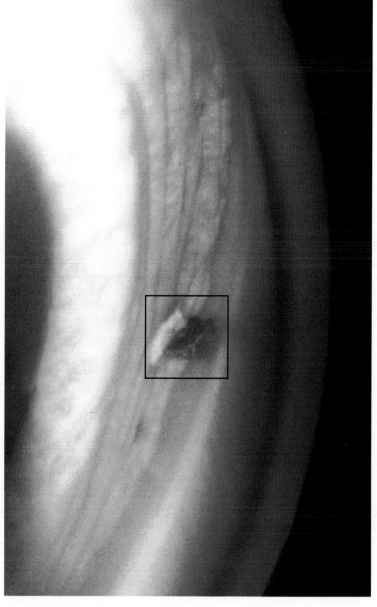

Fig. 15.67 Same patient as in Figs 15.65 and 15.66. The iron foreign body (box) was in the angle and could be appreciated only by gonioscopy.

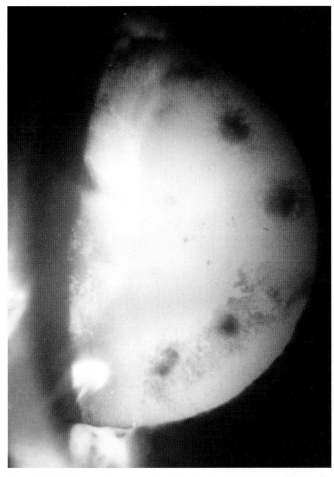

Fig. 15.68 Intraocular iron foreign body. Brown deposits are seen in the lens, and there is a mature cataract.

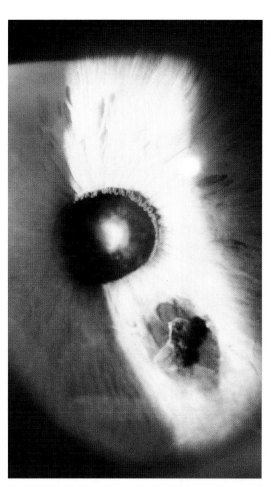

Fig. 15.69 Iron foreign body embedded in the iris. A small central cataract is present.

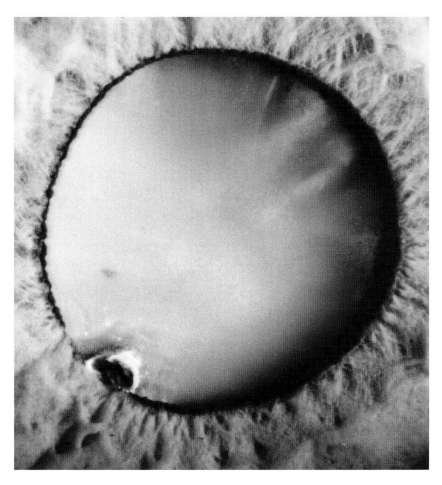

Fig. 15.70 Traumatic cataract resulting from an iron foreign body that penetrated the anterior lens capsule.

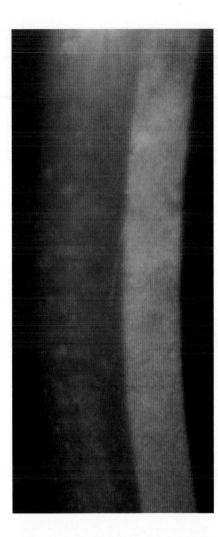

Fig. 15.71 Intraocular copper foreign body (chalcosis). This resulted in a green–yellow discoloration in Descemet's membrane.

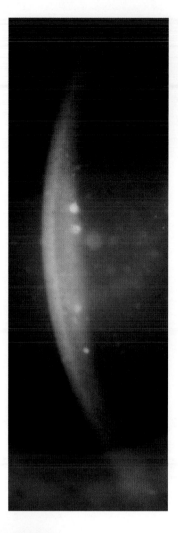

Fig. 15.73 Herpetic keratitis. This 9-year-old girl gave a history of an insect bite on her right eyelid several days before developing disciform keratitis. She had several recurrences that were successfully treated with topical corticosteroids and topical antivirals for a presumed herpetic etiology. Occasionally, patients with herpetic keratitis relate their ocular condition to an episode of trauma.

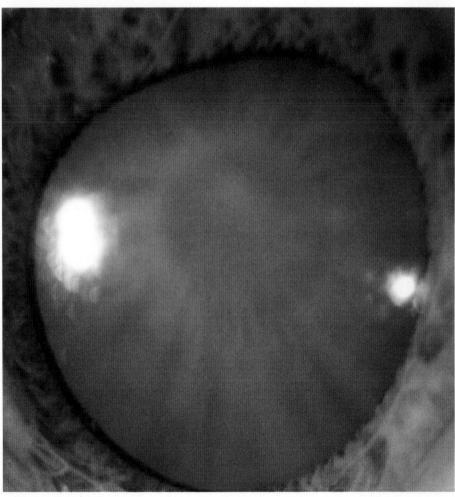

Fig. 15.72 Intraocular copper foreign body causing a sunflower cataract. Foreign bodies that cause chalcosis are usually composed of less than 85% copper. Pure copper produces a suppurative endophthalmitis.

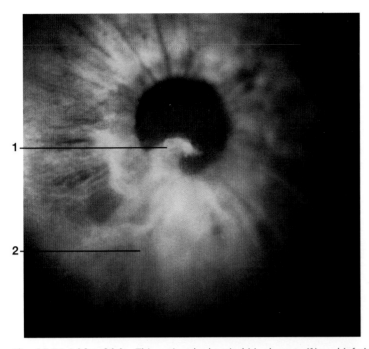

Fig. 15.74 Iridoschisis. This patient had typical iris changes (1) and inferior corneal edema (2). The iris was chronically rubbing on the corneal endothelium.

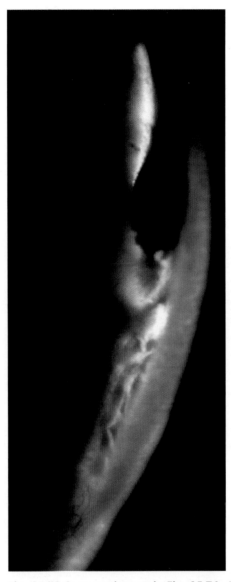

Fig. 15.75 Same patient as in Fig. 15.74. A thin slit-beam view shows corneal edema and iridocorneal touch.

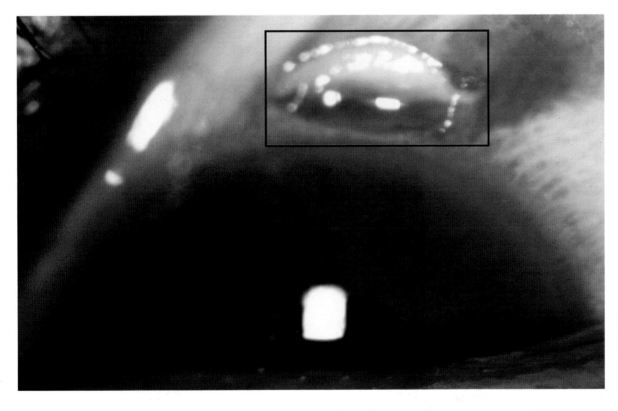

Fig. 15.76 Limbal perforation after blunt trauma. The sclera is thin at the limbus (box) and under the rectus muscle insertions. For this reason, scleral ruptures occur more commonly in these areas.

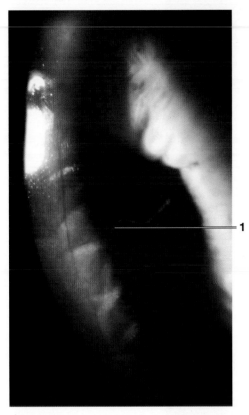

Fig. 15.77 Corneal edema secondary to chronic trauma from a lint foreign body (introduced during cataract surgery) rubbing on the endothelium (1).

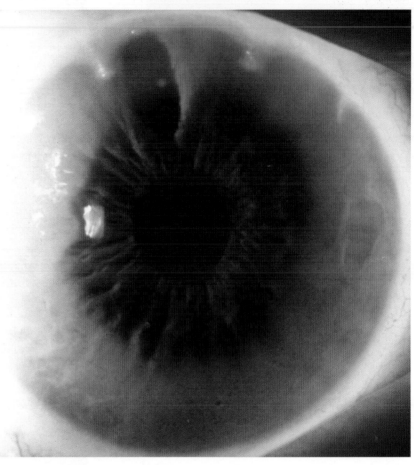

Fig. 15.78 Brown–McLean syndrome. This is characterized by peripheral corneal edema with a relatively clear cornea centrally. The syndrome is seen primarily in aphakic eyes. Many of these eyes have floppy irides, and it is postulated that the mechanical irritation from the iris damages the peripheral endothelium. Peripheral corneal edema is not as extensive in the area overlying a peripheral iridectomy (as seen here).

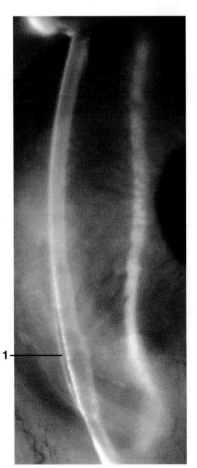

Fig. 15.79 Thin slit-beam view of the Brown–McLean syndrome showing peripheral corneal edema and a large bullae (1).

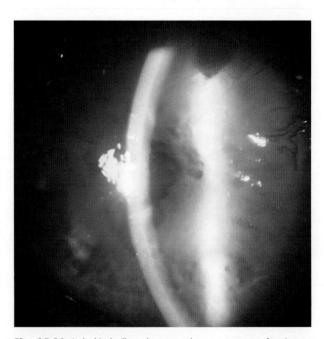

Fig. 15.80 Aphakic bullous keratopathy many years after intracapsular cataract extraction.

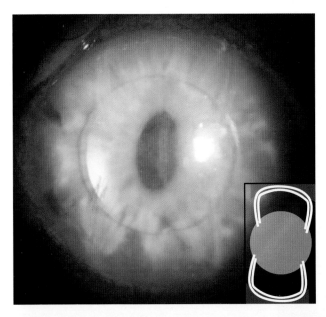

Fig. 15.81 Pseudophakic corneal edema after intracapsular cataract extraction and insertion of a closed looped anterior chamber intraocular lens. The schematic (inset) shows that the haptic loops extend into the angle.

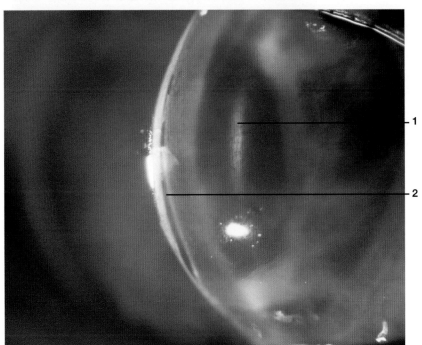

Fig. 15.82 Pseudophakic corneal edema after extracapsular cataract extraction and insertion of a posterior chamber intraocular lens. The posterior chamber intraocular lens (1) is seen behind the iris. There is a large edema cleft within the epithelium (2).

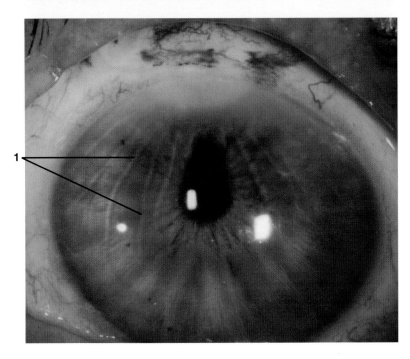

Fig. 15.83 Thermal wound injury during phacoemulsification. Occlusion of irrigation or aspiration during phacoemulsification may result in a rapid rise in the temperature of the phacoemulsification tip. This rise in temperature may cause thermal damage to the cornea, as seen here. The initial injury causes shrinkage of tissue with striae (1). Vision is reduced due to regular and irregular astigmatism.

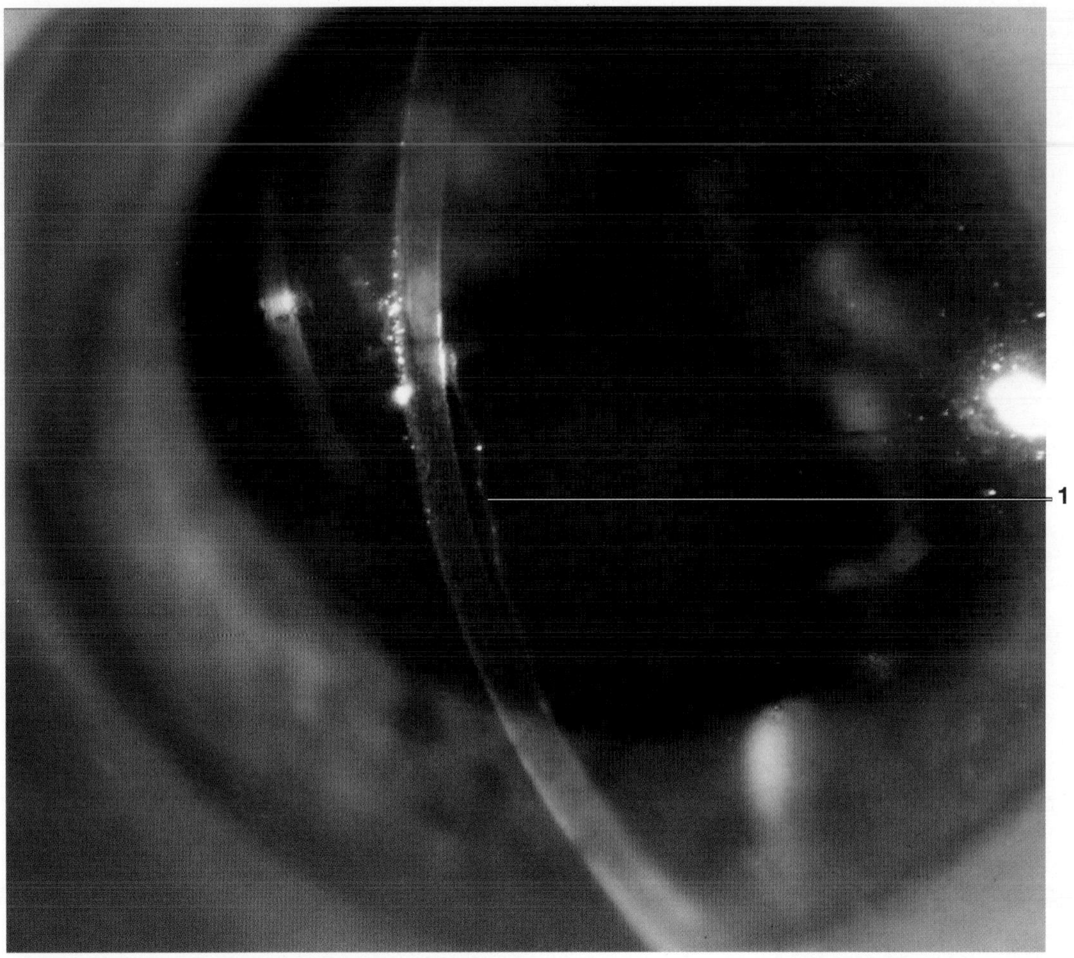

Fig. 15.84 Mild corneal edema after cataract extraction from a detached Descemet's membrane (1).

— 1

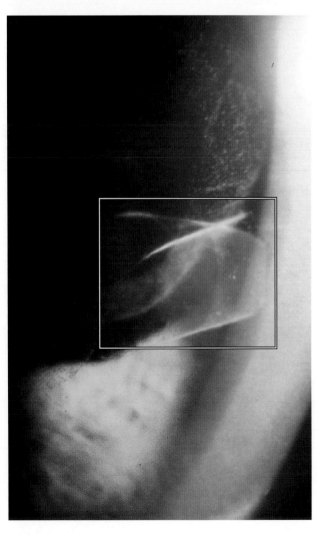

Fig. 15.85 Scrolled Descemet's membrane (box) associated with trauma from cataract surgery.

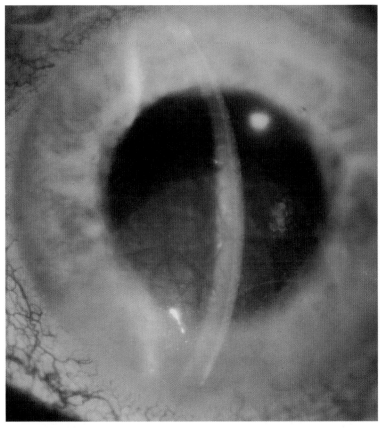

Fig. 15.86 Detachment of Descemet's membrane. This patient has inferior corneal edema due to a focal detachment of Descemet's membrane.

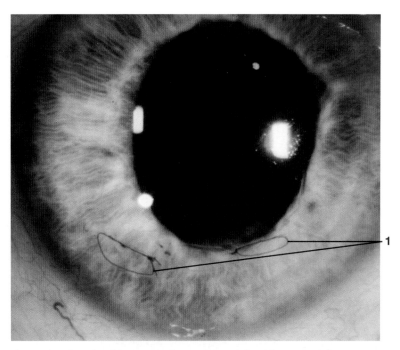

Fig. 15.87 Repair of Descemet's membrane detachment with transcorneal sutures. This is the same patient as seen in Fig. 15.86. Despite attempted repair with intracameral sulfur hexafluoride (SF6) the detachment remained. Two transcorneal polypropylene (Prolene) mattress sutures (1) were used to fixate Descemet's membrane to the cornea.

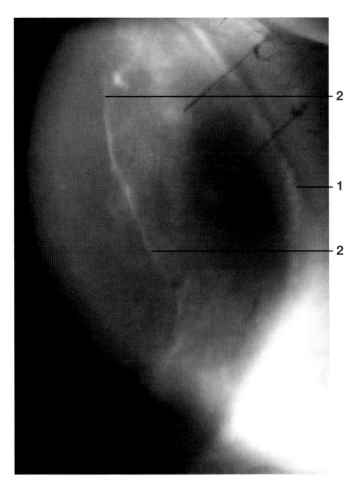

Fig. 15.88 Epithelial ingrowth after cataract surgery. An epithelial membrane can be seen beginning near the limbus (1) with its leading edge (2) into the cornea.

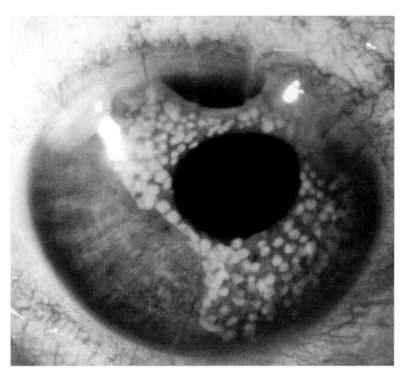

Fig. 15.89 Same patient as in Fig. 15.88. Argon laser photocoagulation has been applied to the surface of the iris to delineate the extent of epithelial growth. Epithelium turns white when treated with the argon laser. The prognosis with extensive epithelial downgrowth is usually poor.

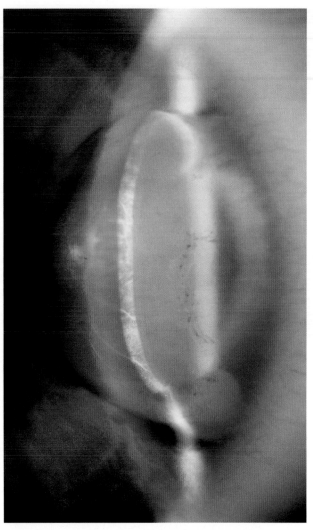

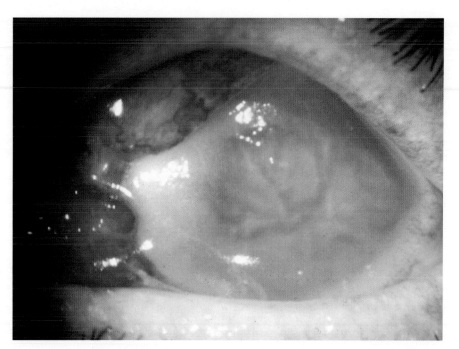

Fig. 15.91 Anterior segment ischemia 3 days after muscle surgery on three rectus muscles. The early signs of anterior segment ischemia include corneal edema and anterior uveitis.

Fig. 15.90 Anterior chamber epithelial inclusion cyst. This was noted several months after penetrating trauma.

Acid Burns

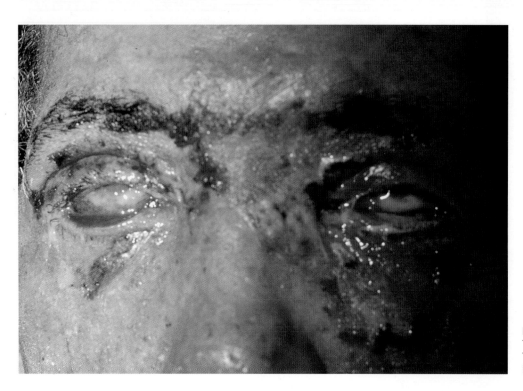

Fig. 15.92 Severe acid burn to the face and eyes. The scarring in the skin has caused a cicatricial ectropion. There is ischemic ulceration of the cornea and sclera in both eyes.

Alkali Burns

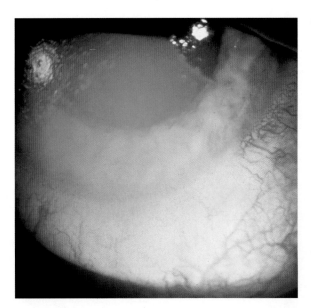

Fig. 15.93 Moderately severe anhydrous ammonia burn to the conjunctiva and cornea.

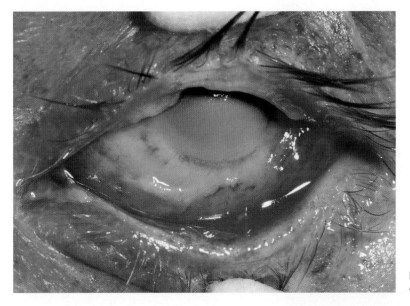

Fig. 15.94 Severe alkali burn with conjunctival and scleral ischemia and marked corneal edema.

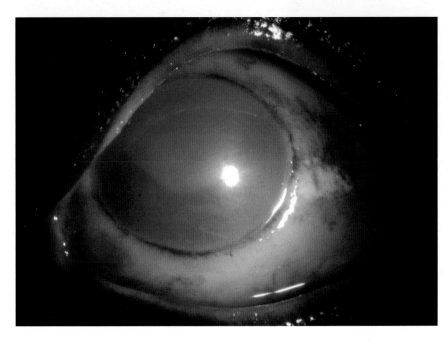

Fig. 15.95 Alkali burn with nonhealing epithelial defect resulting from ischemia. Eyes with severe alkali burns often develop glaucoma and cataracts.

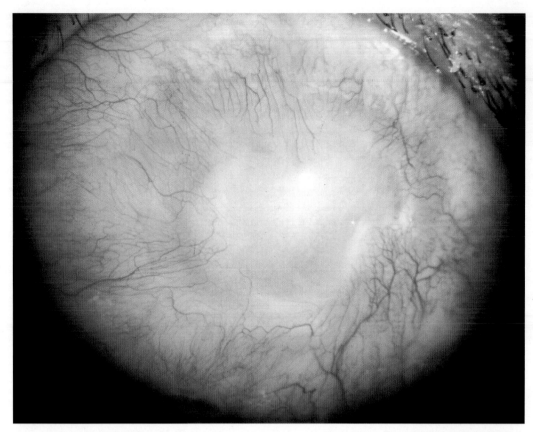

Fig. 15.96 Severe alkali burn after 1 year. The cornea is scarred and there is extensive vascularization. The prognosis for keratoplasty in these patients is poor because of the high risk of rejection from increased stromal vascularization and poor ability to maintain a normal epithelial surface as a result of damaged conjunctival and corneal stem cells.

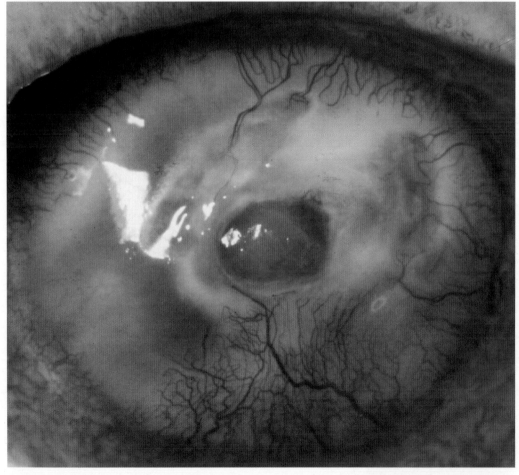

Fig. 15.97 Alkali burn with stromal necrosis and perforation. Alkaline compounds are lipophilic and penetrate deep into the corneal stroma. They cause saponification of fatty acids in cell membranes, which leads to rapid cell death.

Chapter 16

Contact Lens Complications

Contact lens complications are related to three basic mechanisms: (1) mechanical trauma to the conjunctiva and cornea, (2) chronic and acute hypoxia from decreased transmissibility of oxygen in the presence of a contact lens, and (3) allergic reactions from protein deposits in the contact lenses. Many patients who wear contact lenses have dry eyes and/or blepharitis, which further compromise the conjunctival and corneal surface, increasing the chances of complications.

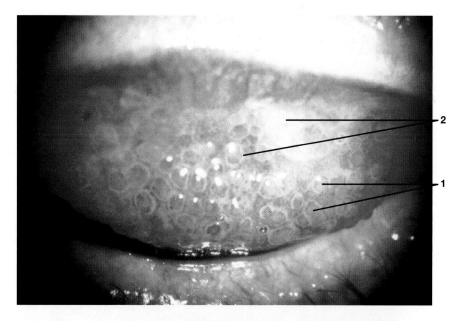

Fig. 16.1 Giant papillary conjunctivitis. The symptoms include itching and mucous discharge. Giant papillae (1) are present on the upper tarsal conjunctiva. Mucus (2) may surround the papillae as seen below or may be floating freely as seen above. The pathophysiology of this disorder is multifactorial and probably relates to chronic trauma from the contact lens and an allergic reaction to proteins that accumulate in the contact lens.

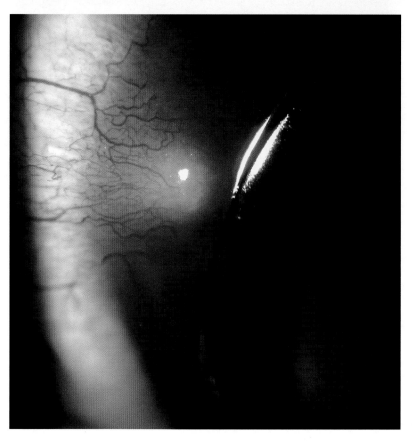

Fig. 16.2 Phlyctenule from a contact lens. Chronic mechanical irritation from the edge of a rigid contact lens can lead to a corneal phlyctenule.

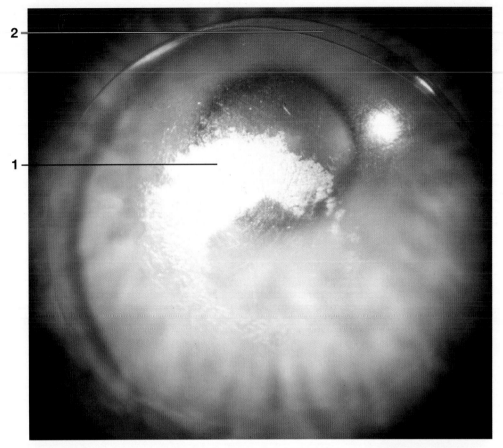

Fig. 16.3 Debris (1) may accumulate on the surface of the contact lens or between the contact lens and the epithelium. If it is on the back of the lens, the debris can rub on the epithelium and increase the risk of infectious keratitis. The superior portion of the lens is lifted away from the cornea, producing a space filled by air (2).

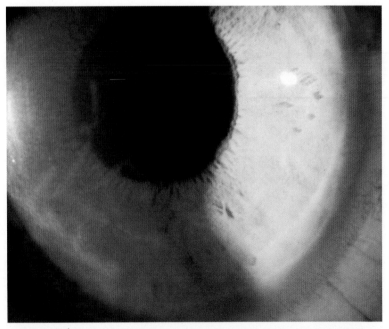

Fig. 16.4 Mechanical irritation from soft contact lenses may produce dendritic epithelial patterns in the corneal epithelium. These patterns should be distinguished from herpes simplex dendrites (see Fig. 11.18) and dendritic forms from *Acanthamoeba* keratitis (see Fig. 11.75).

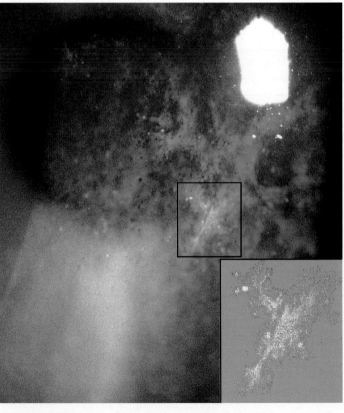

Fig. 16.5 Fluorescein staining of dendritic epithelial patterns in a soft contact lens wearer. In contrast, herpes simplex epithelial keratitis produces an actual ulceration into the superficial cornea.

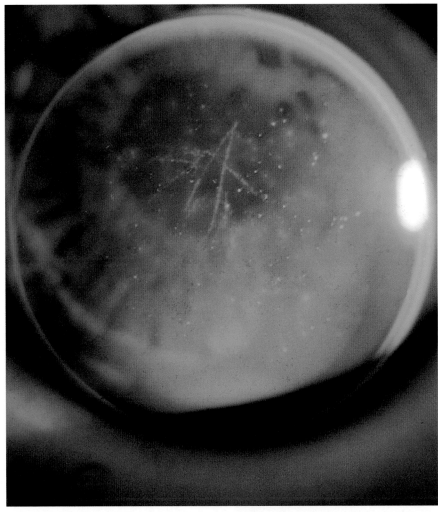

Fig. 16.6 Dust trail linear abrasions from a rigid contact lens. These occur when a foreign body lodges between the contact lens and the patient's cornea.

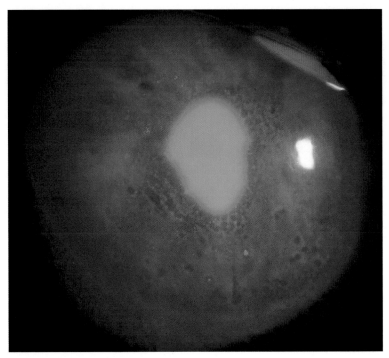

Fig. 16.7 Corneal erosions from a soft contact lens. These should be treated with topical antibiotics rather than pressure patching because the risk of developing infectious keratitis is high.

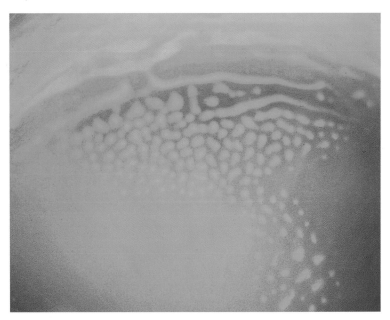

Fig. 16.8 Air bubble indentations with fluorescein pooling in a contact lens wearer.

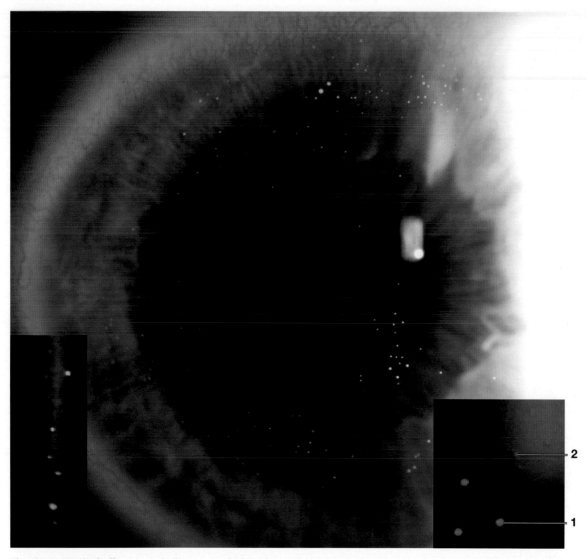

Fig. 16.9 Mucin balls. Mucin balls are round white deposits that accumulate between the posterior surface of a contact lens and the corneal epithelium. When the contact lens is removed, the mucin balls may be blinked away, but in some cases they remain adherent to the cornea (1) for several hours. When they are removed, they leave a depression in the epithelium (2). They are more common with rigid soft contact lens materials such as high-DK silicone lenses.

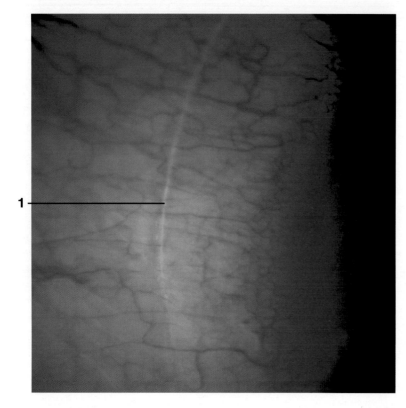

Fig. 16.10 Tight-fitting soft contact lens producing a groove in the conjunctiva (1). Tight lenses decrease the oxygen diffusion to the cornea and can be associated with vascularization, edema, and infiltrates.

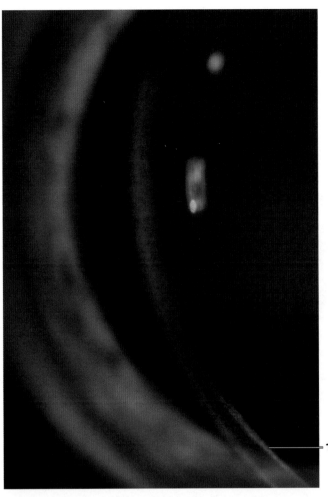

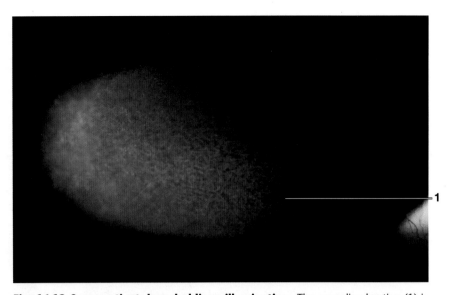

Fig. 16.12 Same patient; broad oblique illumination. The cyan discoloration (1) is seen to be diffuse.

Fig. 16.11 Cyan mottling of the posterior cornea in a soft contact lens wearer; slit-beam view. The etiology of this lesion (1) is unknown.

Fig. 16.13 Epithelial dysplasia. Chronic mechanical irritation from a contact lens can induce epithelial dysplasia, as seen here. This is a benign condition, although treatment is very difficult and may require surgery such as a conjunctival transplant or keratoepithelialplasty.

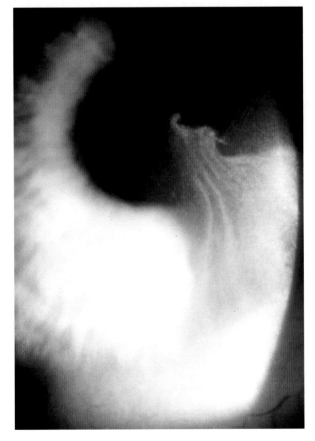

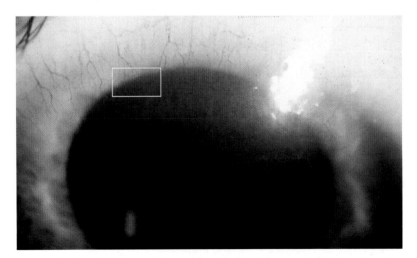

Fig. 16.14 Superficial pannus in a soft contact lens wearer resulting from chronic hypoxia.

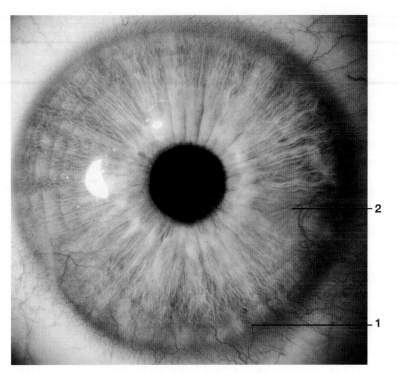

Fig. 16.15 Superficial (1) and stromal (2) vascularization from a low-riding, rigid contact lens.

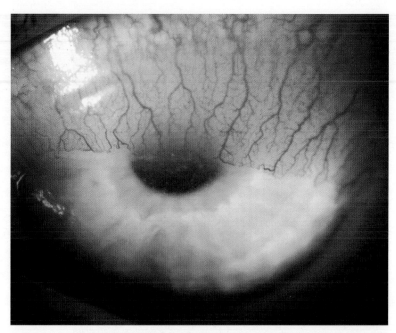

Fig. 16.16 Severe corneal vascularization from a poorly fitted, soft contact lens.

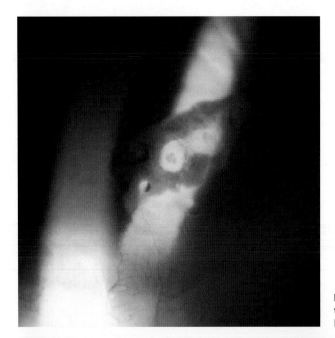

Fig. 16.17 Occasionally a blood vessel in the cornea breaks from contact lens-related trauma. This is an example of a subepithelial hemorrhage in a soft contact lens wearer. Intrastromal hemorrhages can also occur.

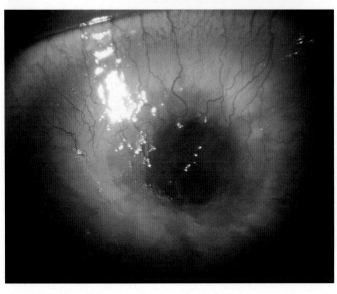

Fig. 16.18 Corneal vascularization and epithelial dysplasia in a soft contact lens wearer. Chronic contact lens wear has altered the epithelium.

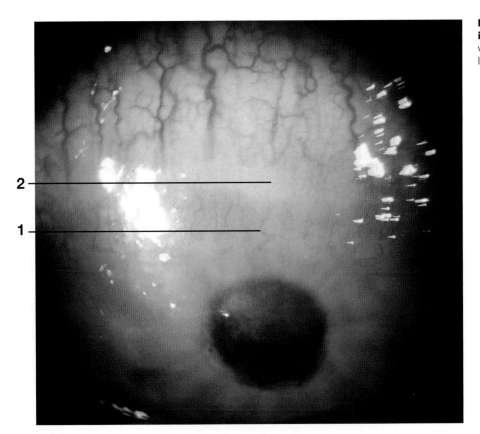

Fig. 16.19 Superior limbic keratoconjunctivitis syndrome in a soft contact lens wearer. There is superficial conjunctival vascularization (1) and limbal thickening (2). Preservatives in contact lens solutions can produce a similar clinical picture.

Fig. 16.20 Mild diffuse anterior stromal infiltrate in a soft contact lens wearer. This infiltrate is sterile and caused by corneal hypoxia.

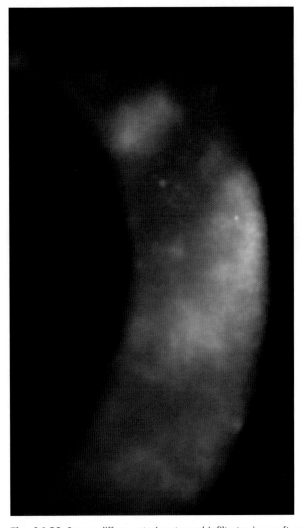

Fig. 16.21 Severe diffuse anterior stromal infiltrates in a soft contact lens wearer.

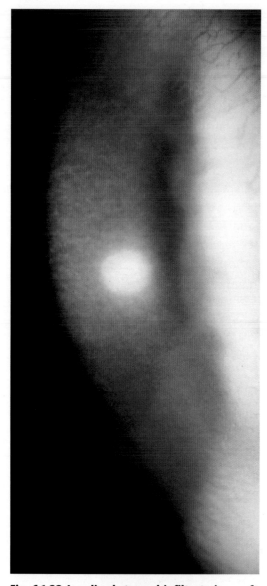

Fig. 16.22 Localized stromal infiltrate in a soft contact lens wearer.
There is no epithelial defect, and this infiltrate was a sterile reaction. Frequent
antibiotic instillation and follow-up examination the next day are indicated.
Corneal cultures are usually not necessary.

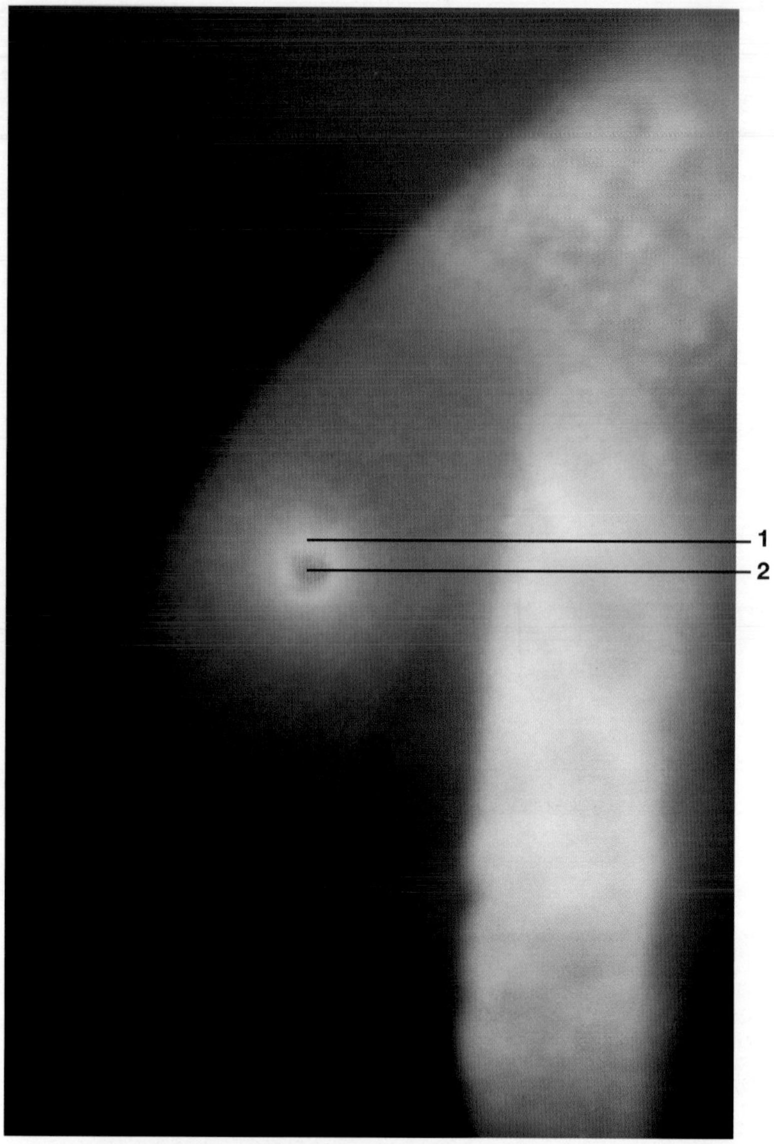

**Fig. 16.23 Localized stromal infiltrate (1) with an overlying epithelial
defect (2) in a soft contact lens wearer.** When an epithelial defect is
present, there should be a high index of suspicion for infectious keratitis. Corneal
cultures are often initiated, depending on the size and extent of the corneal
infiltrate.

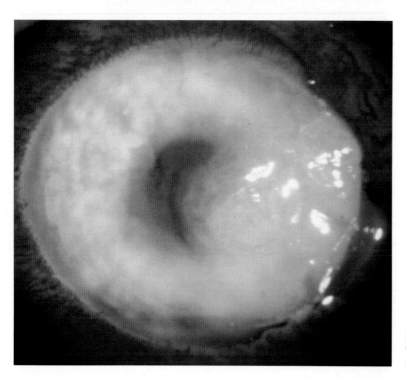

**Fig. 16.24 Extensive pseudomonas bacterial corneal ulcer associated
with soft contact lens use.** Corneal cultures are performed. Frequent fortified
antibiotics are indicated.

Chapter 17

Disorders of the Sclera

Collagen vascular diseases associated with scleritis and keratitis were discussed in Chapter 14. The purpose of this chapter is to demonstrate the clinical features of the different forms of episcleritis and scleritis.

Scleral Thinning

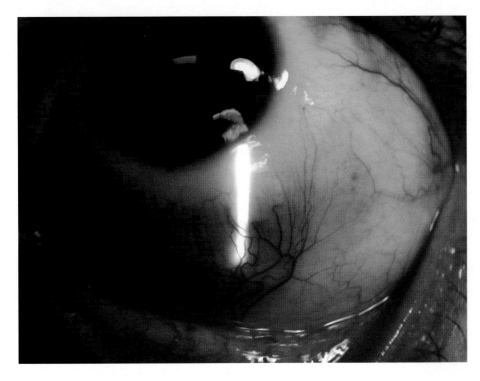

Fig. 17.1 Scleral thinning in a 13-diopter myope. When the sclera thins, the underlying dark uveal pigment begins to become visible.

Episcleritis

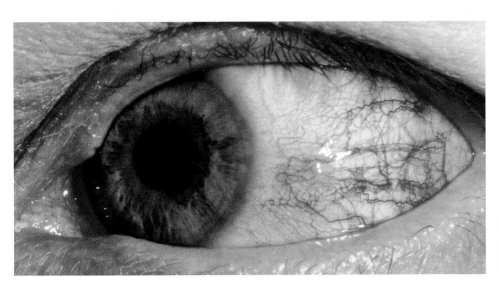

Fig. 17.2 Nodular episcleritis in a patient with gout. The symptoms of episcleritis include redness and mild ocular irritation. There is some blanching of the vessels after the instillation of topical phenylephrine. In many cases, there is no known systemic association.

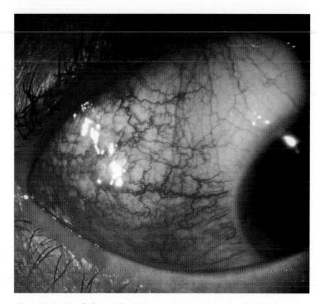

Fig. 17.3 Nodular scleritis. In this variety of scleritis there is an elevated inflamed mass within the area of inflammation.

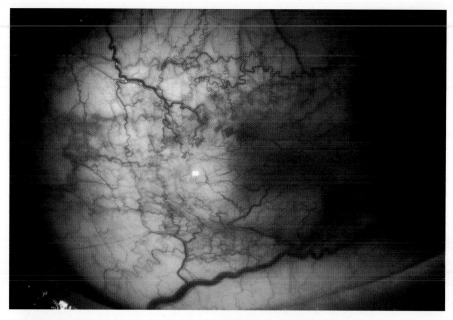

Fig. 17.4 Nodular scleritis. In this patient with nodular scleritis, the nodule is more discrete and elevated. The nodule resolved completely after treatment with oral corticosteroids.

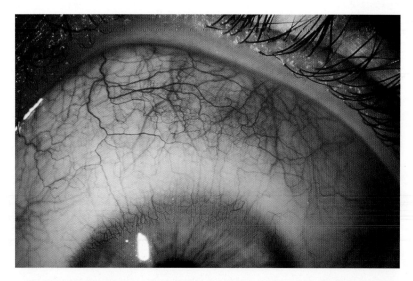

Fig. 17.5 Diffuse scleritis. The hallmark of scleritis is severe ocular and orbital pain. Often there is an associated iritis. There is injection of the conjunctiva and deep episcleral vessels; the inflammation extends into the sclera. Scleritis is often associated with systemic conditions, and systemic treatment is usually required to control the pain and inflammation.

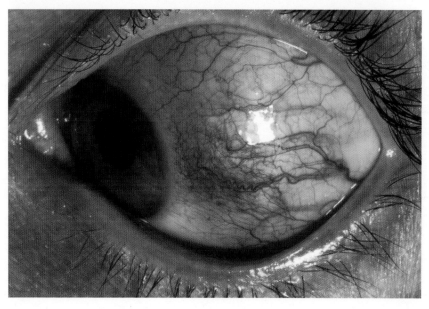

Fig. 17.6 Diffuse scleritis. Dilation of the deep episcleral vessels gives the lesion a bluish-red (violaceous) discoloration.

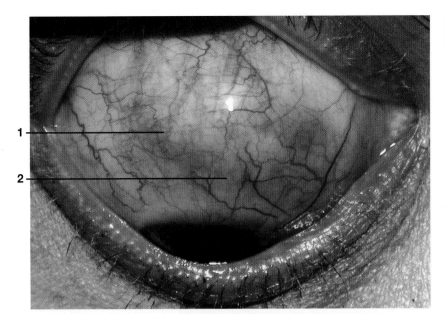

Fig. 17.7 Recurrence of scleritis. In this patient there is an area of active scleritis (1) adjacent to an area of scleral thinning (2) from previous scleral inflammation.

1

2

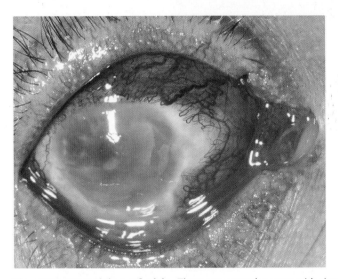

Fig. 17.8 Necrotizing scleritis. There are avascular areas with tissue loss adjacent to areas of active inflammation. This is the most severe form of scleritis and requires aggressive treatment. In this patient the underlying diagnosis was rheumatoid arthritis.

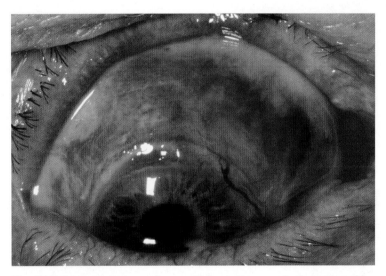

Fig. 17.9 Scleromalacia perforans. This usually occurs in the setting of long-standing rheumatoid arthritis. It is a painless, progressive thinning of the sclera not associated with episodes of acute inflammation. Minor trauma may result in scleral perforation.

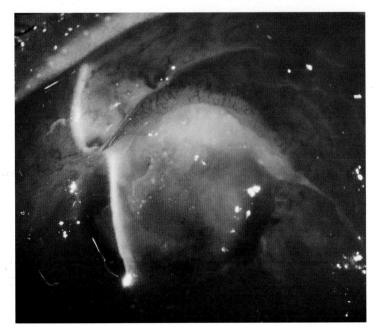

Fig. 17.10 Pseudomonas scleritis that began as a localized keratitis. In all cases of scleritis it is important to exclude an infectious etiology. *Pseudomonas* scleritis is extremely difficult to treat, and the prognosis is poor.

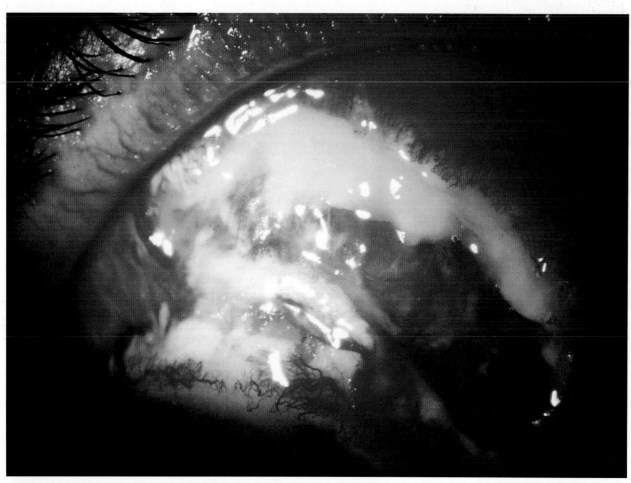

Fig. 17.11 Nocardia scleritis after cataract surgery.

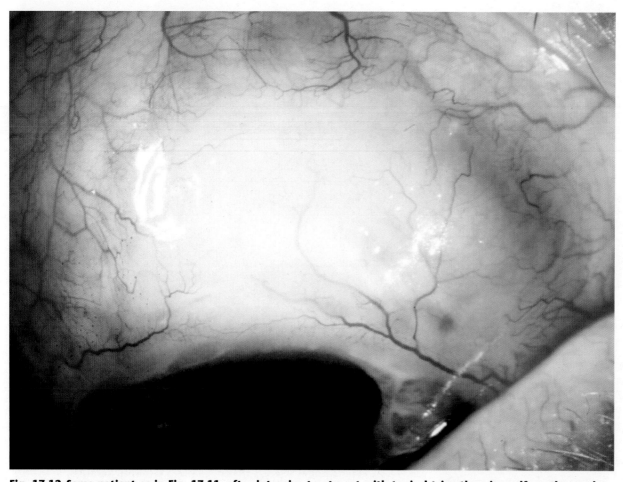

Fig. 17.12 Same patient as in Fig. 17.11, after intensive treatment with topical trimethoprim–sulfamethoxazole.
The sclera has thinned and the patient developed marked against-the-rule astigmatism.

Chapter 18

Iris Tumors

Tumors of the iris are rare. However, it is essential to recognize potentially fatal tumors such as iris melanomas and to be able to differentiate them from benign tumors such as iris cysts.

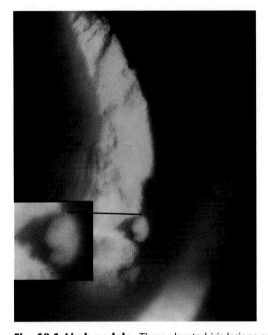

Fig. 18.1 Lisch nodule. These elevated iris lesions are often seen in neurofibromatosis. They are multiple and tan, and composed of nevus cells (inset).

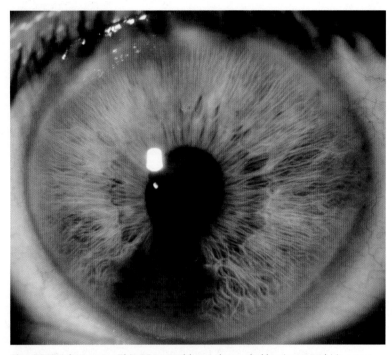

Fig. 18.2 Iris nevus. This 55-year-old man has a darkly pigmented iris nevus. There is distortion of the pupillary border (ectropion uveae).

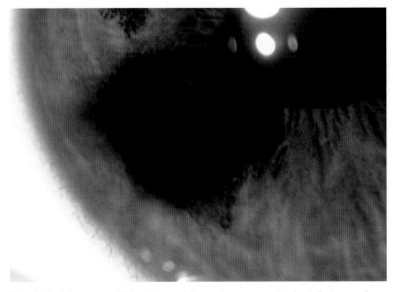

Fig. 18.3 Iris nevus. This 42-year-old man has a nevus in the inferior nasal quadrant of the iris. The lesion has remained stable for the past 8 years.

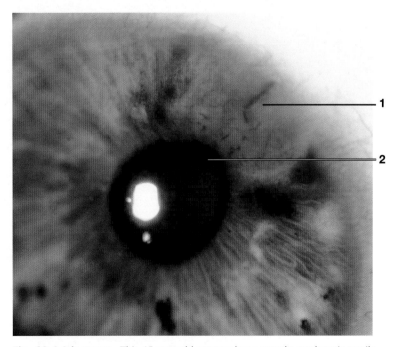

Fig. 18.4 Iris nevus. This 45-year-old woman has a mostly amelanotic sessile mass (1) in the superonasal quadrant of the iris. There are fine vessels, but no feeder vessels. There is a pigment epithelial cyst (2) on the posterior surface of the lesion. The ciliary body is not involved.

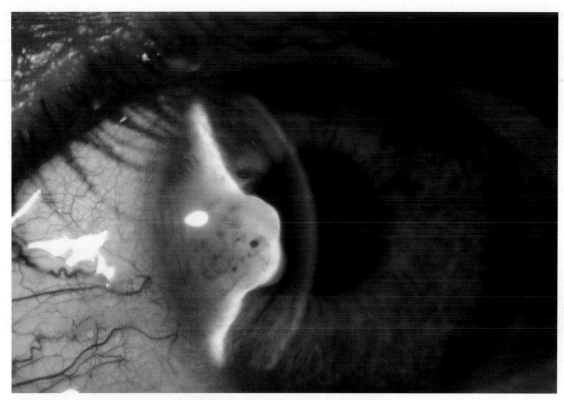

Fig. 18.5 Iris and ciliary body malignant melanoma. Differentiating iris nevi from iris melanomas is often difficult. Features suggestive of melanoma include tumor size, distortion of the iris, ectropion uveae, intrinsic vascularity, and sector cataract. The most important feature is documented growth. This is a mixed cell type of malignant melanoma of the iris and ciliary body. It was removed with an iridocyclectomy procedure.

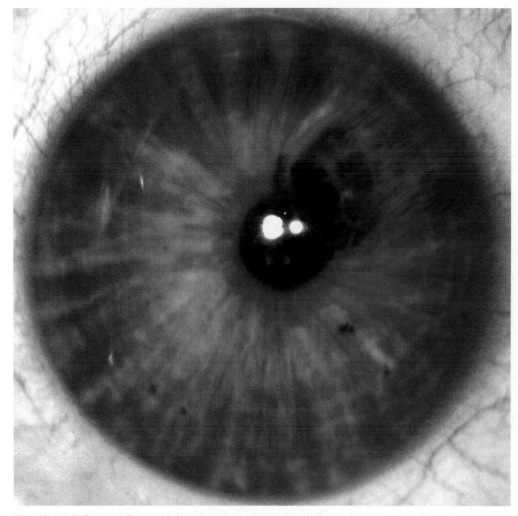

Fig. 18.6 Iris hemangioma. Iris hemangiomas are composed of vascular tufts on the iris surface. Recurrent hyphema is a potential complication.

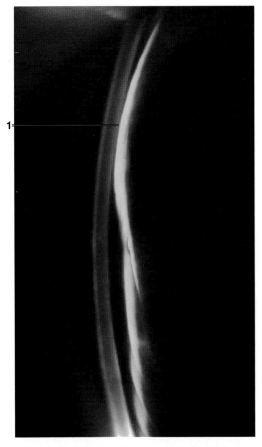

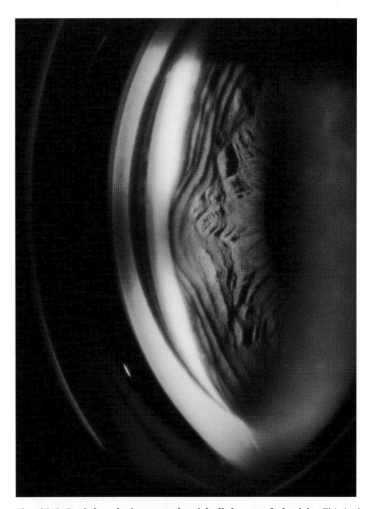

Fig. 18.7 Peripheral pigmented epithelial cyst of the iris. Peripheral pigment epithelial cysts of the iris appear as a bulging of the iris (1) toward the cornea. Because they originate in the iris pigment epithelium, they are often difficult to visualize unless the pupil is widely dilated. The iris stroma overlying the cyst has a normal architecture. These cysts are usually located on the temporal side of the iris, as in this case.

Fig. 18.8 Peripheral pigmented epithelial cyst of the iris. This is the same patient as in Fig. 18.7. Gonioscopy demonstrates the bulging forward of the iris from the underlying cyst.

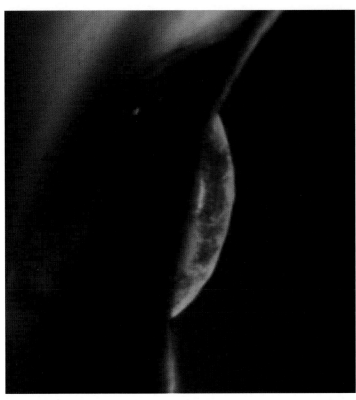

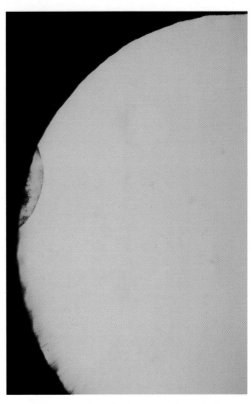

Fig. 18.9 Peripheral pigmented epithelial cyst of the iris. This is the same patient as in Figs 18.7 and 18.8. When the pupil is widely dilated, the cyst is visualized. Peripheral pigment epithelial cysts are usually clear, whereas mid-zonal and pupillary cysts tend to be pigmented.

Fig. 18.10 Peripheral pigmented epithelial cyst of the iris. This is the same patient as in Figs 18.7–18.9. With retinal retro-illumination the cyst is noted to be clear with minimal pigmentation.

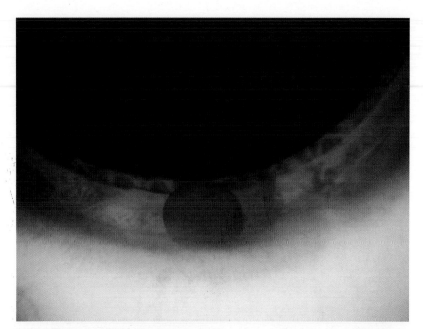

Fig. 18.11 Dislodged anterior chamber pigment epithelial cyst.
Dislodged anterior chamber pigment epithelial cysts are extremely rare. They presumably become dislodged from the iris pigment epithelium and pass from the posterior chamber into the anterior chamber. In some cases they are adherent to the iris and in other cases they float freely in the anterior chamber.

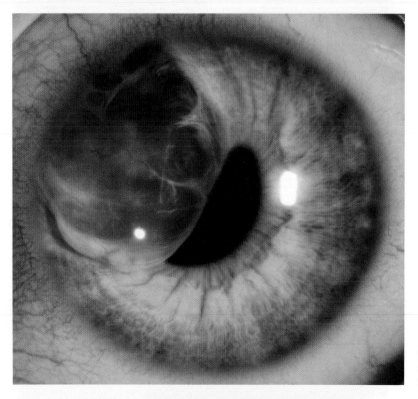

Fig. 18.12 Congenital iris stromal cyst. These are congenital lesions that can remain stable for many years and then suddenly enlarge. The iris is thinned and lacks its normal architecture.

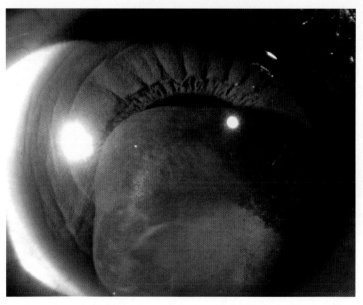

Fig. 18.13 Congenital iris stromal cyst. A large congenital iris stromal cyst almost completely blocks the pupillary aperture.

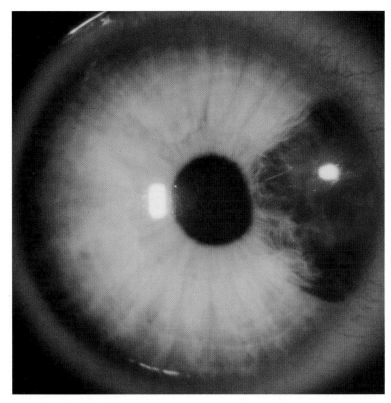

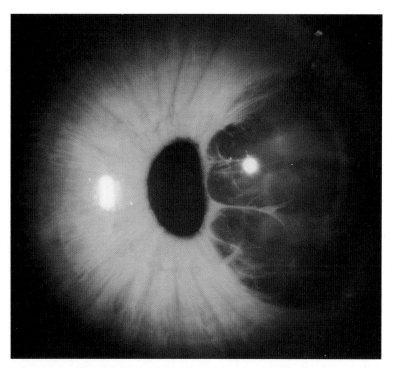

Fig. 18.15 Congenital iris stromal cyst. One month later, the cyst seen in Fig. 18.14 has grown and is causing moderate distortion of the pupil.

Fig. 18.14 Congenital iris stromal cyst. This congenital iris stromal cyst is causing mild distortion of the pupil.

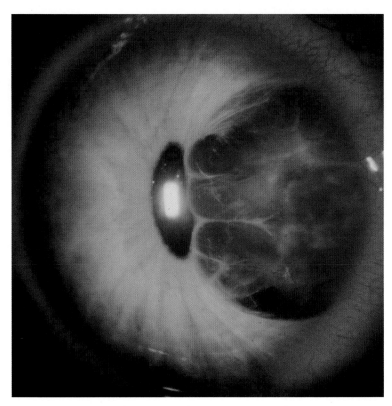

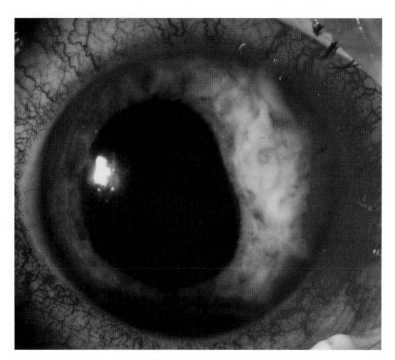

Fig. 18.17 Metastatic small cell lung cancer to the iris. Most metastatic cancers to the eye are found in the choroid, with only 10% occurring in the iris. In men the primary tumor is most often found in the lung, and in women in the breast. In this patient the primary tumor was a small cell lung carcinoma. Metastatic tumors frequently bleed, as seen here, and the presenting sign is often a hyphema.

Fig. 18.16 Congenital iris stromal cyst. Two months later, the cyst seen in Figs 18.14 and 18.15 has grown and is causing severe distortion of the pupil.

Chapter 19

Anterior Uveitis

Anterior uveitis can occur alone or combined with a keratitis or scleritis. This chapter focuses on primary causes of anterior uveitis related to specific etiologies. However, many cases of anterior uveitis are idiopathic and cannot be attributed to any systemic or local disease process.

Sarcoidosis

Sarcoidosis is a systemic inflammatory condition that affects multiple organ systems, including the eyes, skin, central nervous system, and pulmonary system. Sarcoid granulomas can occur in the conjunctiva (see Figs 5.45 and 5.46).

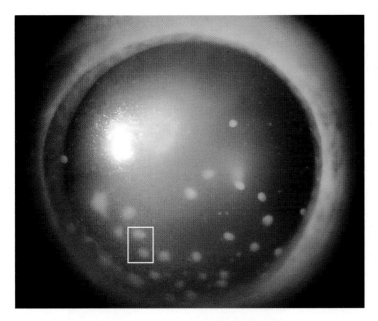

Fig. 19.1 Acute uveitis from sarcoidosis. There are multiple "mutton-fat" keratic precipitates (*box*), as well as microcystic corneal edema caused by a rapid increase in intraocular pressure to 50 mmHg. A chronic granulomatous iridocyclitis is the most common ocular finding in sarcoidosis, although occasionally a nongranulomatous uveitis may occur.

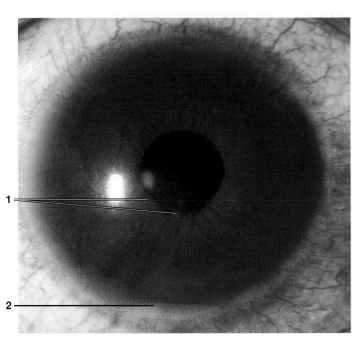

Fig. 19.2 Posterior synechiae (1) and a hemorrhagic hypopyon (2) from an episode of acute sarcoid iridocyclitis.

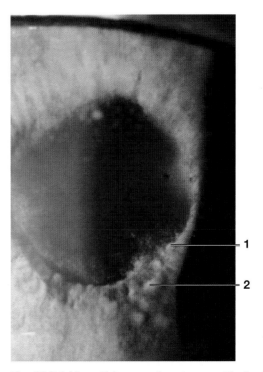

Fig. 19.3 Iridocyclitis secondary to sarcoidosis. Koeppe nodules (1) occur at the pupillary margin, and Busacca nodules (2) occur on the iris surface.

Fuchs' Heterochromic Iridocyclitis

Fuchs' heterochromic iridocyclitis is a unilateral chronic iridocyclitis that causes heterochromia as a result of iris stromal thinning and iris pigment epithelial loss.

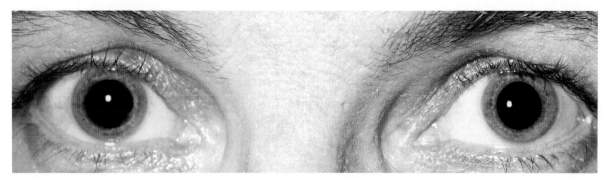

Fig. 19.4 Heterochromia in a patient with Fuchs' heterochromic iridocyclitis in the left eye.

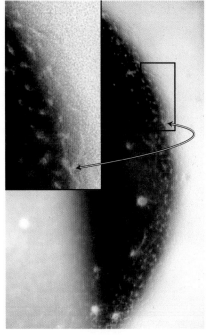

Fig. 19.5 Fuchs' heterochromic iridocyclitis. There are small, white, stellate keratic precipitates on the back of the cornea (inset).

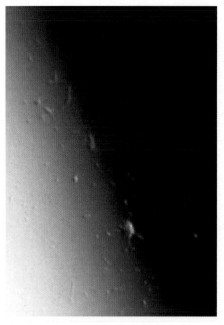

Fig. 19.6 Fuchs' heterochromic iridocyclitis. Stellate precipitates are seen under high magnification. These precipitates are most likely composed of inflammatory cells and fibrin. Usually minimal aqueous cell and almost no flare are associated with these precipitates. Anterior chamber cells do not decrease with corticosteroids.

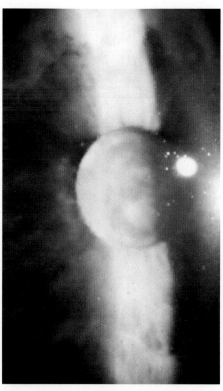

Fig. 19.8 Fuchs' heterochromic iridocyclitis. A posterior subcapsular cataract may be present, and can progress to a mature white cataract (as seen here). Peripheral anterior synechiae and posterior synechiae do not usually develop in this disorder. Cataract surgery is very successful in this condition.

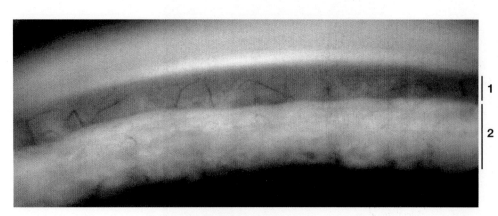

Fig. 19.7 Gonioscopy in Fuchs' heterochromic iridocyclitis. Fine blood vessels course over the trabecular meshwork (1) and iris (2). A paracentesis characteristically produces bleeding from these vessels.

Behçet's Disease

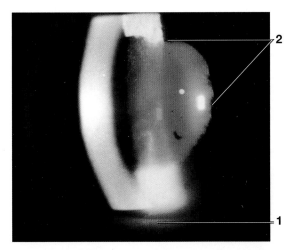

Fig. 19.9 Uveitis with hypopyon (1), characteristic of Behçet's disease. Posterior synechiae (2) are present.

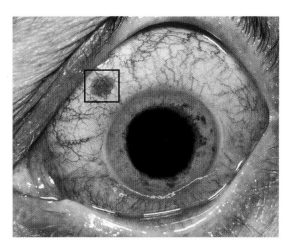

Fig. 19.10 Scleritis in Behçet's disease with a localized erythematous nodule (box).

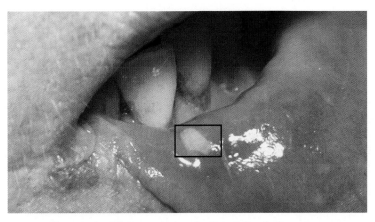

Fig. 19.11 Typical aphthous oral ulcer (box) in Behçet's disease.

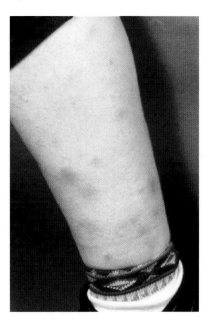

Fig. 19.12 Subcutaneous erythematous nodules in Behçet's disease.

Vogt–Koyanagi–Harada Syndrome

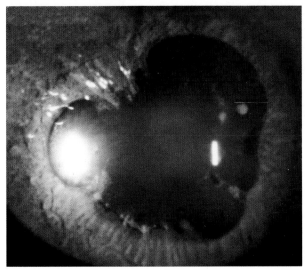

Fig. 19.13 Vogt–Koyanagi–Harada syndrome with posterior synechiae from an anterior uveitis.

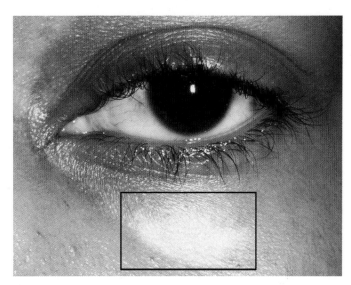

Fig. 19.14 Vogt–Koyanagi–Harada syndrome with vitiligo (box).

Juvenile Rheumatoid Arthritis

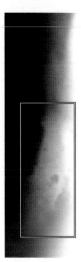

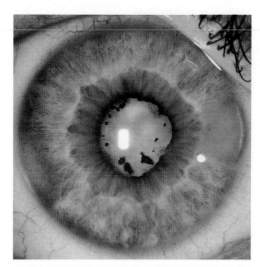

Fig. 19.15 Band keratopathy. This finding may occur in the presence or absence of active inflammation in patients with juvenile rheumatoid arthritis.

Fig. 19.16 Mature white cataracts and extensive posterior synechiae. These findings may occur in patients with juvenile rheumatoid arthritis.

Syphilitic Uveitis

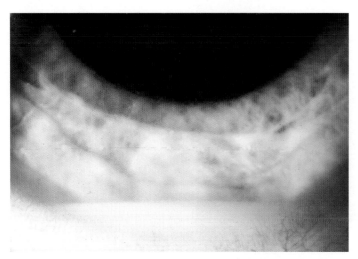

Fig. 19.17 Syphilitic uveitis with hypopyon in a patient with AIDS.

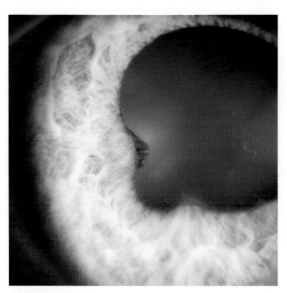

Fig. 19.18 Fellow eye of the patient shown in Fig. 19.17, with posterior synechiae.

HLA-B27-related Uveitis

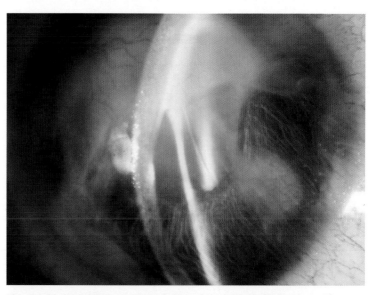

Fig. 19.19 HLA-B27-associated disorders include Reiter's syndrome, ankylosing spondylitis, inflammatory bowel disease, and psoriatic arthritis. This patient with uveitis and ankylosing spondylitis developed a severe inflammatory response after cataract surgery. There is corneal edema associated with a retrocorneal membrane superiorly. The posterior chamber intraocular lens is encased in fibrin.

Chapter 20

Penetrating and Lamellar Keratoplasty

In 1906, Edward Zirm reported the first successful penetrating keratoplasty. Since that time, advances in surgical techniques have greatly improved the prognosis of corneal transplantation. The clinician must recognize the spectrum of postoperative complications that can occur after penetrating keratoplasty.

Preoperative and Postoperative Appearance

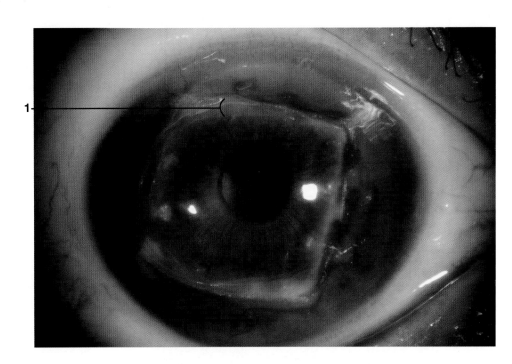

Fig. 20.1 Square corneal transplant performed by Ramon Castroviejo in 1956. Dr Ramon Castroviejo was a pioneer of modern corneal transplantation surgery. His original technique employed a double-edged blade to create a square lamellar incision into the corneal stroma. The incision was then beveled toward the center of the pupil to produce a shelved incision (1). The shelved incision helped prevent postoperative wound leaks and the formation of iridocorneal adhesions. The transplant tissue was obtained from a whole globe in a similar matter, without beveling the incision. The square graft was placed over the square bed and secured into place with overlay sutures (the wound edges were not approximated with sutures, as the suture material at the time was not fine enough to reapproximate delicate corneal tissue). The patient shown here maintained 20/30 visual acuity with a rigid gas-permeable lens 50 years after the date of surgery.

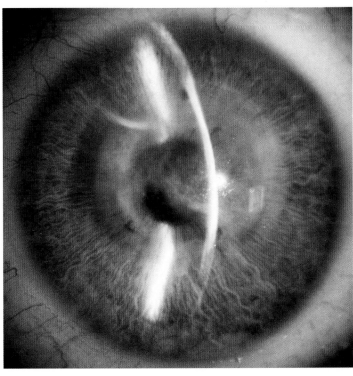

Fig. 20.2 Preoperative view of central corneal scar from a varicella infection.

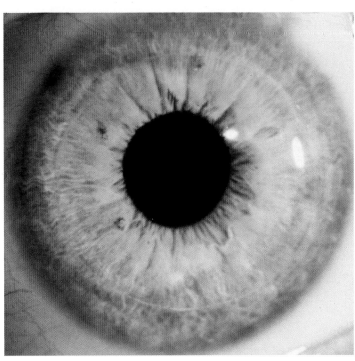

Fig. 20.3 Postoperative appearance of same patient as in Fig. 20.2, 17 months after a penetrating keratoplasty. The graft is clear.

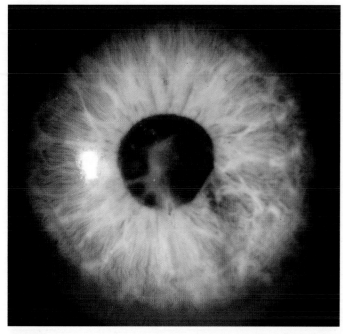

Fig. 20.4 Preoperative appearance of a central corneal scar secondary to trauma.

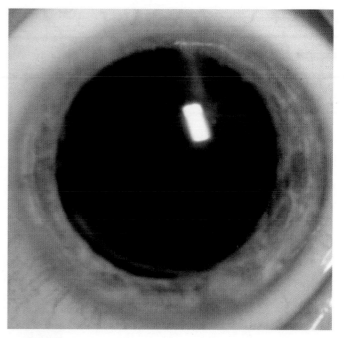

Fig. 20.5 Postoperative appearance 16 months after a rotating penetrating keratoplasty was performed, rotating the scar superiorly.

Intraoperative and Early Postoperative Complications

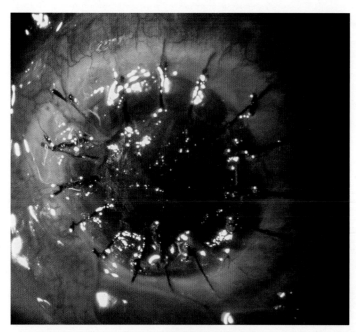

Fig. 20.6 Suprachoroidal hemorrhage that developed intraoperatively. The graft was sutured into place with 8-0 black silk suture because this suture is larger and more visible, and therefore easier to work with in an emergency situation.

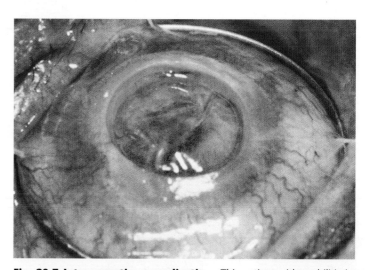

Fig. 20.7 Intraoperative complication. This patient with syphilitic interstitial keratitis underwent a penetrating keratoplasty. A retained Descemet's membrane was noted. This membrane must be removed before suturing the donor cornea.

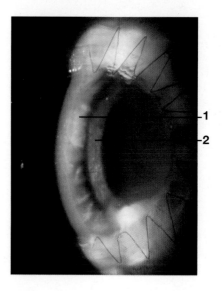

Fig. 20.8 Intraoperative complication. A penetrating keratoplasty was performed for Fuchs' dystrophy. The donor cornea is seen (1) as well as Descemet's membrane from the host cornea (2), which was inadvertently left behind.

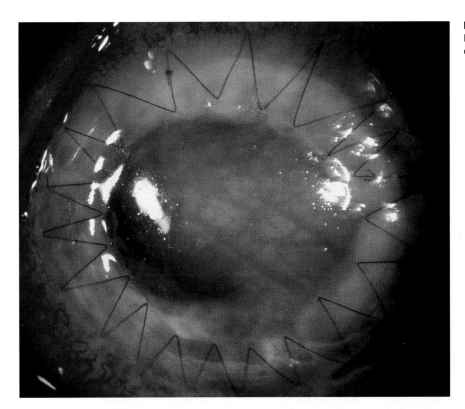

Fig. 20.9 Postoperative complication. A large detachment of Descemet's membrane developed after penetrating keratoplasty. There is diffuse stromal edema.

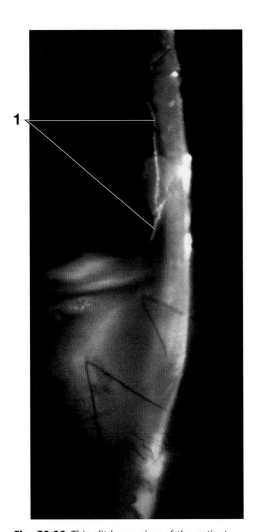

Fig. 20.10 Thin slit-beam view of the patient in Fig. 20.9, showing detached Descemet's membrane (1).

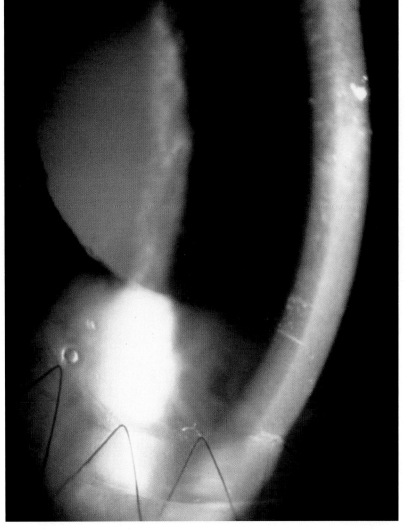

Fig. 20.11 Same patient as in Figs 20.9 and 20.10. Air was injected into the anterior chamber to repair the detached Descemet's membrane. The graft is clear 2 weeks after the air injection.

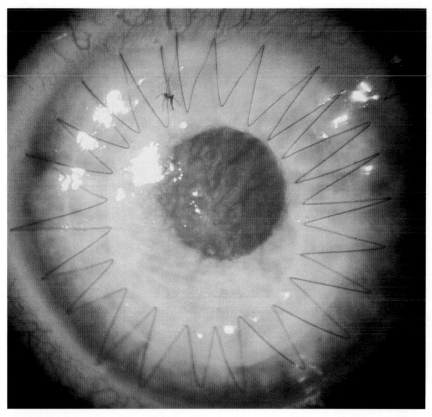

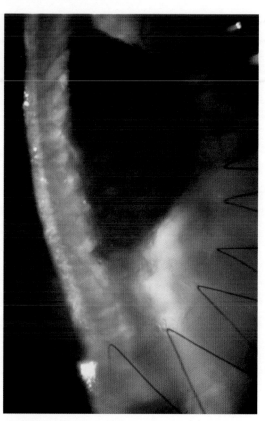

Fig. 20.12 Postoperative complication. Primary donor failure occurs when a graft remains edematous over the entire postoperative period. It is believed to be secondary to endothelial cell dysfunction or surgical trauma. Pathologic examination usually shows the endothelium to be nearly or completely absent.

Fig. 20.13 Thin slit-beam view of the same patient as in Fig. 20.12. There is diffuse stromal edema and folds in Descemet's membrane.

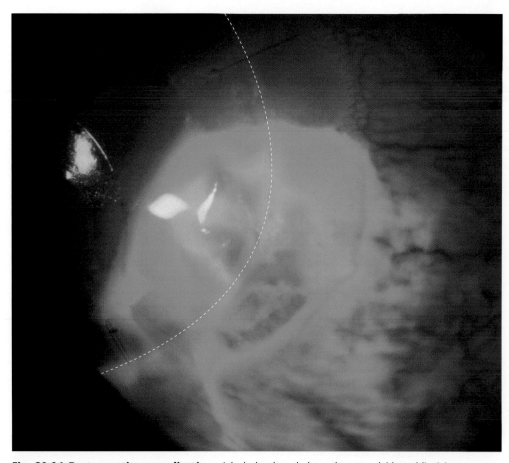

Fig. 20.14 Postoperative complication. A leak developed along the wound (dotted line) in an area of poor tissue apposition after penetrating keratoplasty. Wound leaks may also occur along suture tracks.

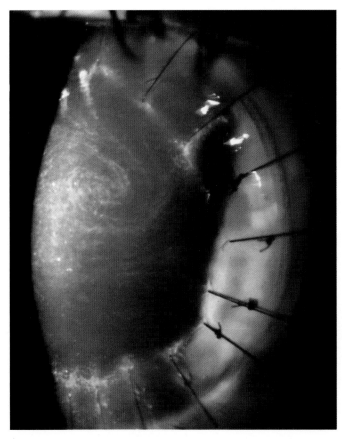

Fig. 20.15 Hurricane keratitis. Swirls of irregular epithelium often occur in the first few weeks after a penetrating keratoplasty. This pattern of healing is thought to be due to toxicity from topical medications and the intrinsic pattern of epithelial healing that occurs as a sliding of the epithelium in a spiral or whorl-shaped pattern.

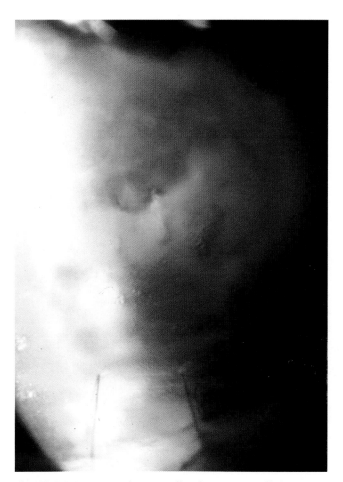

Fig. 20.16 Postoperative complication. A severe fibrin response in the anterior chamber developed in a patient with a history of Mooren's ulcer who underwent a penetrating keratoplasty.

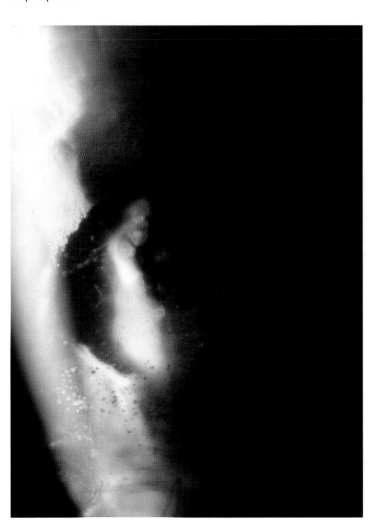

Fig. 20.17 Same patient as in Fig. 20.16. Several hours after the injection of 6 μg of tissue plasminogen activator into the anterior chamber, the eye showed marked resolution of the anterior chamber fibrin, and the intraocular lens can now be visualized.

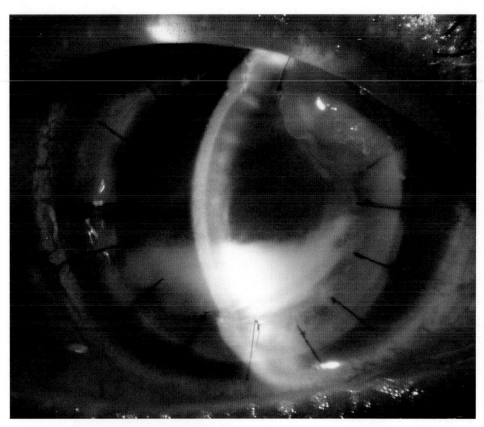

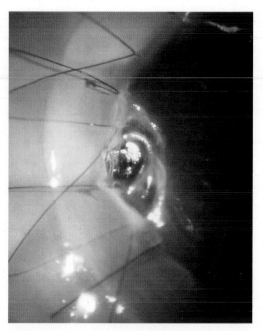

Fig. 20.19 Postoperative complication. A delle has developed on the host tissue secondary to an edematous, elevated, wound margin.

Fig. 20.18 Postoperative complication. Endophthalmitis is a rare but serious complication after penetrating keratoplasty. The causative agent was *Streptococcus pneumoniae*.

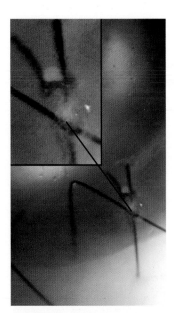

Fig. 20.20 Filaments. These are commonly found attached to sutures (inset). They should be removed with forceps because they can induce a foreign body sensation and may predispose to infection.

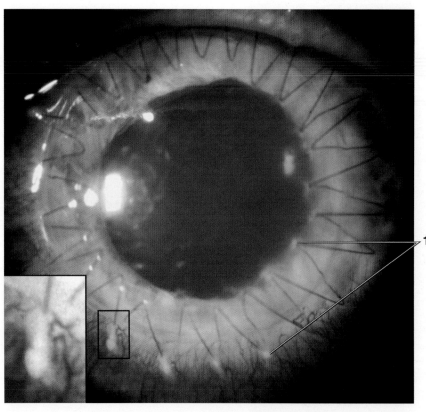

Fig. 20.21 Multiple sterile abscesses surrounding corneal sutures (1). A high-magnification view is seen (inset). These infiltrates are often composed of eosinophils and are more common in young patients with marked peripheral inflammation.

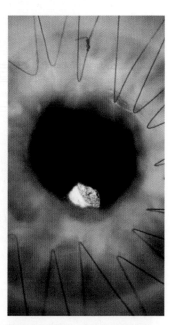

Fig. 20.22 Postoperative complication. A metallic foreign body was found in this graft during a routine examination. The patient did not feel it because of decreased sensation in the graft. Corneal sensation in grafts returns slowly over the course of 2 years, but typically does not reach normal levels.

Late Complications

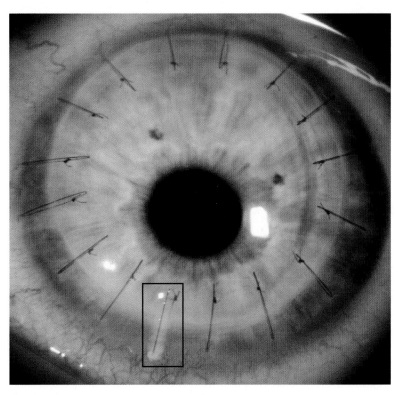

Fig. 20.23 Suture erosion, a common late complication of penetrating keratoplasty. In this case, an inferior suture has become loose and is covered with mucus (box).

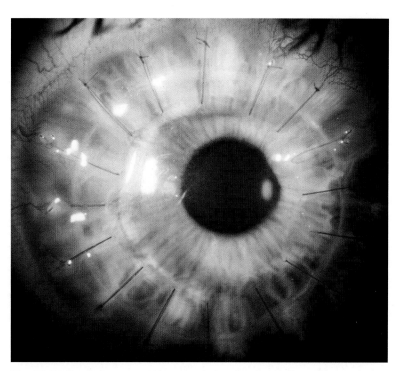

Fig. 20.24 Eroded sutures. These can induce localized inflammation and vascularization. This graft is clear; however, it is not unusual for patients to have multiple eroded sutures, corneal vascularization, and acute allograft rejection.

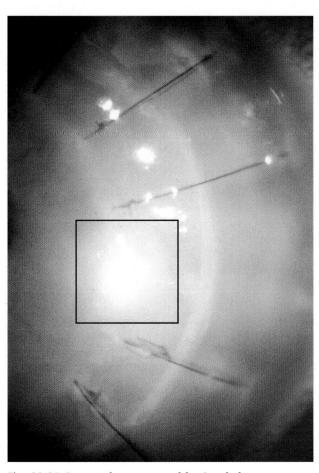

Fig. 20.25 Suture abscess caused by Staphylococcus aureus infection (box). Sutures can provide an entry tract for microorganisms into the stroma.

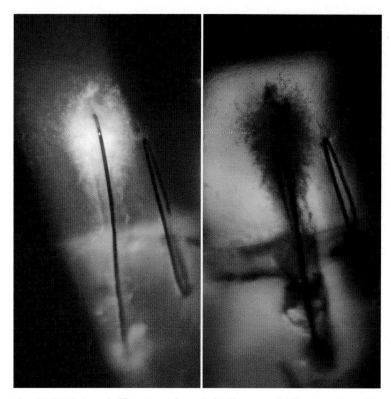

Fig. 20.26 Suture infiltrate with an infectious crystalline keratopathy appearance 1 year after keratoplasty. Direct illumination (left) and indirect illumination (right). The suture was removed and cultured. The culture showed no growth. The patient was treated empirically with vancomycin, and the infiltrate eventually cleared.

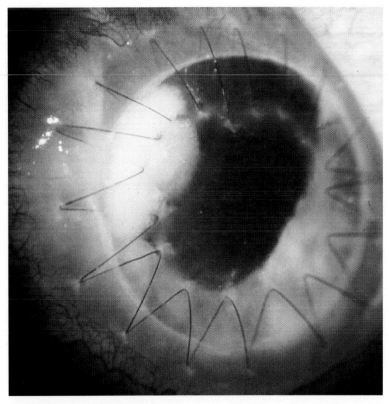

Fig. 20.27 Late complication. This patient developed a *Streptococcus pneumoniae* infection several years after penetrating keratoplasty.

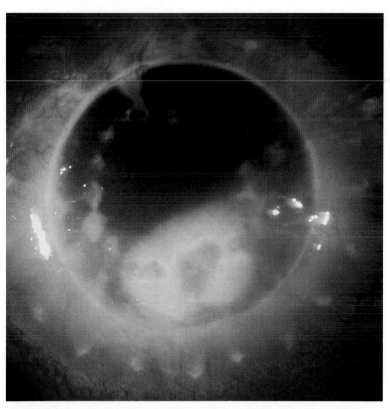

Fig. 20.28 Fellow eye of the same patient as in Fig. 20.27. There is an infiltrate resulting from *Proteus* species in the inferior graft. This infection occurred several months after the infection shown in Fig. 20.27.

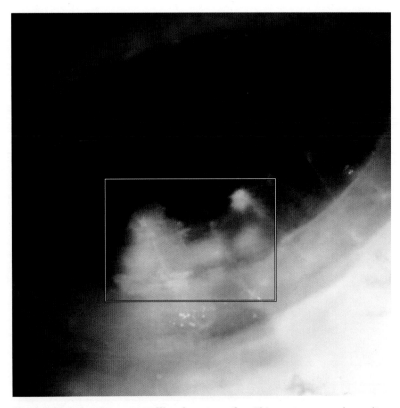

Fig. 20.29 Infectious crystalline keratopathy. This most commonly results from an infection with *Streptococcus viridans* group (specifically, nutritionally variant streptococci). The organism forms a crystalline pattern in the corneal stroma (box), and the overlying epithelium is often intact. There is minimal host response to the infection, and for this reason the stroma surrounding the infiltrate is relatively clear. The infection is typically located at the wound site. This condition is associated with chronic immunosuppression with topical corticosteroids.

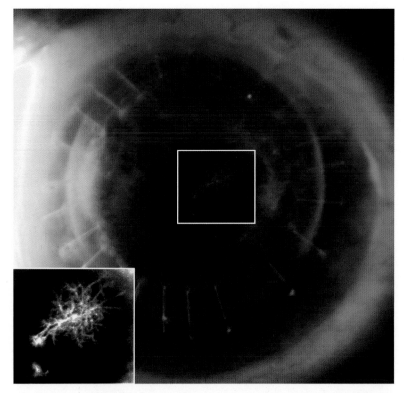

Fig. 20.30 Infectious crystalline keratopathy in the central portion of a graft.

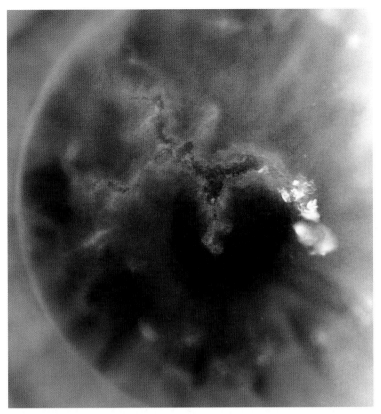

Fig. 20.31 Recurrence of active herpes simplex infection in a graft performed for scarring secondary to herpes simplex keratitis. Antiviral agents should be used along with topical corticosteroids after penetrating keratoplasty to lessen the risk of recurrent herpes simplex infection. Systemic acyclovir may decrease the chance of this occurrence.

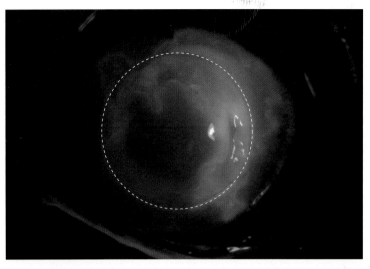

Fig. 20.32 Recurrence of active herpes simplex infection in a graft. The geographic pattern of the epithelial defect, and the location on the graft and the host tissue, should alert the examiner to the strong suspicion of recurrent herpes simplex infection. The dotted circle is the penetrating keratoplasty wound.

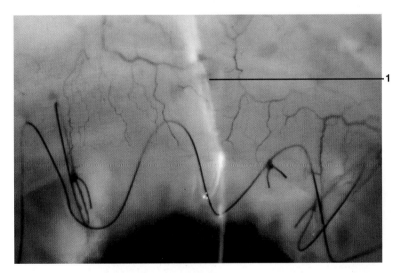

Fig. 20.33 Suture track fistula. An epithelialized fistula (1) has formed along a suture tract. The suture has been removed.

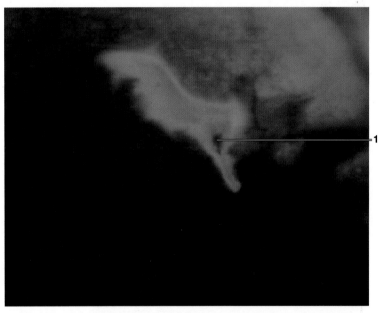

Fig. 20.34 Same patient as in Fig. 20.33. The fistula is Seidel positive (1).

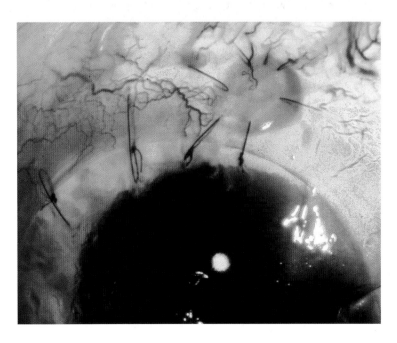

Fig. 20.35 Same patient as in Figs 20.33 and 20.34. Fistulous tracts can be difficult to repair. In this case, cryotherapy was applied to the area to destroy active epithelial cells. A circular lamellar dissection was performed and a circular corneal patch graft was used to seal the hole.

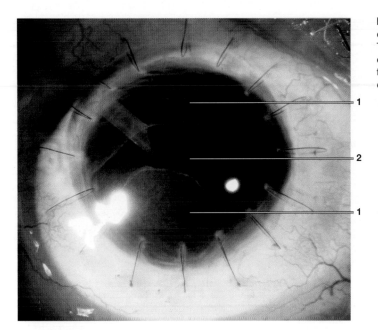

Fig. 20.36 Epithelial ingrowth after penetrating keratoplasty. Epithelial ingrowth on the posterior cornea appears as a faint gray membrane with scalloped, rolled edges. The leading edge can be stable over years, or may progress rapidly over several weeks. The overlying cornea is usually not edematous. The anterior chamber often contains large, free-floating, epithelial cells and an absence of flare. In this example, there are two areas of epithelial ingrowth (1) surrounding a central area of normal cornea (2).

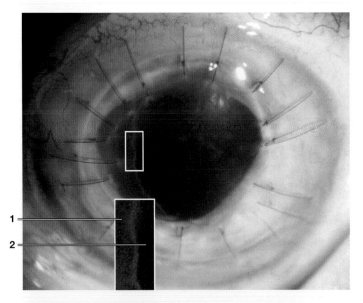

Fig. 20.37 Epithelial ingrowth. The inset demonstrates an area of epithelium on the posterior cornea (1) next to an area of normal endothelium (2).

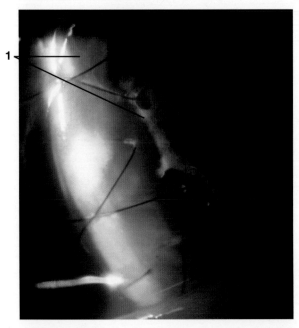

Fig. 20.38 Calcium deposits (1) found near sutures after penetrating keratoplasty. In some cases, topical phosphate corticosteroids (e.g., Inflamase Forte) rather than topical acetate corticosteroids (e.g., Pred-Forte) may be responsible.

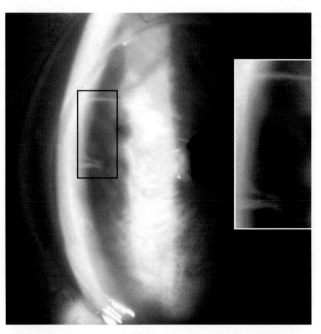

Fig. 20.39 Late complication. This patient with cystoid macular edema had strands of vitreous extending to the keratoplasty wound (inset). The pupil is peaked toward the wound.

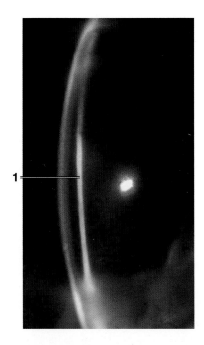

Fig. 20.40 Avascular retrocorneal membrane (1).

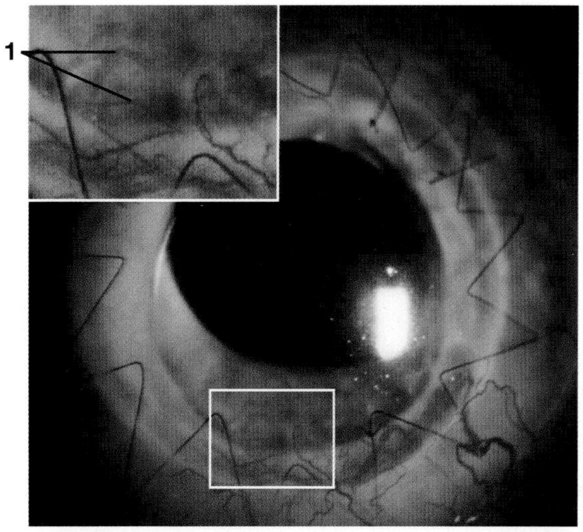

1

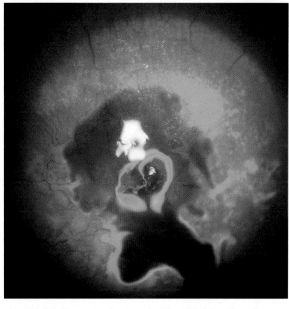

1

Fig. 20.41 Late complication. A dense, circumscribed, white, retrocorneal membrane is present for 360° inside the keratoplasty wound. Fine vessels (1) extend into the membrane. Poor wound apposition may predispose to this complication. The membrane grows slower than epithelial ingrowth, and the prognosis is better.

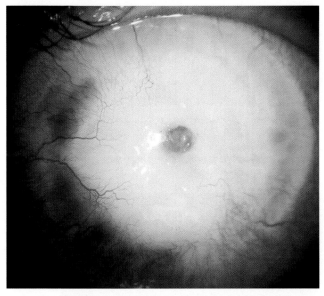

Fig. 20.42 Failed graft with a central filtering cicatrix. This complication can develop when a scarred graft slowly thins over time.

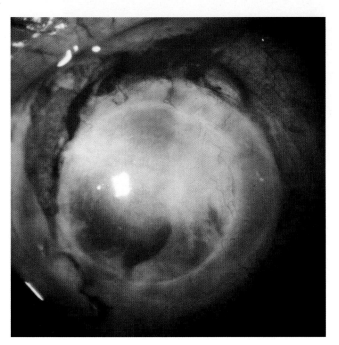

Fig. 20.43 Same patient as in Fig. 20.42. When fluorescein dye is applied, the central area is Seidel positive.

Fig. 20.44 Blunt trauma sustained 22 years after a penetrating keratoplasty. Uveal tissue is protruding from the outer keratoplasty wound. The inner wound is intact. (This patient had two penetrating keratoplasties.)

Rejection Reactions

Allograft rejection occurs in up to one-third of eyes undergoing corneal transplantation. Most commonly it occurs in the first 6 months after transplantation, but may occur any time in the life of the graft. Corneal vascularization dramatically increases the risk of rejection. Fortunately, most rejection reactions can be reversed with local and systemic corticosteroids. Rejection must be recognized early, and patients should seek immediate attention if they experience one of the three danger signals: decreased vision (the most common and frequently recognized signal), redness, or discomfort.

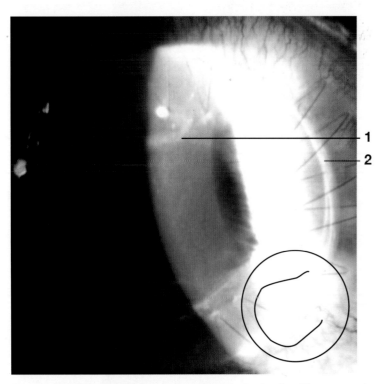

Fig. 20.45 Epithelial rejection. An epithelial rejection line (1) occurs as the recipient epithelium replaces the donor epithelium. It moves in centrally from the corneal transplant wound (2). The shape of the epithelial rejection line is shown in the schematic, lower right. In this case, the epithelial rejection line was seen 3 weeks after surgery.

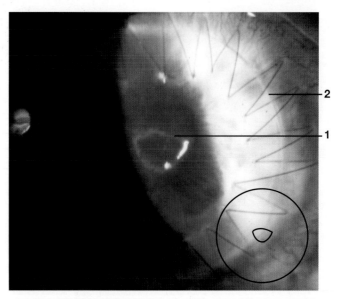

Fig. 20.46 Same patient as in Fig. 20.45, 4 days later. The epithelial rejection line (1) has moved almost to the center of the donor from the wound (2). The shape of the epithelial rejection line is shown in the schematic, lower right.

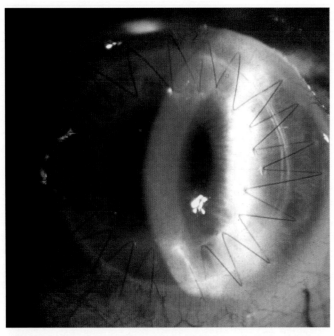

Fig. 20.47 Same patient as in Figs 20.45 and 20.46, 11 days later. The epithelial rejection has cleared. Host epithelium covers the graft.

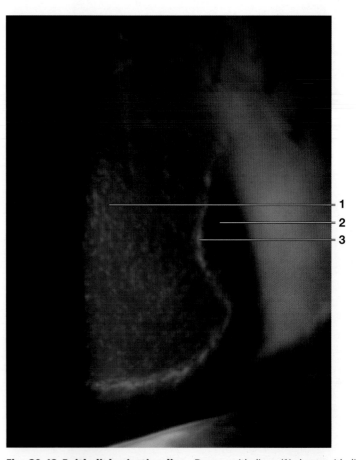

Fig. 20.48 Epithelial rejection line. Donor epithelium (1), host epithelium (2), and an epithelial rejection line (3) composed of inflammatory cells and donor epithelium are shown.

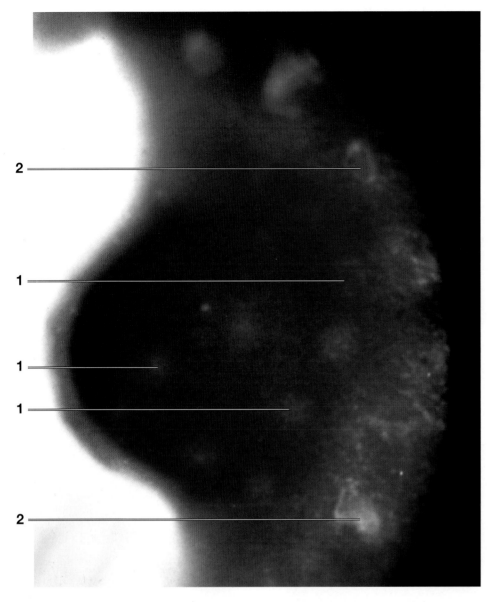

2 —————————

1 —————————

1 —————————

1 —————————

2 —————————

Fig. 20.49 Subepithelial infiltrates. These can occur as an isolated form of graft rejection or may accompany other forms. They resemble the subepithelial infiltrates seen after adenoviral infection. As an isolated finding, they represent a mild form of graft rejection and usually clear with moderate doses of topical corticosteroids. Illustrated are subepithelial infiltrates (1) and corneal suture scars (2).

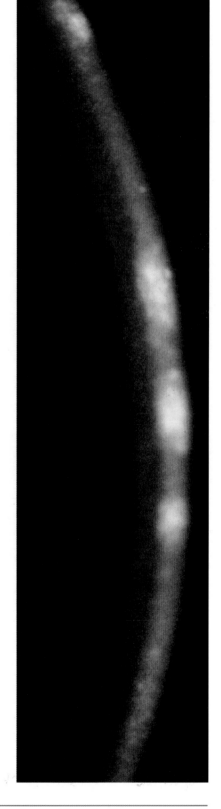

Fig. 20.50 Thin slit-beam view showing subepithelial infiltrates in the anterior stroma.

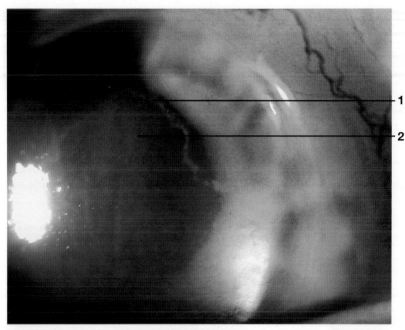

Fig. 20.51 Endothelial rejection line. Endothelial rejection lines begin at the graft host interface and "march" across the cornea. In this example, the rejection line (1) began inferiorly and has progressed to cover almost the entire graft, except for a small superior area. The rejection line is composed of inflammatory cells and in some cases is seen as distinct keratic precipitates. The graft overlying the area of rejection is usually edematous (2), owing to stress or damage to the endothelium. Prompt treatment with corticosteroids may salvage the graft.

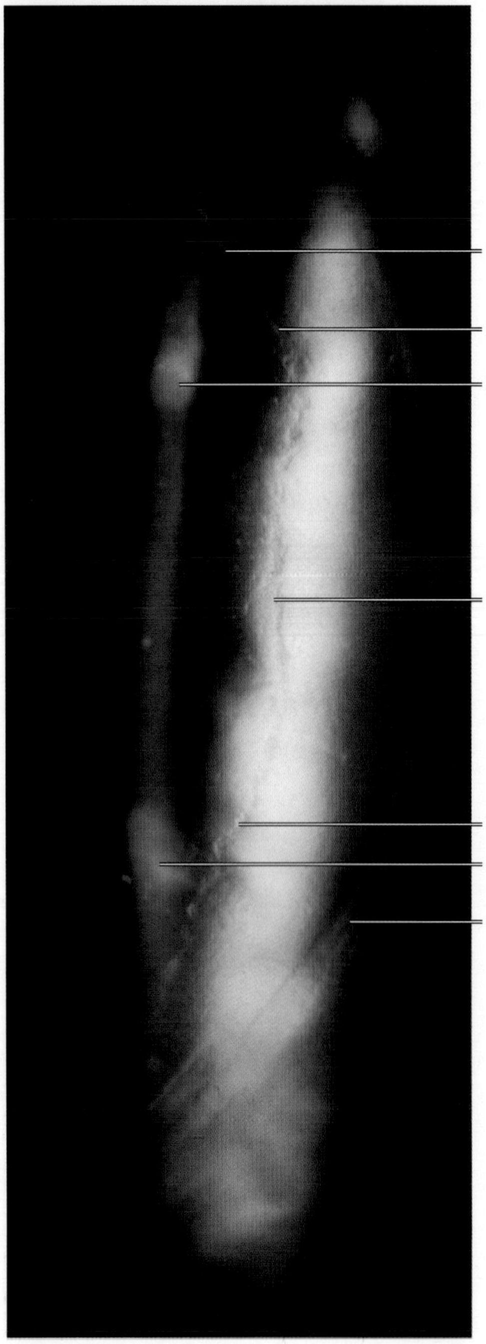

Fig. 20.52 Endothelial rejection line. The rejection line is composed of white keratic precipitates in direct light (1). The rejection line is translucent in indirect light (2). Suture tract scars (3) and the penetrating keratoplasty wound (4) are also seen.

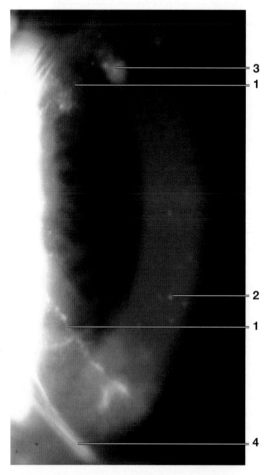

Fig. 20.53 Endothelial rejection line (1), keratic precipitates (2), suture tract scars (3), and the penetrating keratoplasty wound (4) are shown.

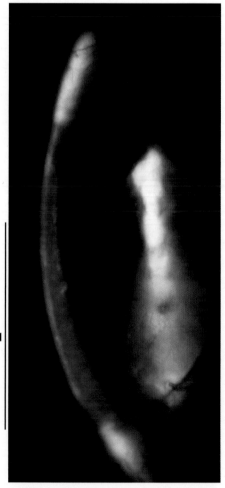

Fig. 20.54 Endothelial rejection line. As the endothelial rejection line progresses across the endothelium, corneal edema develops. Here the rejection line began inferiorly and has extended near the central cornea. Stromal edema is seen inferiorly (1), corresponding to the path of the rejection line.

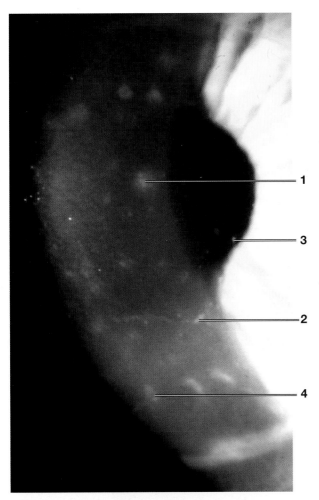

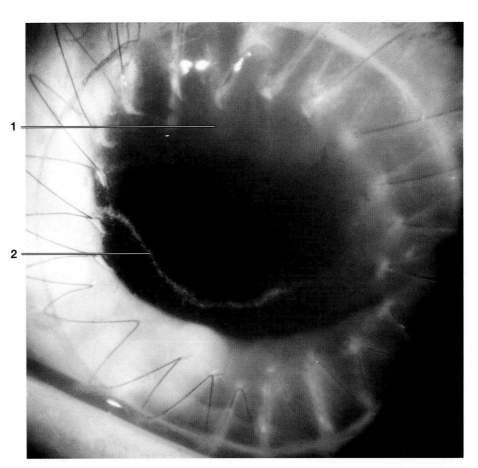

Fig. 20.55 Subepithelial infiltrates (1), endothelial rejection line (2), keratic precipitates (3), and corneal scars (4). This case demonstrates the simultaneous occurrence of two forms of rejection: endothelial and subepithelial infiltration.

Fig. 20.56 Stromal rejection (1). This appears as a diffuse stromal haze or infiltrate, usually associated with stromal vascularization. If the rejection occurs without endothelial involvement, as in this case, the corneal thickness remains relatively normal. An epithelial rejection line (2) is present.

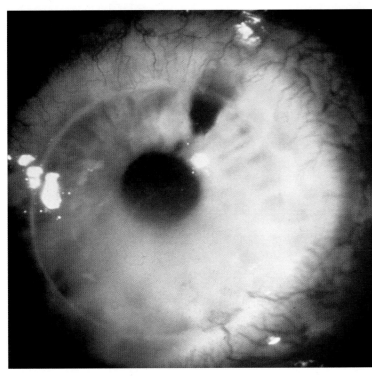

Fig. 20.57 Diffuse endothelial rejection with corneal edema.

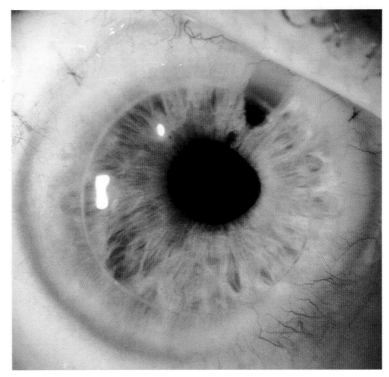

Fig. 20.58 Same patient as in Fig. 20.57 after intensive treatment with topical and systemic corticosteroids. The rejection has resolved, and the graft is clear.

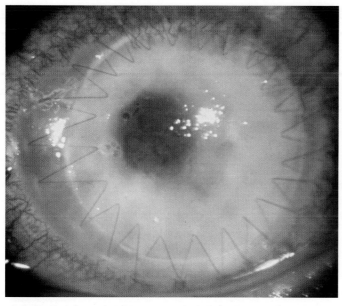

Fig. 20.59 Severe endothelial rejection with stromal and epithelial edema.

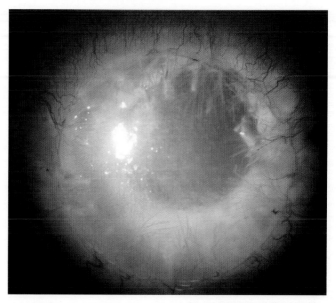

Fig. 20.60 Graft failure because of rejection. There is marked stromal vascularization.

High Astigmatism

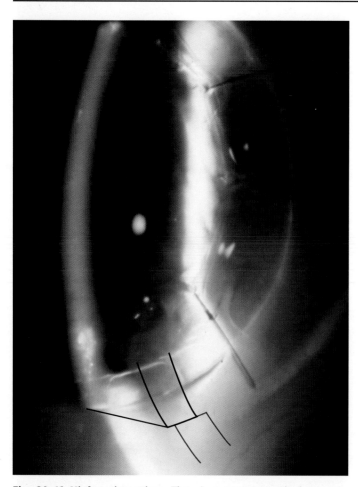

Fig. 20.61 High astigmatism. There is severe anterior displacement of the graft inferiorly. This leads to flattening of the graft in the meridian of the anterior wound displacement.

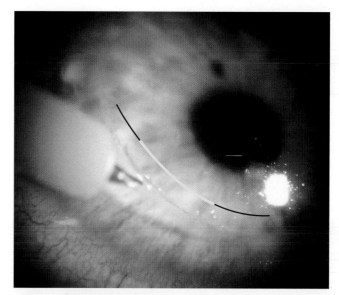

Fig. 20.62 High astigmatism (6 diopters) after penetrating keratoplasty. A relaxing incision was performed within the wound. The incision is made in the meridian of greatest corneal curvature. The area of the incision is represented by a yellow band, and the wound is represented by a black line above and to the right of the actual incision.

Fig. 20.63 Extremely high astigmatism (10 diopters) after penetrating keratoplasty. A wedge resection was performed in this case. The area of resected tissue is outlined in black, and the sutures have re-approximated the new wound edges. The wedge resection is performed in the meridian of least corneal curvature.

Deep Optical Lamellar Keratoplasty

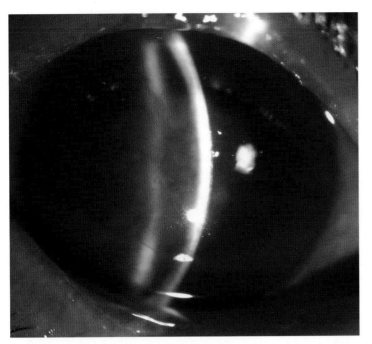

Fig. 20.64 Deep optical lamellar keratoplasty. This 68-year-old woman has lattice dystrophy type I (Arg124Cys mutation). This is a preoperative photograph, prior to a deep optical lamellar keratoplasty. The vision is 0.02 (20/1000).

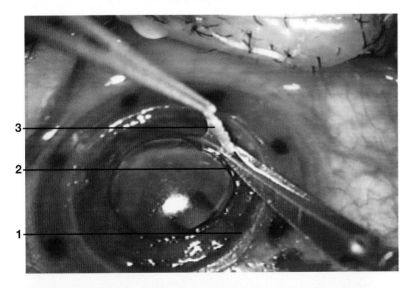

Fig. 20.65 Deep optical lamellar keratoplasty; same patient as in Fig. 20.64. In this procedure, a 70% trephination (1) is performed and the overlying stroma removed. A plane is established between the remaining stroma and Descemet's membrane (2). The removal of the remaining stroma (3) is facilitated by relatively poor adhesion of the stroma very posterior to Descemet's membrane. The donor tissue is prepared by removing Descemet's membrane and endothelium. The donor tissue can then be sutured into the host bed.

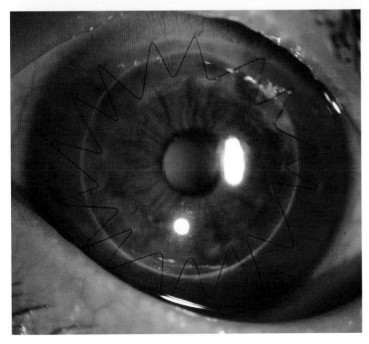

Fig. 20.66 Deep optical lamellar keratoplasty; same patient as in Figs 20.64 and 20.65. This is the appearance of the eye at 10 months after operation. The vision has improved to 0.6 (20/30). Four years later the vision had declined to 0.15 (20/133) owing to recurrent erosions and recurrence of the dystrophy.

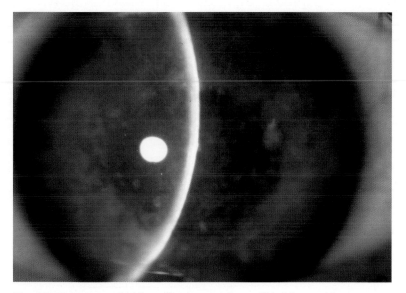

Fig. 20.67 Deep optical lamellar keratoplasty. This 54-year-old woman had macular dystrophy. This is a preoperative photograph prior to a deep optical lamellar keratoplasty. The vision is 0.01 (20/2000).

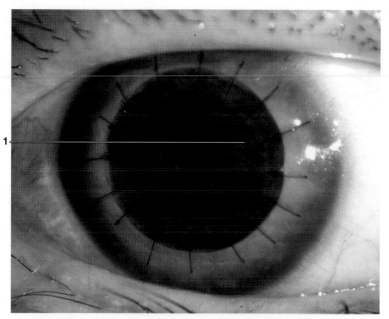

Fig. 20.68 Deep optical lamellar keratoplasty; same patient as in Fig. 20.67. This is the appearance of the eye 4 months after surgery. Residual haze (1) is seen in the peripheral graft because not all of the pathologic material could be removed from the host cornea (the deposits of macular dystrophy are found throughout the cornea, including Descemet's layer). The vision improved only to 0.1 (20/100) and was limited by diabetic retinopathy.

Deep Lamellar Endothelial Keratoplasty (DLEK)

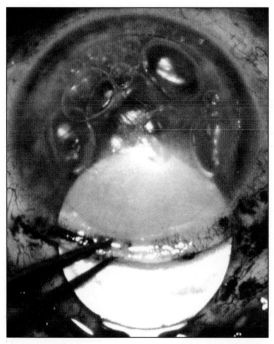

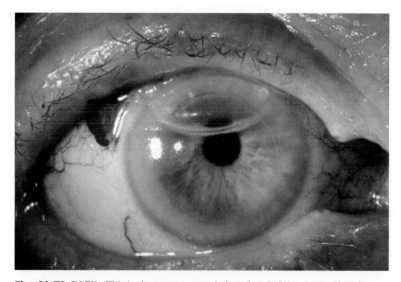

Fig. 20.70 DLEK. This is the appearance 1 day after DLEK surgery. The air bubble is still in place and the cornea is remarkably clear.

Fig. 20.69 Deep lamellar endothelial keratoplasty (DLEK). DLEK is indicated for conditions that damage the corneal endothelium, such as Fuchs' corneal dystrophy. In this procedure, a disk of endothelial tissue with a thin layer of stromal tissue is dissected from a donor cornea. A deep lamellar trephination of the host tissue is performed with a Terry trephine to remove the damaged endothelium and a thin layer of posterior stroma. The donor disk of endothelium is inserted on an Ousley spatula and lifted to coapt with the recipient bed. The spatula is removed (as seen here). The donor disk is held in position with an air bubble. Advantages to this procedure, compared with traditional penetrating keratoplasty, include more rapid visual rehabilitation and less corneal astigmatism. Interface optical clarity is variable and can lead to a reduction in best spectacle-corrected visual acuity.

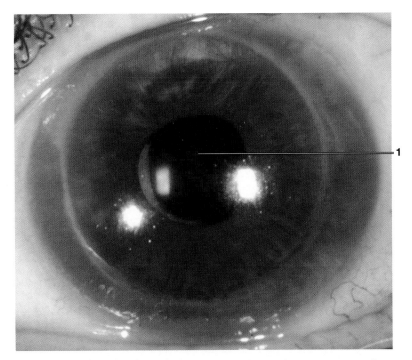

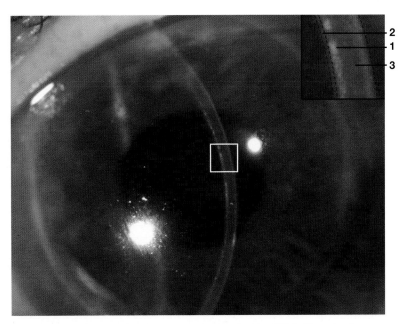

Fig. 20.72 DLEK. This is the same patient seen in Fig. 20.71. There is pigment in the interface (1) between the donor tissue (2) and the host tissue (3).

Fig. 20.71 DLEK. This patient had a layered hyphema after DLEK surgery. On the first postoperative day, no blood was seen in the interface. The next day, blood started accumulating in the interface. This photograph was taken 18 months after the surgery. The blood has fully resorbed, but there is pigment (1) in the interface. The patient's best corrected visual acuity is 20/60, considered to be due to the disturbed interface.

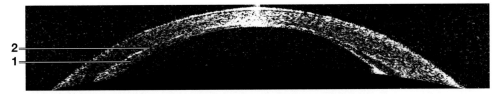

Fig. 20.73 DLEK. This is a modified optical coherence tomogram (OCT) of the same patient seen in Figs 20.71 and 20.72. The deep lamellar tissue (1) and the interface opacification (2) caused by the blood are seen.

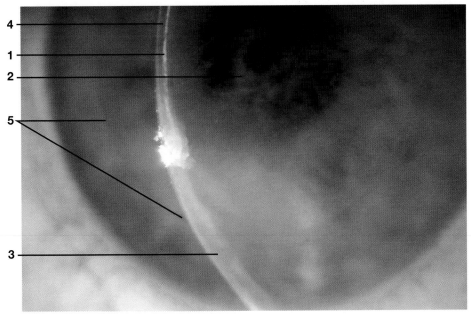

Fig. 20.74 DLEK. This patient developed diffuse lamellar keratitis after a deep lamellar endothelial keratoplasty procedure. Inflammatory cells are seen in the deep lamellar interface with thin slit-beam illumination (1) and with diffuse illumination (2). The inflammation resolved with intensive topical corticosteroid treatment and the best corrected visual acuity is now 20/50. Note that the peripheral cornea is edematous and thickened (3), and the central cornea is thinner (4), indicating that the transplanted endothelial cells are functioning properly. The deep wound (5) from the lamellar endothelial keratoplasty is also seen.

Chapter 21

Therapeutic and Reconstructive Procedures

This chapter discusses conjunctival and corneal surgical procedures other than penetrating keratoplasty.

Conjunctival Flaps

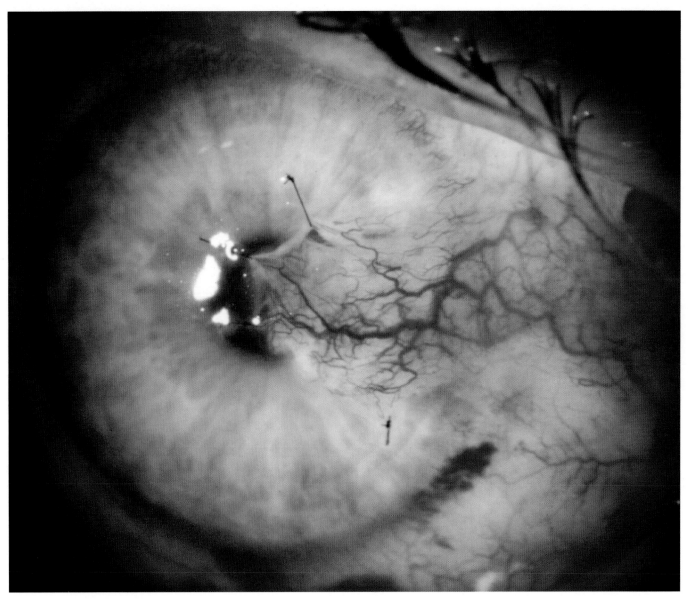

Fig. 21.1 Conjunctival flap. This patient with chronic progressive external ophthalmoplegia developed an exposure ulcer near the nasal limbus. The etiology of the ulcer was related to poor lid closure from an overcorrected ptosis repair and an absent Bell's reflex. (The preoperative appearance is seen in Fig. 13.23.) The area of ulceration was controlled with a small conjunctival pedicle flap, as seen here. The flap retracted slightly with time, and the visual acuity returned to the preoperative level once the sutures were removed.

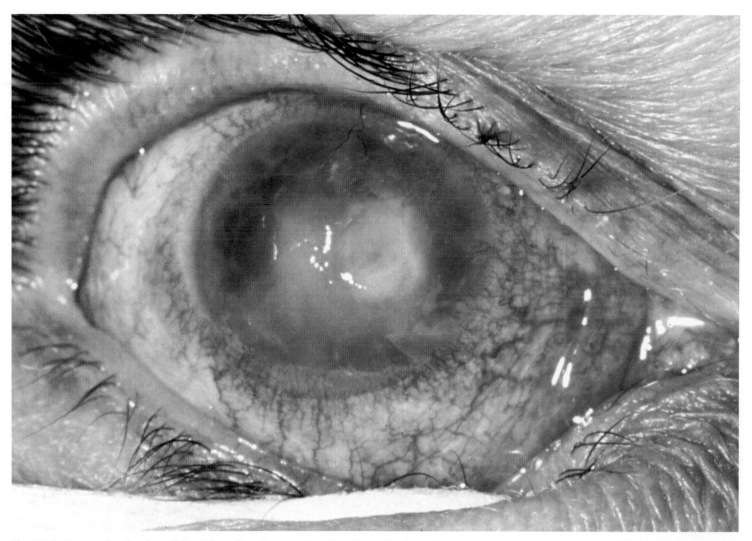

Fig. 21.2 Herpes simplex keratitis with a chronic neurotrophic ulcer. The ulcer did not respond to conservative therapy. This is the appearance of the eye before a Gunderson conjunctival flap procedure.

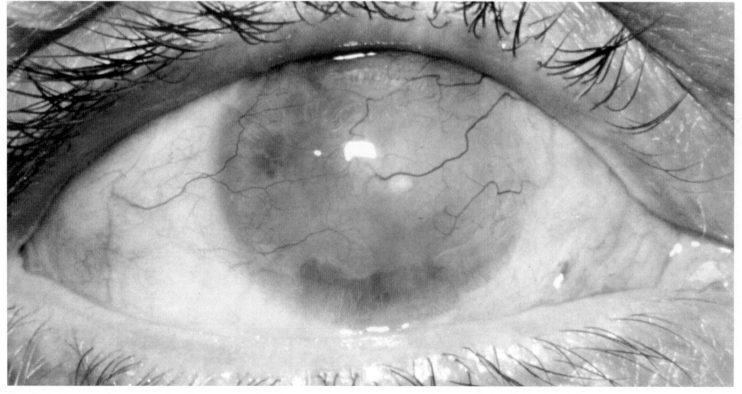

Fig. 21.3 Same patient as in Fig. 21.2, 10 months after surgery. The eye is quiet and the conjunctival flap has healed.

Surgery for Pterygia

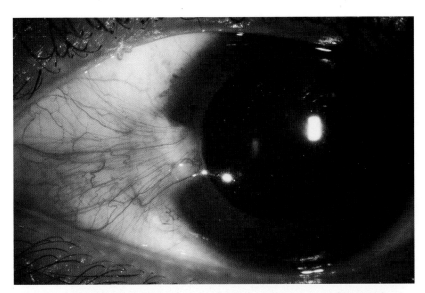

Fig. 21.4 Pterygium before excision.

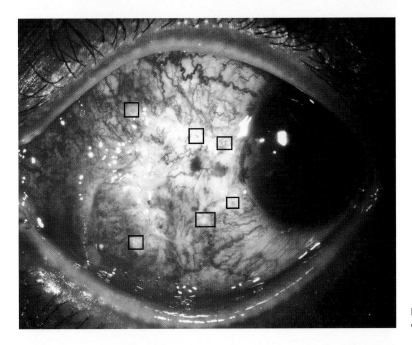

Fig. 21.5 Same patient as in Fig. 21.4, 1 week after surgery with conjunctival autograft. The boxes show the position of the buried sutures.

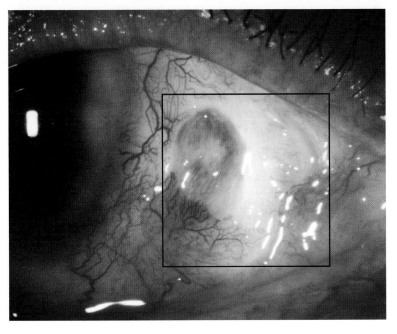

Fig. 21.6 Pterygium excision with mitomycin application to the scleral bed. Approximately 1 year after the excision there was continued scleral melting and a lack of vascularity in the necrotic scleral bed. Uveal tissue is seen at the base of the ulcer.

Glue Application for Corneal Perforation

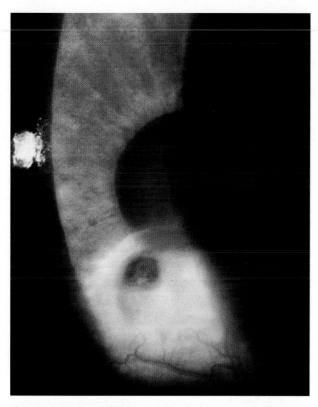

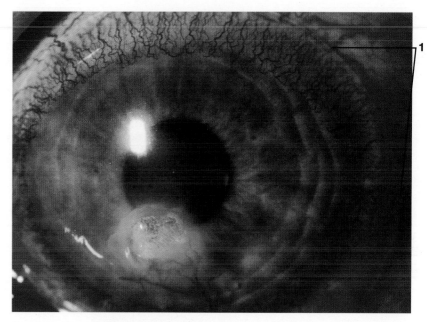

Fig. 21.8 Tissue adhesive application. This is the same patient as seen in Fig. 21.7, 1 hour after the application of cyanoacrylate glue and a bandage contact lens (1). The perforation site is well sealed and the anterior chamber has reformed.

Fig. 21.7 Tissue adhesive application. This patient had a corneal perforation related to chronic acne rosacea keratitis. The anterior chamber is flat and iris plugs the wound.

Mechanical Keratectomy

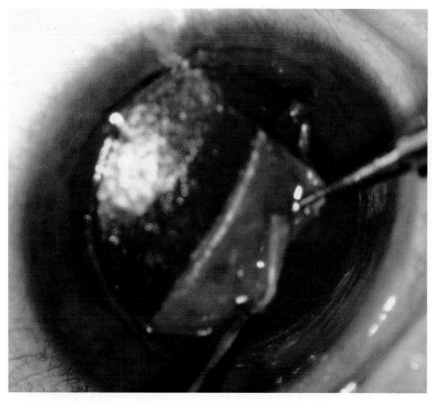

Fig. 21.9 Superficial keratectomy. A superficial lamellar dissection can be performed to remove anterior corneal opacities.

Phototherapeutic Keratectomy

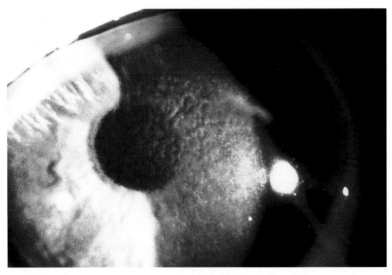

Fig. 21.10 Phototherapeutic keratectomy. This is a 31-year-old woman with Reis–Bucklers' dystrophy and a preoperative best corrected vision of 20/200.

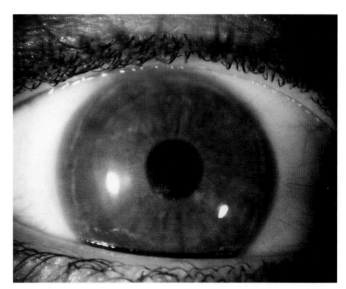

Fig. 21.11 Phototherapeutic keratectomy; same patient as in Fig. 21.10. Six months after phototherapeutic keratectomy, the cornea is mostly clear and the visual acuity with correction is 20/30.

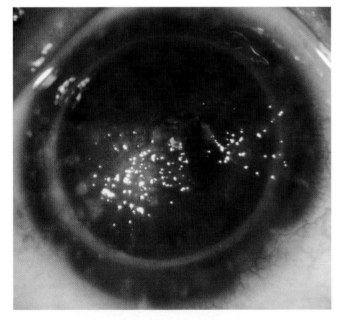

Fig. 21.12 Phototherapeutic keratectomy. This patient had recurrent gelatinous drop-like corneal dystrophy after penetrating keratoplasty.

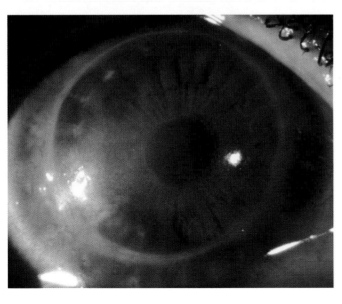

Fig. 21.13 Phototherapeutic keratectomy; same patient as in Fig. 21.12. After phototherapeutic keratectomy, the corneal surface is smooth and there is less corneal opacity.

Keratolimbal Allograft (KLAL)

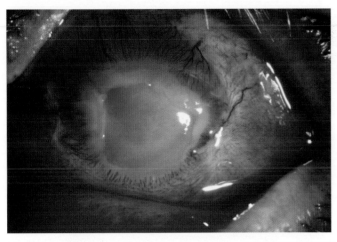

Fig. 21.14 Chronic nonhealing corneal ulcer after a severe alkali burn. Preoperative appearance of the eye before a keratolimbal allograft.

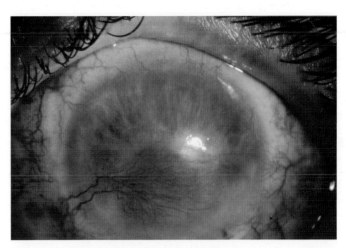

Fig. 21.15 Same patient as in Fig. 21.14. Keratolimbal allograft is a procedure in which donor limbal tissue is transplanted to provide a new source of stem cells. In this patient, the corneal epithelium is more normal and there is less neovascularization 3 months after keratolimbal allograft.

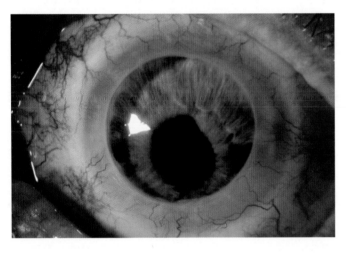

Fig. 21.16 Same patient as in Figs 21.14 and 21.15 after penetrating keratoplasty. Successful penetrating keratoplasty was performed 3 months after keratolimbal allograft.

Conjunctival Limbal Autograft (CLAU)

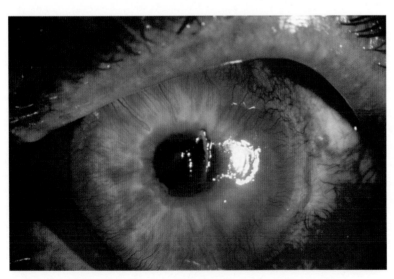

Fig. 21.17 Conjunctival limbal autografting. This patient sustained a unilateral chemical injury. There is corneal neovascularization and a nonhealing epithelial defect.

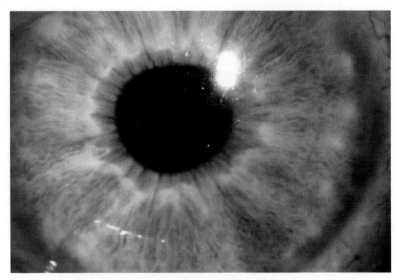

Fig. 21.18 Conjunctival limbal autografting. Conjunctival limbal autografting is a procedure in which donor conjunctiva from the fellow eye is used as a source of stem cells. This is the same patient as seen in Fig. 21.17, several months after conjunctival limbal autografting. The corneal surface is more normal and there is minimal neovascularization.

Surgery for Recurrent Erosions

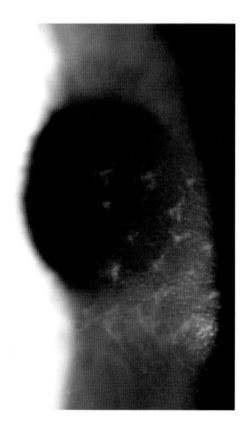

Fig. 21.19 Recurrent erosion syndrome. There is defective adhesion of the epithelium and basement membrane complex to the underlying corneal stroma. (See Figs 13.1–13.7 for clinical description.) With anterior stromal puncture, a hypodermic needle is passed through the epithelium into the anterior stroma to create a focal area of scarring. Multiple punctures are performed, and the scars formed serve to "spot weld" the epithelium to the underlying stroma.

Reconstuctive Lamellar Keratoplasty

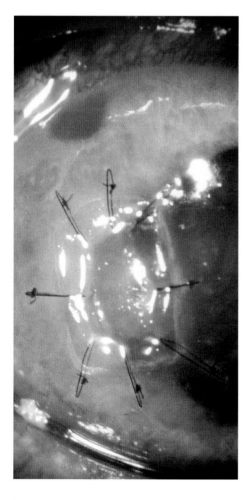

Fig. 21.20 Rectangular lamellar graft for a peripheral perforation in a patient with rheumatoid arthritis.

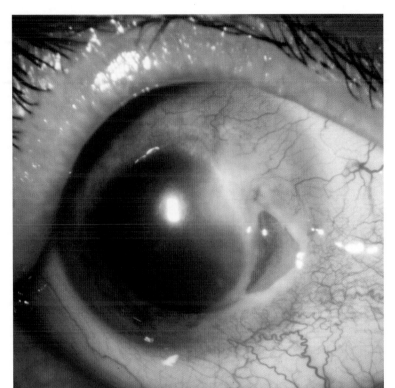

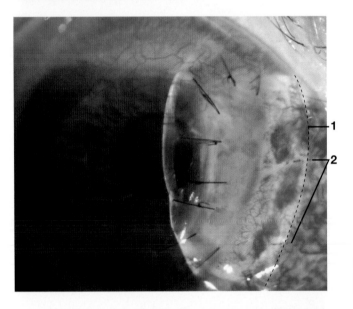

Fig. 21.22 Same patient as in Fig. 21.21 after surgery. A crescentic lamellar graft was performed. The peripheral edge of the graft is identified (1), as well as two peripheral sutures (2).

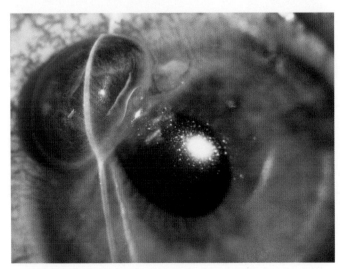

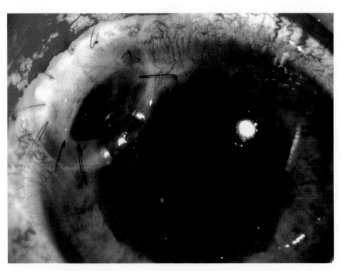

Fig. 21.23 Patch graft, preoperative. Iris tissue is protruding from this large peripheral corneal perforation.

Fig. 21.24 Same patient as in Fig. 21.23. The perforation was treated with a full-thickness corneal patch graft following full-thickness corneal dissection centrally and partial-thickness scleral dissection peripherally.

Anterior Segment Reconstruction

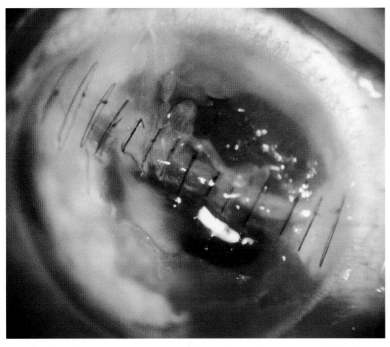

Fig. 21.25 Repaired corneal laceration. Peripheral, long, powerful sutures and shorter central sutures are used to minimize the potential for central corneal flattening.

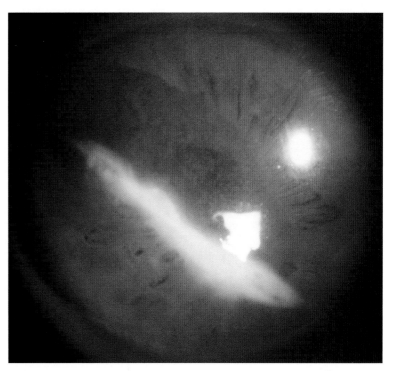

Fig. 21.26 Corneal laceration. This is the appearance 20 years after a traumatic self-sealing laceration with scarring and extensive incorporation of iris into the wound.

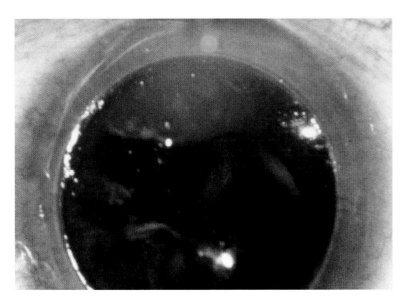

Fig. 21.27 Same patient as in Fig. 21.26. This photograph was taken during penetrating keratoplasty and shows extensive loss of iris tissue.

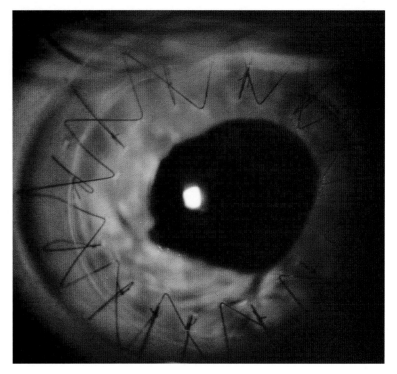

Fig. 21.28 Same patient as in Figs 21.26 and 21.27 after penetrating keratoplasty with iris repair.

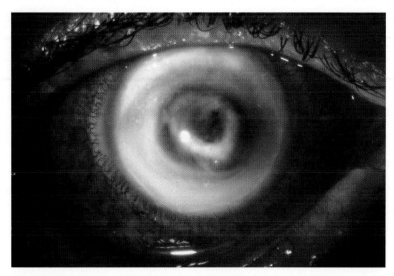

Fig. 21.29 Tectonic penetrating keratoplasty. This patient had an extensive *Pseudomonas* corneal ulcer encompassing the entire cornea. There is a central corneal perforation.

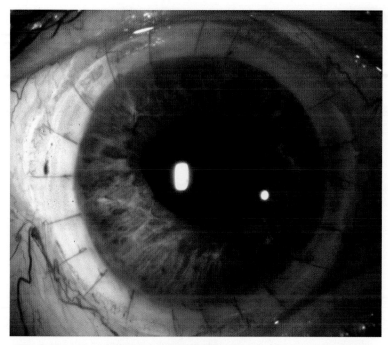

Fig. 21.30 Same patient as in Fig. 21.29. Several months after tectonic corneal transplantation, the graft is clear. This patient has maintained 20/40 vision with a contact lens with over 5 years of follow-up.

Tattooing

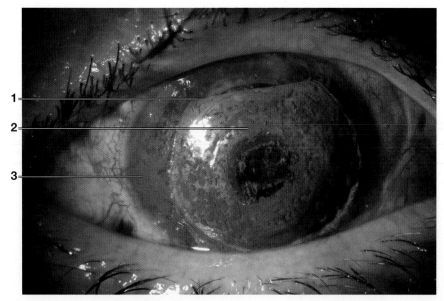

1
2
3

Fig. 21.31 Corneal tattooing. This patient with traumatic aniridia had corneal tattooing 8 years previously. Because of photophobia, a further tattooing procedure was performed. A refractive surgery microkeratome was used to create a flap with a superior hinge (1). Pigment (2) was applied to the bed of the wound. Some previously applied pigment (3) remains.

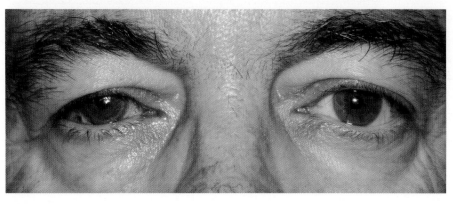

Fig. 21.32 Corneal tattooing; same patient as in Fig. 21.31. The treated right eye cosmetically matches the normal left eye.

Temporary Keratoprosthesis

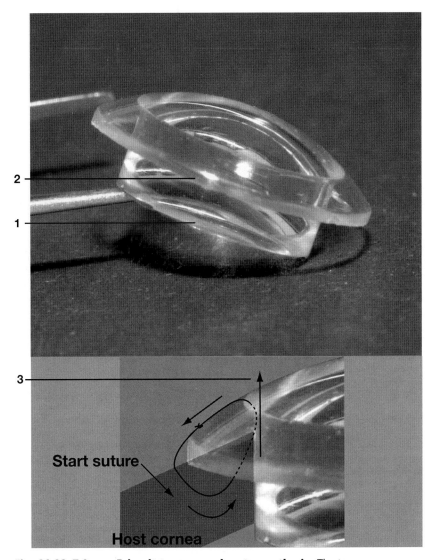

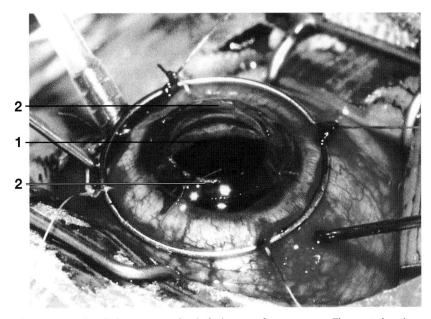

Fig. 21.33 7.0-mm Eckerdt temporary keratoprosthesis. The temporary keratoprosthesis is composed of an optic (1) and a flange (2). The fixation suture is passed through the corneal tissue and exits at the junction of the stem and the flange (3).

Fig. 21.34 Eckerdt keratoprosthesis being used at surgery. The central optic (1) is surrounded by a peripheral flange (2).

Permanent Keratoprosthesis

Prosthokeratoplasty should be considered in patients in whom all other therapeutic options have been exhausted, including multiple attempts with penetrating keratoplasty, or in cases where keratoplasty would certainly fail. Indications for prosthokeratoplasty include severe chemical burns, ocular cicatricial pemphigoid, Stevens–Johnson syndrome, and recurrent graft failure. Preoperative visual function should be bare ambulatory or nonambulatory in both eyes.

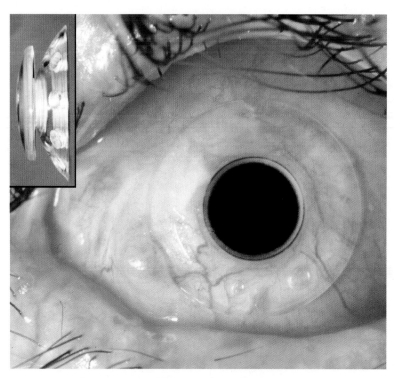

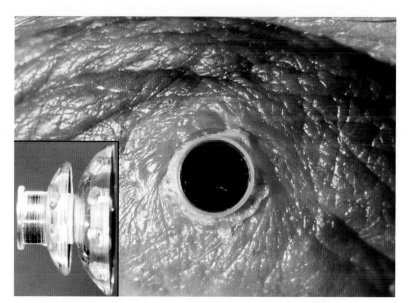

Fig. 21.36 Dohlman–Doane (Boston) type II keratoprosthesis performed for Stevens–Johnson syndrome. The prosthesis is similar in design to the type I prosthesis, but there is a longer optical cylinder that protrudes through the lid skin. Here, total ankyloblepharon necessitated the use of a through-the-lid design. The visual acuity has improved to 20/20 at 15 months of follow-up. The inset shows the prosthesis before insertion.

Fig. 21.35 Dohlman–Doane (Boston) type I intracorneal keratoprosthesis performed 30 years after an explosion injury. The cornea between the anterior and posterior supporting plates of the keratoprosthesis is well vascularized, and there is no sign of necrosis around the optical cylinder. The visual acuity has improved to 20/20 at 20 months of follow-up. The inset shows the prosthesis before insertion.

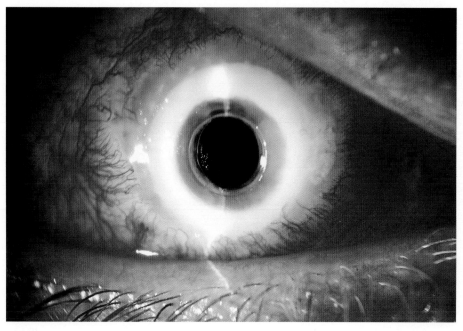

Fig. 21.37 AlphaCor™ keratoprosthesis. The AlphaCor™ keratoprosthesis is manufactured from the hydrogel, poly 2-(hydroxymethacrylate) (PHEMA) polymer. The outer skirt is composed of a high water content PHEMA sponge, and the porosity of the sponge promotes bio-integration with the host tissue. The central optical core is composed of a transparent PHEMA gel. In stage I of the procedure, the keratoprosthesis is inserted deep in a lamellar pocket within the cornea. The central 3.5 mm of the posterior cornea is removed. The entire device is left within the lamellar pocket for 3 months to allow for bio-integration of the porous skirt with the corneal tissue. In stage II of the procedure, a 3-mm central trephination is performed through the anterior cornea to expose the optical core. This picture was taken 1 day after the optical core was exposed. Visual acuity is 20/50.

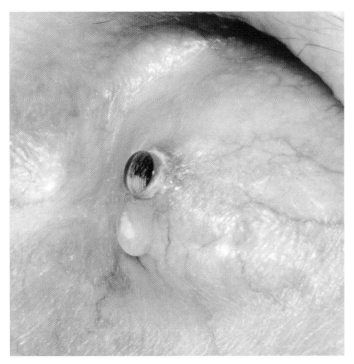

Fig. 21.38 Nut-and-bolt keratoprosthesis with aqueous leak around the optical cylinder. This complication requires immediate surgical repair.

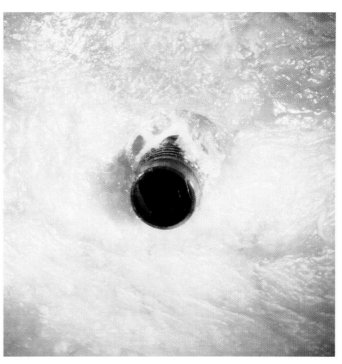

Fig. 21.39 Nut-and-bolt keratoprosthesis with partial unscrewing of the optical cylinder and exposed Dacron mesh superiorly. This was repaired successfully, and the patient has maintained 20/200 vision at more than 3 years of follow-up.

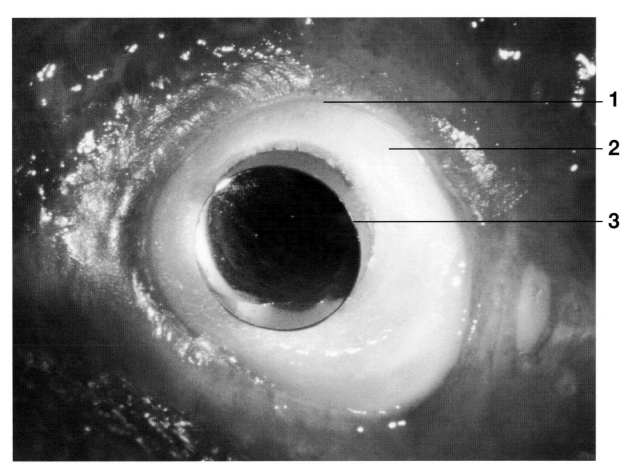

Fig. 21.40 Skin retraction around the optical cylinder of a nut-and-bolt keratoprosthesis. Skin (1) has retracted from an underlying layer of Gortex (2), which was used to support the keratoprosthesis. The optical cylinder (3) is in a relatively good position. The Gortex was removed, and the keratoprosthesis was successfully repaired. The patient has maintained 20/40 vision at more than 10 years of follow-up.

Chapter 22

Refractive Surgery

Refractive surgery is a rapidly evolving field, and new procedures are continually being developed. This chapter highlights several refractive procedures including the most commonly performed refractive procedure: laser-assisted in situ keratomileusis (LASIK). Many procedures performed today will become obsolete as new and improved techniques are developed.

Incisional Refractive Surgery

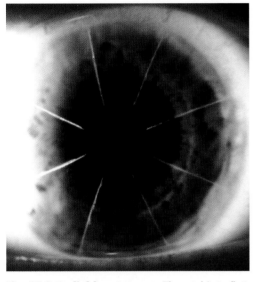

Fig. 22.1 Radial keratotomy. The goal is to flatten the central cornea with deep peripheral radial incisions. The degree of flattening is related to many factors, including the number of incisions, the size of the central optical zone, the depth of incisions, and wound healing. This is an excellent postoperative result following radial keratotomy. The visual acuity is 20/20 uncorrected.

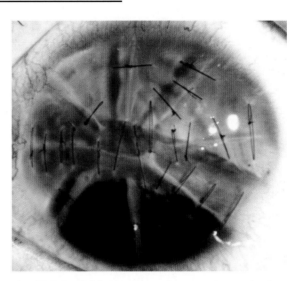

Fig. 22.3 Radial keratotomy. Postoperative repair of a traumatic wound rupture follows the lines of corneal incisions and extends through the visual axis. Much of the iris was lost.

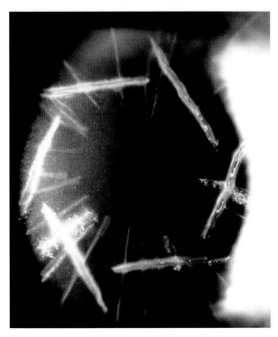

Fig. 22.2 Combined hexagonal and radial keratotomy. Multiple crossed incisions result in irregular astigmatism with resultant poor vision.

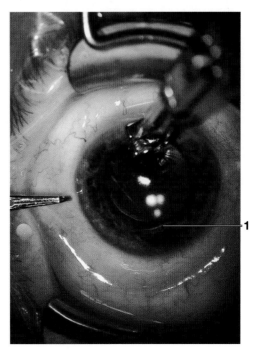

Fig. 22.4 Astigmatic keratectomy. A diamond knife is used to create an arcuate incision (1) into the peripheral cornea to reduce astigmatism at the time of cataract surgery.

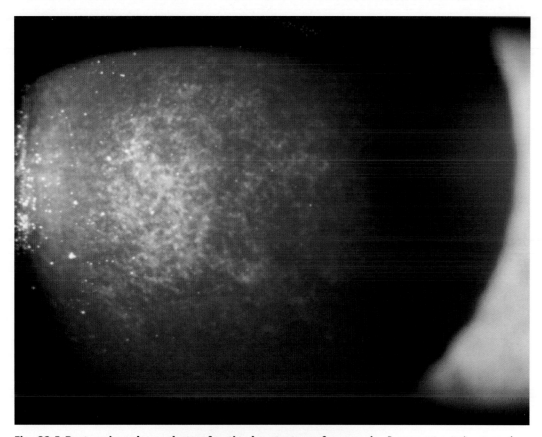

Fig. 22.5 Post-excimer laser photorefractive keratectomy for myopia. Permanent anterior stromal scarring is demonstrated by a broad oblique beam.

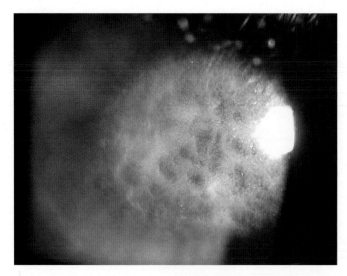

Fig. 22.7 Dense haze at 6 months after photorefractive keratectomy for high myopia.

Photorefractive Surgery: Laser-Assisted In Situ Keratomileusis (LASIK)

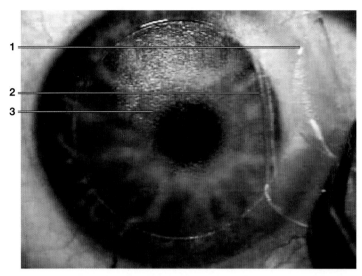

Fig. 22.8 LASIK. The superficial corneal flap (1) is attached to the underlying cornea by the hinge (2). The laser treatment is performed on the stromal bed (3). At completion of the laser treatment, the corneal flap is repositioned.

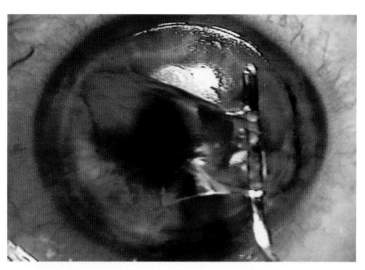

Fig. 22.9 LASIK, buttonhole in the flap. Buttonholes have been associated with loss of suction during flap preparation, excessively steep corneas, and abnormalities in the microkeratome blade. In this case a canula is protruding through the buttonhole.

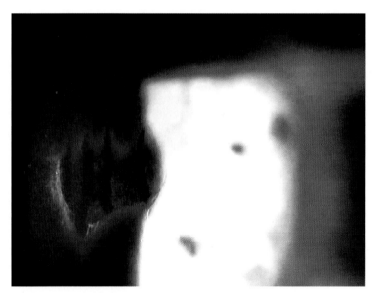

Fig. 22.10 LASIK, buttonhole in the flap. One month after an intraoperative buttonhole there is haze surrounding the area of the buttonhole.

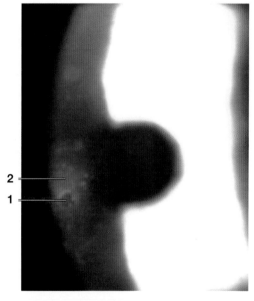

Fig. 22.11 LASIK, buttonhole in the flap. In this case a buttonhole (1) was associated with epithelial ingrowth (2).

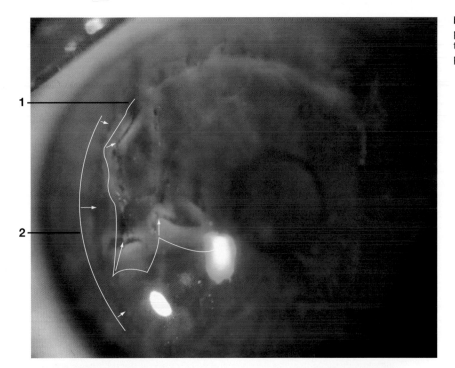

Fig. 22.12 LASIK, torn flap. Lifting of the flap for an enhancement procedure resulted in a torn flap. The schematic white line (1) delineates the tear in the flap, and the schematic white line (2) delineates the position of the flap edge prior to the enhancement procedure.

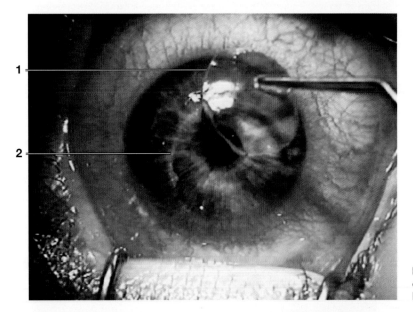

Fig. 22.13 LASIK, free cap. Free caps are associated with a loss of suction during flap preparation and excessively flat corneas. In this case, the free flap (1) is being held by forceps. The wound edge (2) is seen.

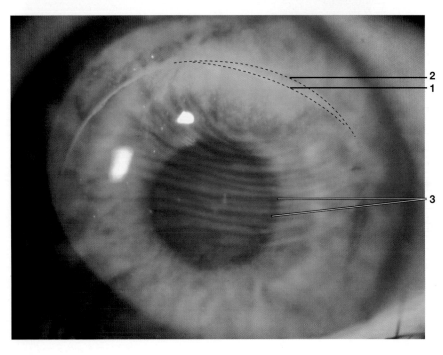

Fig. 22.14 LASIK, flap dislocation. The edge of the flap (1) is dislocated from its proper position (2). There are striae (3) visible in the central cornea.

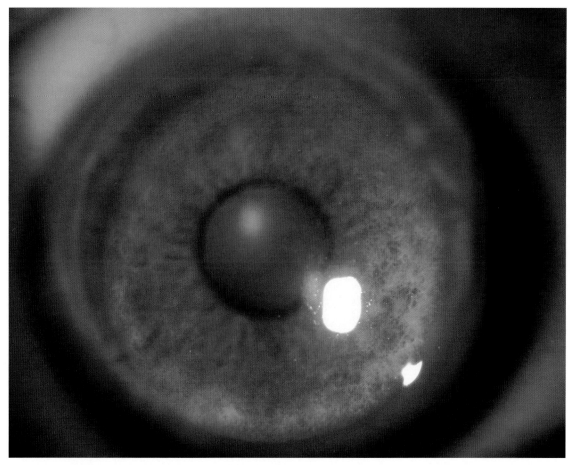

Fig. 22.15 LASIK, lost flap. This patient developed a free cap during LASIK surgery. The flap was replaced and a bandage contact lens was placed. On the first postoperative day the flap was missing. This picture was taken 6 months after surgery. There is corneal scarring that is more prominent in the peripheral cornea. The vision is 20/20 with spectacle correction of moderate hyperopia and astigmatism.

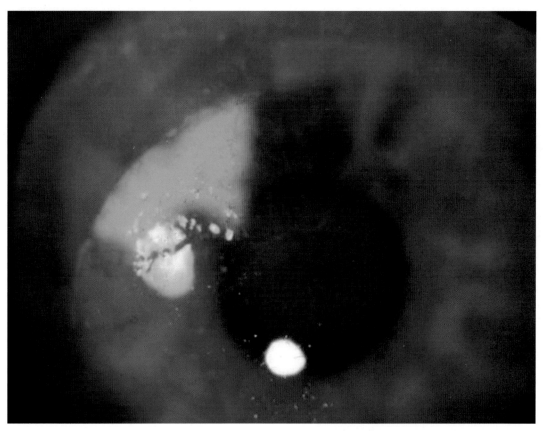

Fig. 22.16 LASIK, epithelial defect. Epithelial defects can occur during flap creation. They are often associated with preexisting epithelial basement membrane disease. Improved microkeratome design has lessened the frequency of this complication.

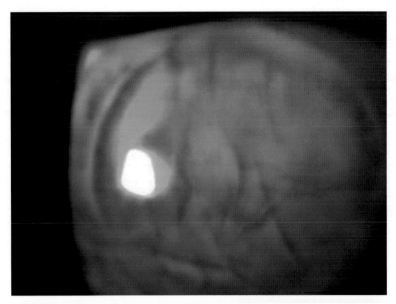

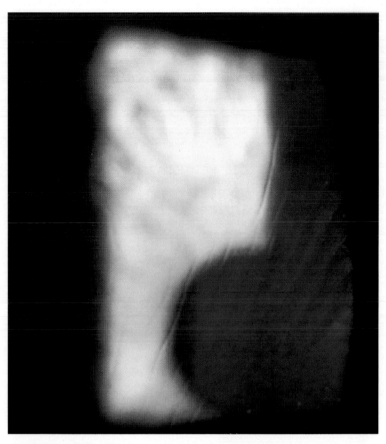

Fig. 22.17 LASIK, striae. Multiple vertical and horizontal striae are noted with fluorescein stain.

Fig. 22.18 LASIK, striae. Vertical striae are seen through the visual axis. Early reposition of flaps with striae improves the long-term visual prognosis.

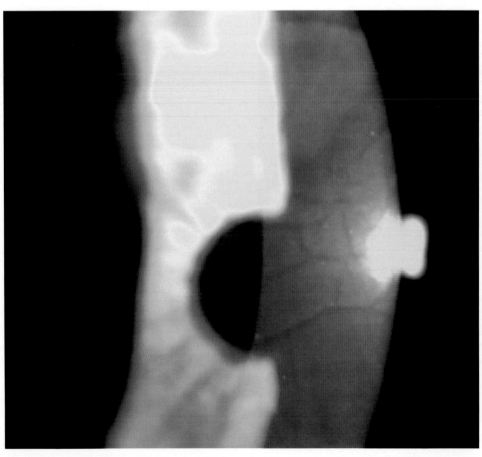

Fig. 22.19 LASIK, striae. "Basket weave" striae can also reduce the best corrected visual acuity.

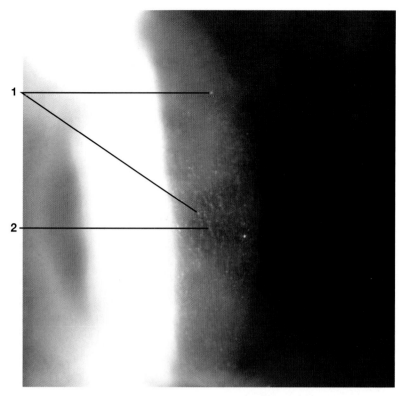

Fig. 22.20 LASIK, grade 1 diffuse lamellar keratitis (DLK). DLK is due to inflammatory cells in the lamellar interface. Various inciting agents have been suggested, including epithelial defects, endotoxins that build up in wet autoclave reservoirs, cleaning solutions, talc from gloves, meibomian gland secretions, microkeratome oil, rust on instruments, blade debris, iodine skin cleaners, and carboxymethylcellulose lubrication drops. In this example of grade 1 DLK, there is focal white granular material (1) and linear granular material (2) in the lamellar interface. Grade 1 DLK is confined to a small area in the cornea and usually resolves with topical corticosteroid treatment.

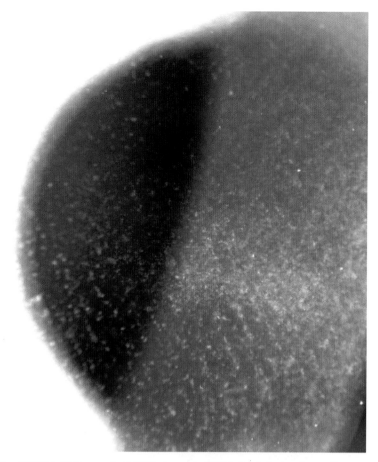

Fig. 22.21 LASIK, grade 2 DLK. In grade 2 DLK, the inflammatory cells are more diffusely distributed throughout the lamellar interface. This process usually resolves with intensive topical corticosteroid, and in some cases oral corticosteroid therapy. Interface irrigation is sometimes necessary.

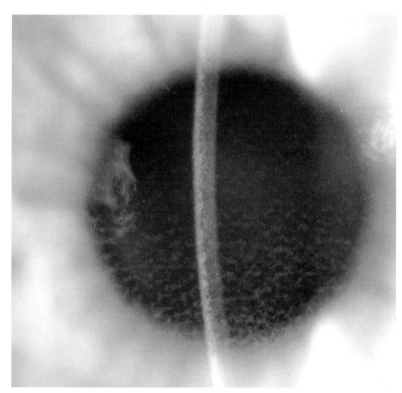

Fig. 22.22 LASIK, grade 3 DLK. In grade 3 DLK, there is diffuse lamellar inflammation with clumping of cells. Intensive treatment with topical and oral corticosteroids is necessary to prevent possible damage to the cornea. Interface irrigation is indicated.

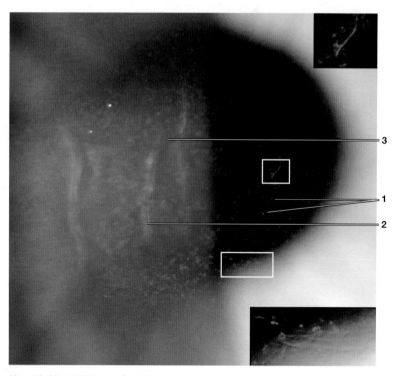

Fig. 22.23 LASIK, grade 4 DLK. Two weeks after grade 4 DLK there are a few inflammatory cells (1) in the interface. Large striae (2) develop as a result of localized tissue loss. There is a diffuse haze in the cornea (3). Interface debris (square box) and fine horizontal striae (rectangular box) are also noted. Following resolution of the inflammation there is irregular astigmatism, hyperopia due to localized flattening of the cornea, and resultant loss of best corrected visual acuity.

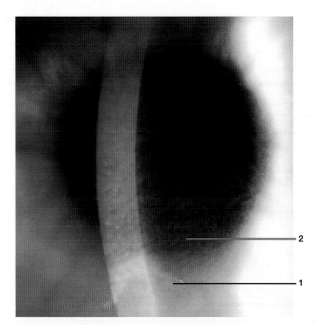

Fig. 22.24 LASIK, recurrent erosion. Late-onset recurrent erosion developed in this patient after LASIK. The epithelium is irregular and stains with fluorescein (1). DLK is noted in the interface due to an accumulation of inflammatory cells (2).

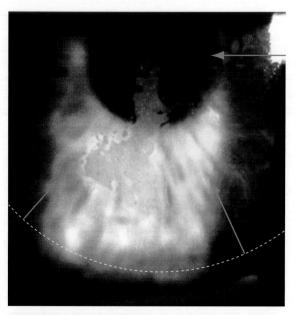

Fig. 22.25 LASIK, epithelial ingrowth. Epithelial ingrowth occurs when epithelium grows into the stromal interface. It is more common after enhancement surgery but may occur after primary surgery, especially if there was an epithelial defect at the time of operation. Extensive epithelial ingrowth, as seen here, can cause irregular astigmatism and loss of spectacle-corrected visual acuity. The blue arrows depict the direction of ingrowth from the wound toward the central cornea.

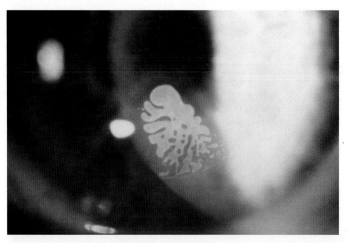

Fig. 22.26 LASIK, epithelial ingrowth. A frond of epithelium from the inferior LASIK wound extends into the interface.

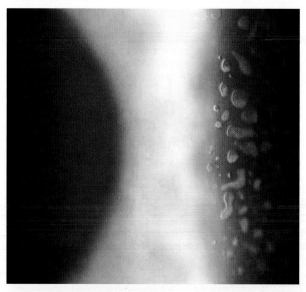

Fig. 22.27 LASIK, epithelial ingrowth. There are islands of epithelium surrounded by relatively clear areas.

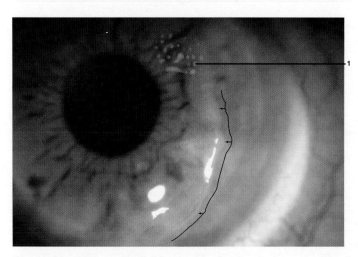

Fig. 22.28 LASIK, epithelial ingrowth. Peripheral edge melt of the flap (seen from 3 o'clock to 5 o'clock) occurs in some cases of epithelial ingrowth (1).

Fig. 22.29 LASIK, epithelial ingrowth. This patient had recurrent epithelial ingrowth that was removed four times. There is residual epithelial ingrowth (1) and stromal scarring (2). Scraping and the placement of flap sutures to prevent recurrence are recommended for recalcitrant cases of epithelial ingrowth.

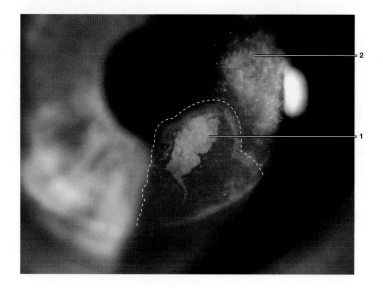

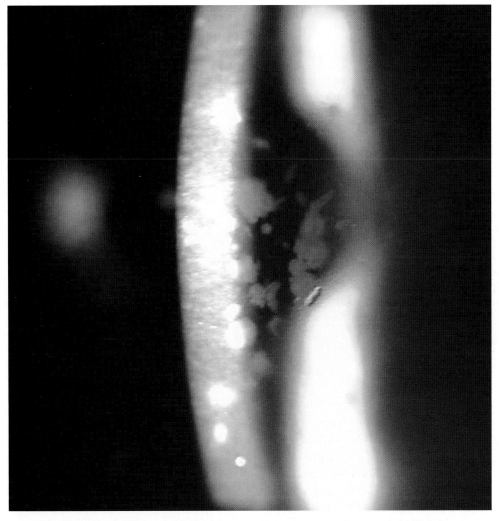

Fig. 22.30 LASIK, mycobacterial keratitis. Two weeks after Lasik, this patient developed *Mycobacterium chelonae* keratitis. There are well defined infiltrates in the LASIK interface.

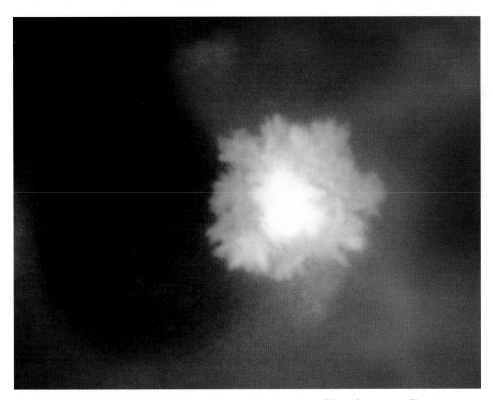

Fig. 22.31 LASIK, mycobacterial keratitis. In this case, the infiltrate has a crystalline appearance.

Photorefractive Surgery: Laser-Assisted Subepithelial Keratectomy (LASEK)

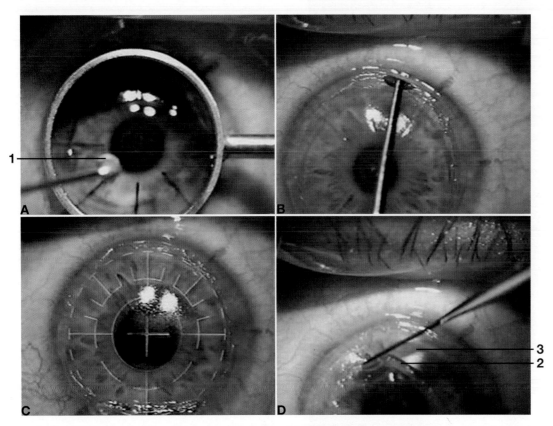

Fig. 22.32 Surgical procedure of laser-assisted subepithelial keratectomy (LASEK). A, Alcohol (1) being dropped into a well. **B,** Pulling back the epithelial flap. **C,** Laser applied to the bed. **D,** Epithelial flap (2) being pulled over the bed (3).

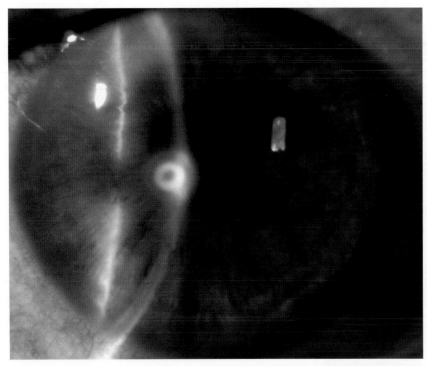

Fig. 22.33 LASEK. This 52-year-old woman developed an *Aureobasidium pullulans* fungal corneal ulcer 1 month after LASEK surgery. *Aureobasidium* is a dematiaceous or "pigmented" fungus commonly isolated from plant debris, soil, wood, textiles, and indoor air environment. It was believed that the fungus had been introduced into the cornea by self-inoculation, rather than at the time of surgery. The infiltrate resolved with antifungal treatment and the visual acuity improved to 20/32.

Intrastromal Rings

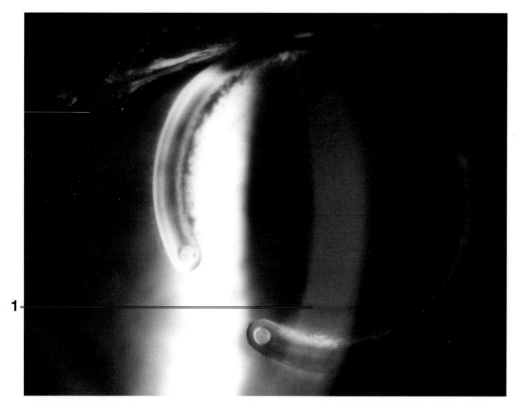

Fig. 22.34 Intrastromal rings for keratoconus. Intrastomal ring segments have been used to reduce corneal steepening and astigmatism associated with keratoconus. An iron line (1) is seen due to an irregular tear film distribution in this area.

Thermal Keratoplasty

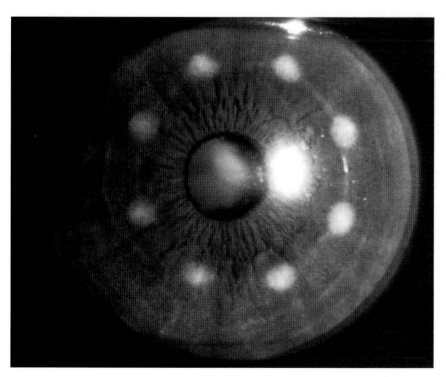

Fig. 22.35 Thermal keratoplasty. The noncontact holmium:YAG laser was used to create eight treatment areas in the peripheral cornea. Shrinkage of tissue peripherally results in central steeping of the cornea with a resultant reduction in hyperopia.

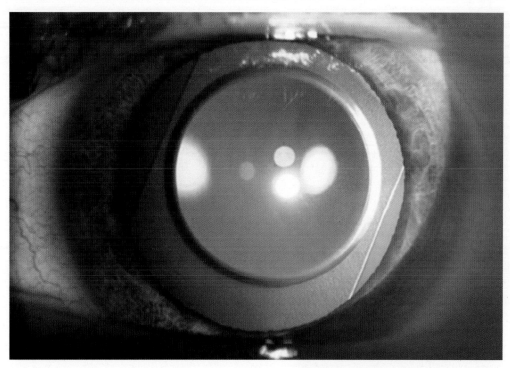

Fig. 22.36 Posterior chamber phakic intraocular lens for the correction of myopia. A posterior chamber phakic intraocular lens is placed posterior to the iris and anterior to the lens capsule.

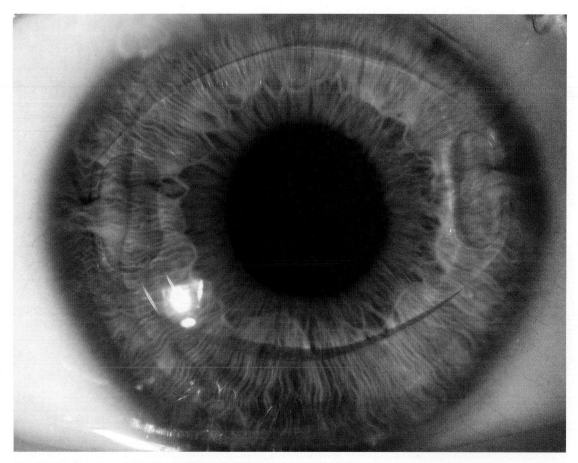

Fig. 22.37 Anterior chamber iris-fixated phakic intraocular lens for the correction of myopia. An Artisan® lens is fixated to the mid-peripheral iris with claw haptics.

Index

A

Abscess
  conjunctiva, 65
  sterile suture, 322
Acanthamoeba
  corneal ulcer, 230
  cysts, 233, 234
  epitheliopathy, 230
  keratitis, 230–4
  in penetrating keratoplasty, 231, 233
  pseudodendrites, 230
  radial neuritis, 232
  ring infiltrate, 231
  scleritis, 232
  stromal keratitis, 230
  trophozoites, 234
Acanthosis nigricans, 129
Acetylcysteine, 35
Acid burn of cornea, 292
Acid-fast bacillus, 132
Acne, 23
Acrochordon, 12
Actinic keratosis, 12
Actinomyces israelii, 40
Adenoviral conjunctivitis, 66–8
Adenovirus, 66–8
  laboratory diagnosis, 208
Adrenochrome deposits, 136
Adult inclusion conjunctivitis, 69–70
AIDS, 25, 55, 316
Air bubble indentations, 297
AK *see* Astigmatic keratectomy
Alkali burn of conjunctiva, 293–4, 342
Alkali burn of cornea, 293–4, 342
Alkaptonuria, 106
Allergic conjunctivitis, 27, 28, 76, 79
Allergic inflammation, 27–8
Alopecia, 28
AlphaCor keratoprosthesis, 348
Amblyopia, 10, 94
Amiodarone deposits, 138, 139
Amyloidosis, 7, 121–2
Anesthetic abuse, 232, 248, 249
Angular blepharitis, 24
Aniridia, 206
Ankyloblepharon, 128, 348
Anterior blepharitis, 19, 20
Anterior chamber
  epithelial inclusion cyst, 292
  phakic intraocular lens, 262
Anterior chamber cleavage syndromes, 97–101
  flat nasal bridge, 100
  hypospadias, 100
  maxillary hypoplasia, 100
  microdontia, 100
  nasal bridge, 100
Anterior eyelid margin, 19, 20, 24
Anterior membrane dystrophies, 145–52
  see also individual dystrophies
Anterior segment ischemia, 292
Anterior segment reconstruction, 345, 346
  intraoperative, 345
  postoperative, 345
  preoperative, 345
Anterior stromal puncture, 343
Anterior stromal scarring, 213
  photorefractive keratectomy, 351
Anthrax, 143
Antimetabolites, 141

Aphakic corneal edema, 288
Aphthous oral ulcer, 315
Aqueous leak around optical cylinder, 369
ARA-C, 141
Arcus juvenilis, 194
Arcus senilis, 93, 106, 113, 167, 168, 194
Arg124Cys, 165
Arg124His, 165
Arg124Leu, 165
Arg555Gln, 165
Arg555Trp, 165
Argon laser
  delineation of epithelial ingrowth, 291
  photocoagulation injury, 275, 291
Argyrosis, 136
Arlt's line, 72
Arthritis, 85, 305
Artisan® lens, 362
Aspergillus, 226
  corneal ulcer, 226
  lactophenol cotton blue stain, 226
Astigmatic keratectomy, 351
Astigmatism, 94, 186, 187, 306, 332
Atopic keratoconjunctivitis, 78, 79
Aureobasidium pullulans, 360
  keratitis, 360
Autonomic, 38
Avellino dystrophy, 163, 164, 165
Axenfeld-Rieger syndrome, 100
Axenfeld's anomaly, 97–101
Axenfeld's intrascleral nerve loop, 51
Axenfeld's nerve loop, 51

B

Bacillus anthracis, 143
Bacterial conjunctivitis, 63–5, 73
Bacterial corneal ulcer, 209
Bacterial infections, 25, 209–20, 302, 324, 346, 359
Bacterial keratitis, 209, 210
Bacterial laboratory diagnosis, 208
Bacterial ulcer, 219
Band keratopathy, 172, 200, 201, 316
  JRA, 316
Band-shaped and whorled microcystic dystrophy, 149
Bandage contact lens, 260, 262
Bartonella henselae, 74
Basal cell carcinoma, 14–15
Basement membrane stain, 81
Basket weave, LASIK, 356
BDUMP, 52
Beading of corneal nerves, 132
Behçet's disease, 315
Benign eyelid tumors, 7–14
Benign intraepithelial dyskeratosis, 43
Benign lymphoid hyperplasia, 54
Benign monoclonal gammopathy, 123–4
  sludging in conjunctival vessels, 124
Benign pigmented lesions, 48
Bietti's crystalline corneal-retinal dystrophy, 169
BigH3, 153–8, 160, 163, 164, 165, 340, 341
  corneal dystrophy, Bowman's layer type I, 150, 151
Bilirubin deposits, 113
Bitot spot, 118
Blanching, 303
Blast injury, 269
Bleb-like, 148
Blebs, 65, 148, 198

Blepharitis, 16, 17, 19–24, 26, 27
  angular, 24
  herpes simplex, 211
  mixed, 24
  seborrheic, 19, 21, 22, 23, 24
  staphylococcal, 19
Blepharoconjunctivitis, 210
Blepharokeratoconjunctivitis, 78
Blood, intraocular, long-standing, 271
Blood staining, 271
Blue sclera, 114, 115
Bluish-red discoloration, 304
Blunt trauma, 264, 287
Borrelia burgdorferi, 131
Break-up time, 31
Brown-McLean syndrome, 288
Buccal mucosal lesions
  in cicatricial pemphigoid, 81
  in linear IgA disease, 82
Buphthalmos, 96
Busacca nodules, 313
BUT *see* Break-up time
Buttonhole flap, LASIK, 353, 354

C

Calcific band keratopathy, 172, 200, 201, 316
Calcific degeneration, 172, 200, 201
Calcified scleral plaques, 205
Calcium deposits, 126, 200, 326
Canaliculitis, 40
Candida
  keratitis, 225
  puff ball, 225
Canthus, 24
Capillary hemangioma, 10
Castroviejo, Ramon, 317
Cat scratch disease, 74
Cataract, 104, 206, 267, 285, 314
  JRA, 316
  surgical complications, 206, 288–91, 306
Cavernous hemangioma, 11
CDBI, 150, 151
CDBII, 151
Cellulitis
  orbital, 25
  preseptal, 25
Central cloudy dystrophy of François, 196
Central corneal ulcer, 252, 253
Cephalosporium, 228, 229
  corneal ulcer, 228, 229
  culture, 228, 229
  fungal culture, 228, 229
Cercopithecine herpesvirus, 74
Chalazion, 20
Chalcosis, 286
Chandler's syndrome, 190–2
  gonioscopy, 190
  specular microscopy, 191
CHED *see* Congenital hereditary endothelial dystrophy
Chelation, 200
Chemical and biological warfare, 143–4
Chemical injury, 263, 292, 293–4, 342
Chemosis, 76
Chickenpox, 130
  conjunctival pock, 130
  disciform keratitis, 130
Chlamydia, 69–73
Chlamydial conjunctivitis, 69–73

Rhinophyma, 22
Rieger's anomaly, 98–100
Riley-day syndrome, 38
River blindness, 133
Rizutti's sign, 179
Rosacea, 22
    chronic, 22–3
    keratitis, 23, 340
Rose bengal staining, 33, 34, 84, 220
Rotating keratoplasty, 318
Rust ring, 277–9

S

S-shaped lid, 34, 39
Salzmann's nodular degeneration, 198, 203, 204
Sandfly, 27
Sarcoid, 56
Sarcoid iridocyclitis, 313
Sarcoid nodules, 56
Sarcoidosis, 34, 313
Sarcoma, 55
Scales, 19
    of skin, 127
Scarring see Cicatricial
Scheie's syndrome, 108
    clawlike hands, 108
    histopathology, 110
    pigmentary retinopathy, 108
Schirmer's test, 32
Schnyder's crystalline dystrophy, 167, 168, 169
Schwalbe's line, 97–99
Schwann cells, 14
Scissoring reflex, 179
Sclera
    degeneration, 205
    granulomatous mass, 256
    infection, 210
    ischemia, 293
    perforation, 304
    plaques, 205
    thinning, 114, 303
Scleral buckle, 65
Scleritis, 255, 304–6, 315
    Acanthamoeba, 232
    active, 305
    diffuse, 304
    herpes simplex, 219
    herpes zoster, 225
    inactive, 305
    necrotizing, 251, 257, 305
    Nocardia, 306
    nodular, 304
    old, 305
    previous, 305
    Pseudomonas, 305
Sclerocornea, 93, 94
Sclerokeratitis, 116
Scleromalacia perforans, 251, 305
Sclerosing keratitis, 133
Sclerouveitis, 255
Sebaceous cell carcinoma, 17
Sebaceous gland, 21, 22
    dysfunction, 21, 22
Sebaceous secretions, 20
Seborrheic blepharitis, 19, 21, 22, 23, 24
Seborrheic keratosis, 11, 12
Secondary bacterial ulcer, 219
Secondary ectasias, 189
Seidel's test, 37, 215, 224, 253, 320, 325, 327
SEIs see Subepithelial infiltrates
Senile ectropion, 1, 3
Senile entropion, 3
Sessile papilloma, 41
Shield ulcer, 77
Silicone plugs, 37

Silver (GMS) stain, 234
Sinus, 25
Skeletal disorders, 114–25
Skin, scales, 126
Skin foreign body, 269
Skin lesions
    in cicatricial pemphigoid, 80
    from forceps, 272
    Stevens-Johnson syndrome, 83
Skin retraction around optical cylinder, 369
Skin tag, 12
SLK see Superior limbic keratoconjunctivitis
Sludging in conjunctival vessels, 124
Small cell lung cancer, iris tumor, 311
Smallpox, 131, 317
Smallpox vaccination, 144
Spastic entropion, 4
Specimen collection, 207
Specular microscopy, 89, 173, 174, 273
    Chandler's syndrome, 191
    posterior polymorphous dystrophy, 173
    technique, 89, 90
Spheroidal degeneration, 202, 203
Spindle cells, 18
Spirochete, 131
SPK see Superficial punctate keratopathy
Spondyloepiphyseal dysplasia tarda, 115
Spontaneous subconjunctival hemorrhage, 270
Squamous carcinoma, 48
Squamous cell carcinoma, 15–16, 47–8
Squamous cell tumor, 15–16
Squamous neoplasms, 41–8
Square penetrating keratoplasty, 317
Staphylococcal blepharitis, 19, 24
Staphylococcal marginal infiltrate, 259
Staphylococcus, 19, 24
Staphylococcus aureus, 24, 209, 323
    corneal ulcer, 209
Staphyloma, 251, 280
Stellate keratic precipitates, 134, 314
Stellazine, 140
Stellazine deposits, 140
Stem cell deficiency, 137, 299, 300
Stem cells, 51
Sterile corneal ulcer, 252, 253
    central, 252, 253
    peripheral, 252, 253
Sterile suture abscess, 322
Stevens-Johnson syndrome, 83–5
    fingernails, 83
    keratinization, 84, 85
    skin lesions, 83
Stocker line, 198
Strabismus surgery, 57
Streptococcus pneumoniae, 322
    corneal ulcer, 324
Streptococcus viridans, 209
Striae, LASIK, 356
Striate melanokeratosis, 51
Stromal dystrophies, 153–64
Stromal haze, photorefractive keratectomy, 352
Stromal keratitis, 133
Stromal puncture, 343
Stromal rejection reaction, 331
Stye, 20
Subconjunctival hemorrhage, 270
Subconjunctival lymphoma, 55
Subepithelial infiltrates, 68, 70, 220–1, 329, 331
Subepithelial mucinous dystrophy, 152
Subepithelial neoplasms, 52–60
    benign lymphoid hyperplasia, 54
    cyst, 60
    ectopic, 60
    eyelid lymphangioma, 54
    lymphoid tissue, 53
Sulfamethoxazole, 306

Sulfur granules, 40
Sunflower cataract, 286
Superficial keratectomy, 340
Superficial punctate keratitis of Thygeson, 243
Superficial punctate keratopathy, 33
Superficial variant granular corneal dystrophy, 150, 340, 341
Superior limbic keratoconjunctivitis, 86–7
    contact lens, 301
Suprachoroidal hemorrhage, 318
Surgical complications, 206, 288–91, 306, 339
Surgical lint, intraocular foreign body, 288
Suture abscess, 322–3
Suture erosion, 323
Suture foreign body, 79
Suture granuloma, 57
Suture infiltrate, 323
Suture track fistula, 162, 325
Sutured corneal laceration, 264
Suturing technique, 265
Symblepharon, 68, 80, 81, 84, 250
Syphilis, Descemet's scrolls, 235
Syphilitic facies, 235
Syphilitic interstitial keratitis, 235–6
    ghost vessels, 235
Syphilitic uveitis, 315
Systemic amyloidosis, 7, 121, 157
Systemic lupus erythematosus, 255
Systemic lymphoma, 18, 53

T

T-cell lymphoma, 18
Tangier disease, 107
Tarantula hairs in cornea, 281
Tear break-up time, 31, 118
Tear film, 31, 147
Tear lake, 31
Tears, 31
Tectonic penetrating keratoplasty, 346
Telangiectasia, 23
Temporary keratoprosthesis, 347
Terrien's marginal degeneration, 204, 205
TGFBI, 150–64, 340, 341
Theodore's superior limbic keratoconjunctivitis, 86–7
    contact lens, 301
Therapeutic keratoplasty, 229
Thermal burn, 29
Thermal cataract wound injury, 289
Thermal corneal injury, 275
Thermal keratoplasty, 362
Thiel-Behnke dystrophy, 151, 165
Thiel-Behnke honeycomb dystrophy, 151, 165
Thimerosal, 28
Thorazine, 140
Thorazine deposits, 140
Thygeson's superficial punctate keratitis, 243
Thyroid eye disease, 125–6, 247
    corneal ulcer, 125
    infected corneal ulcer, 126
    proptosis, 125
Ticks, 131
Tight-fitting contact lens, conjunctival groove, 298
Tissue adhesive, 340
Tissue plasminogen activator, 321
Topical medication, 27, 28
    ephinephrine, 303
Torturous retinal vessels, 104
Toxic follicular conjunctivitis, 86
Toxicity, 248
TPA see Tissue plasminogen activator
Trabeculectomy, 137
Trachoma, 71–2
    scarring, 71–2
    vascularization, 71–2